A Clinician's Guide to Contemporary Healthcare

A Clinician's Guide to Contemporary Healthcare

Editor: Kelly Ward

FOSTER ACADEMICS

www.fosteracademics.com

www.fosteracademics.com

FOSTER ACADEMICS

Cataloging-in-Publication Data

A clinician's guide to contemporary healthcare / edited by Kelly Ward.
p. cm.
Includes bibliographical references and index.
ISBN 978-1-63242-474-7
1. Medical care. 2. Medicine--Case studies. 3. Public health. 4. Medicine, Preventive.
5. Health services administration. I. Ward, Kelly.
RA776.5 .C55 2017
613--dc23

Foster Academics,
118-35 Queens Blvd., Suite 400,
Forest Hills, NY 11375, USA

ISBN 978-1-63242-474-7 (Hardback)

Printed and bound in the United States of America.

Contents

Preface

The main aim of this book is to educate learners and enhance their research focus by presenting diverse topics covering this vast field. This is an advanced book which compiles significant studies by distinguished experts. This book addresses successive solutions to the challenges arising in the area of application, along with it; the book provides scope for future developments.

This book unfolds the innovative aspects of healthcare facilities which will be crucial for the progress of this field in the future. Healthcare facilities are basic requirement of the society in today's world. Providing people with better healthcare facilities like better hospitals, cheap medications, inexpensive treatments, emergency medication, etc. is essential for a good quality of life and a region's prosperity. This book attempts to understand the multiple branches that fall under this discipline and how such concepts have practical applications. The topics included herein on healthcare are of utmost significance and bound to provide incredible insights to readers. Researchers and students in this field will be greatly assisted by this text.

It was a great honour to edit this book, though there were challenges, as it involved a lot of communication and networking between me and the editorial team. However, the end result was this all-inclusive book covering diverse themes in the field.

Finally, it is important to acknowledge the efforts of the contributors for their excellent chapters, through which a wide variety of issues have been addressed. I would also like to thank my colleagues for their valuable feedback during the making of this book.

Editor

1

Time Series Analysis of Trends in Malaria Cases and Deaths at Hospitals and the Effect of Antimalarial Interventions, 2001–2011, Ethiopia

Maru Aregawi[1]*, Michael Lynch[1], Worku Bekele[2], Henok Kebede[2], Daddi Jima[3], Hiwot Solomon Taffese[3], Meseret Aseffa Yenehun[3], Abraham Lilay[3], Ryan Williams[1], Madeleine Thomson[4], Fatoumata Nafo-Traore[2], Kesetebirhan Admasu[3], Tedros Adhanom Gebreyesus[3], Marc Coosemans[5]

1 World Health Organization, Global Malaria Program, Geneva, Switzerland, **2** World Health Organization, Country Office, Addis Ababa, Ethiopia, **3** Federal Ministry of Health, Addis Ababa, Ethiopia, **4** International Research Institute for Climate and Society (IRI), Earth Institute, Columbia University, New York, New York, United States of America, **5** Institute of Tropical Medicine, Antwerp, Belgium

Abstract

Background: The Government of Ethiopia and its partners have deployed artemisinin-based combination therapies (ACT) since 2004 and long-lasting insecticidal nets (LLINs) since 2005. Malaria interventions and trends in malaria cases and deaths were assessed at hospitals in malaria transmission areas during 2001–2011.

Methods: Regional LLINs distribution records were used to estimate the proportion of the population-at-risk protected by LLINs. Hospital records were reviewed to estimate ACT availability. Time-series analysis was applied to data from 41 hospitals in malaria risk areas to assess trends of malaria cases and deaths during pre-intervention (2001–2005) and post-interventions (2006–2011) periods.

Findings: The proportion of the population-at-risk potentially protected by LLINs increased to 51% in 2011. The proportion of facilities with ACTs in stock exceeded 87% during 2006–2011. Among all ages, confirmed malaria cases in 2011 declined by 66% (95% confidence interval [CI], 44–79%) and SPR by 37% (CI, 20%–51%) compared to the level predicted by pre-intervention trends. In children under 5 years of age, malaria admissions and deaths fell by 81% (CI, 47%–94%) and 73% (CI, 48%–86%) respectively. Optimal breakpoint of the trendlines occurred between January and June 2006, consistent with the timing of malaria interventions. Over the same period, non-malaria cases and deaths either increased or remained unchanged, the number of malaria diagnostic tests performed reflected the decline in malaria cases, and rainfall remained at levels supportive of malaria transmission.

Conclusions: Malaria cases and deaths in Ethiopian hospitals decreased substantially during 2006–2011 in conjunction with scale-up of malaria interventions. The decrease could not be accounted for by changes in hospital visits, malaria diagnostic testing or rainfall. However, given the history of variable malaria transmission in Ethiopia, more data would be required to exclude the possibility that the decrease is due to other factors.

Editor: Yoel Lubell, Mahidol-Oxford Tropical Medicine Research Unit, Thailand

Funding: The author(s) received no specific funding for this work.

Competing Interests: The authors have declared that no competing interests exist.

* Email: aregawim@who.int

Background

Malaria affects over 68% of the population in Ethiopia, a country of 94 million people in 2013 [1]. The disease is highly seasonal with varying intensity of transmission owing to altitudinal and climatic variations [2]. Across the nine administrative regions, areas that lie below 2000 m altitude are considered as malarious (Figure 1) [3]. The occurrence of malaria epidemics in the past indicates that there is little immunity in the majority of the population, owing to few infective mosquito bites per person per year [4,5]. The high transmission season coincides with the cultivation months; hence malaria has a deleterious effect on agricultural production. *Plasmodium falciparum* accounted for nearly 55% of all malaria cases during 2008–2012 [6].

Malaria control has been one of the major components of the country's National Heath Sector Development and Poverty Reduction Strategy, put forth since 2004 in different phases, the most recent plan being for the period 2010–2015. With investment by the Global Fund to Fight HIV/AIDS, Tuberculosis and Malaria, the USA President's Malaria Initiative, World Bank and other development partners, the government has employed three key antimalarial interventions: i) distribution of long-lasting insecticidal nets (LLINs) through mass campaigns, to the entire population at risk; ii) indoor residual spraying (IRS) in designated

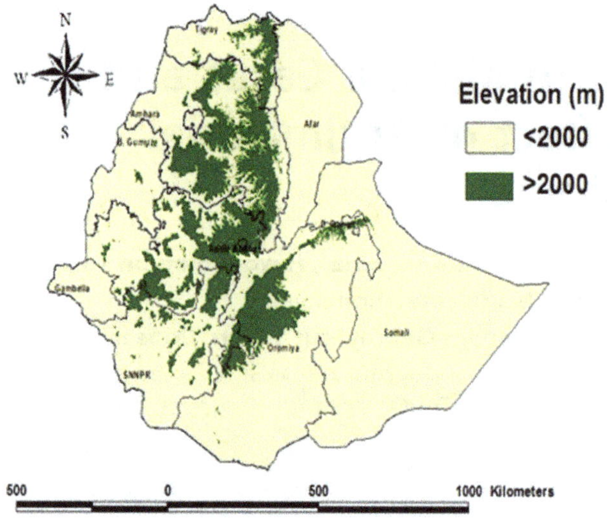

Figure 1. Administrative regions and areas below and above 2000 meters elevation in Ethiopia.

epidemic-prone areas; and iii) increased diagnostic testing through rapid diagnostic tests (RDT) and microscopy, along with deployment of artemisinin-based combination therapy (ACT). Distribution of LLINs started in 2005. ACT was introduced to all public health facilities, free-of-charge to all age groups, as the first-line treatment for uncomplicated malaria in July 2004 [7].

Malaria control efforts have benefited from the national health sector development strategy which aims to increase access to effective health care by deploying health extension workers (HEWs) to provide integrated health promotion and treatment at peripheral health posts and at community level. By 2009 over 30,000 HEWs had been deployed. Treatment provided by HEWs targets the leading causes of death in children: malaria, pneumonia, and diarrhoea [8]. For malaria, the HEWs verify ownership and encourage use of LLINs; diagnose malaria with RDTs and treat confirmed cases; then refer suspected severe malaria cases to the health centres and hospitals.

This study aimed to (i) investigate the proportion of the population benefiting from malaria control interventions, (ii) assess trends in malaria cases and deaths in hospitals in malaria risk areas between 2001 and 2011, and (iii) examine the relationship between malaria interventions and the occurrence of malaria cases and deaths during 2001–2011. Attempts were made to take into account other factors which may affect malaria cases and deaths in hospitals and to employ statistical approaches focused on assessing changes in trends of malaria cases and deaths before and after the major scale up of malaria interventions since 2005. The results are discussed in light of international goals and targets for reducing malaria burden.

Methods

Ethical clearance

Ethical clearance was not required as the retrospective data used from the health facilities were monthly aggregates and anonymous counts of clinical cases and deaths.

Intervention coverage

Information on malaria control interventions (LLINs, IRS, and ACTs) was obtained from national malaria control program (NMCP) records. As the programme started implementation of LLINs in 2005, the number of LLINs distributed to each region during 2005–2011 was recorded. The number of insecticide treated mosquito nets available before 2005 was assumed to be small. Regional population estimates were taken from the 2007 Ethiopian census and adjusted using the population growth of United Nations population estimates for all the study years [9]. The proportion of the population potentially protected by LLINs in a given year was calculated by assuming that each LLIN protected 1.8 persons and lasted three years (number of LLINs distributed during the 3 year period ×1.8/population). The proportion of the population protected with IRS nationwide was calculated by dividing the number of persons in households protected by IRS by the population at risk. The availability of ACT treatment was assessed by reviewing records of stock-outs at hospitals that were visited to access trends in malaria cases and deaths. ACTs were counted as available for a given month if ACTs were in stock for more than three weeks in a month.

Malaria cases and deaths

Data on malaria outpatient cases, admissions and deaths were obtained from health facilities that provided inpatient services and were located below 2000 m or served catchment populations predominantly below 2000 m elevation (Figure 1). Of the total 120 inpatient facilities in Ethiopia, 62 facilities met the above criteria; 55 hospitals were visited, including three located in highland areas that predominantly serve populations from low land areas, while six hospitals were not visited for logistical reasons. Surveillance data were considered adequate if data on all indicators were available for more than 70% of months. Of 56 facilities visited, 41 facilities that had data for >70% of months between 2001–2011 were included in the final analysis.

At each visited hospital, monthly totals of outpatient visits, hospital admissions and deaths, and laboratory tests performed were reviewed. The total numbers of outpatient visits, admissions and deaths for all-causes and for malaria were recorded by two age groups (less than 5 years of age and 5 years old or greater). A suspected outpatient malaria case was defined as a visit in which malaria was the preliminary diagnosis in the outpatient record. A confirmed malaria case was defined if malaria parasites were demonstrated by microscopy (RDT results were not considered as they are used at the lower health facilities and community level by the HEWs). The slide positivity rate (SPR) was defined as the number of microscopy slides with malaria parasites divided by the number of microscopy slides reviewed. Laboratory records could not be broken down by age, nor could they be linked individually to outpatient or inpatient cases. Inpatient malaria cases and deaths were based on the diagnosis at discharge. The non-malaria cases and deaths, used for comparisons, were generated by subtracting malaria from the corresponding all-cause outpatient, admissions and deaths.

Meteorological data

Enhanced National Climate Services (ENACTS) rainfall data that is quality controlled and blended satellite and observational data [10] from the National Meteorological Agency of Ethiopia was obtained by the International Research Institute for Climate and Society, Columbia University, New York, USA. These precipitation data (estimate of rainfall in mm) were aggregated for five major regions of the country and were used as the principal short-term predictor to assess the effect of climate on the trends of malaria cases and deaths [11].

Statistical methods

Stata 11 was used to compile data by year and month and perform statistical analysis [12]. Trends in confirmed malaria cases and SPR, malaria inpatient cases, and malaria deaths were assessed by region. Malaria inpatient cases and malaria deaths were assessed by the two age groups. Confirmed malaria cases and SPR were assessed for all ages as these could not be disaggregated by age. Change in indicators over time was evaluated in three ways: i) by comparing the mean of annual values of cases and deaths during 2001–2005 (considered the pre-intervention period) to the observed value for 2011; ii) using a segmented regression model of an interrupted time series [13], comparing observed 2011 to predicted values in 2011, assuming a continuation of the pre-intervention time trend through 2006–2011; and iii) comparing the average for the observed values for 2006–2011 with the midpoint level predicted using segmented regression, assuming a continuation of the pre-intervention time trend through 2006–2011. The magnitude of changes in indicators was expressed as the relative percent change. For (ii) and (iii), the model adjusts the estimate for (1) possible time trend of the indicator during the pre-intervention period; (2) a possible immediate drop or rise of the indicator following the start of the intervention, and (3) a time trend on the indicator post-intervention. The 95% confidence intervals (CI) around the estimates were computed using the CIs around the regression coefficient estimates. A relative percent change in an indicator for which the CI does not include zero was considered statistically significant. In the time-series regression model for (ii) and iii), an Autoregressive Integrated Moving Average (ARIMA) model was used. A correlogram and partial autocorrelation plots were used to guide selection of the best ARIMA model [14].

To provide insight into whether changes in malaria cases and deaths were related to the introduction of malaria interventions in time, a sensitivity analysis was done by dividing the time series into two segments, a pre-intervention and post-intervention period, and varying the dividing point and evaluating the segmented regression model for each break point. The optimal breakpoint, or the month with the maximum change in the trend line, was considered to be the point where the amount of variation accounted for by the segmented regression model (R^2) was greatest [15].

Month-to-month variability in indicators was evaluated using monthly values of the indicators during pre-and post-intervention periods using sinusoidal functions. To observe and remove short-term seasonal fluctuations, the monthly trends were extracted using a Hodrick-Prescott filter with monthly smoothing parameter [16]. Spectral analysis was done to detect the fundamental frequency components of the series. Additionally, month effects were parametrically modeled by using sinusoidal functions (Indirect Discrete Fourier Transform (IDFT).

The time trend in monthly rainfall, the principal short-term predictor of malaria burden [17], was plotted by region.

Results

Interventions

The national malaria control programme distributed a total of 43.1 million LLINs during 2005–2011 targeting all populations in malarious areas, of which 23.8 million LLINs were distributed during 2005–2007, 2.1 million were distributed 2008–2009 and 17.1 million nets during 2010–2011 (Figure 2).

The proportion of population potentially protected by LLINs increased from nearly zero in 2005 to 78% in 2007, and 51% in 2011 (Figure 3). The proportion of population protected with IRS

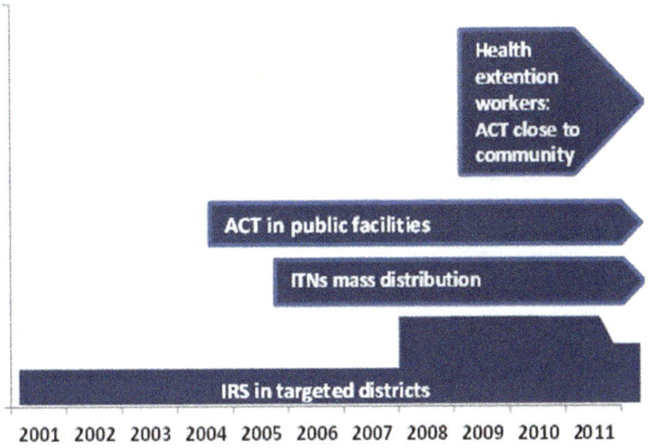

Figure 2. Timeline of implementation of antimalarial interventions, 2001–2011, Ethiopia.

increased from 10% in 2007 to 35% in 2011. In 40 hospitals, ACT stock records were complete for 80% of the months during 2006–2011 (no ACT stock records were available for 2004 and 2005). Stock out of ACT for any age group was very low during 2006–2011 and therefore availability of ACT was >99% during 2006–2009, 97% in 2010 and 87% in 2011. Over 50% of the stock outs in 2011 were in Oromia region.

Yearly trends of malaria cases, admissions and deaths

Of the sampled 62 hospitals, 55 hospitals were visited but only 49 hospitals met the criteria for collection of historical data. Data covering 2001–2011 was complete in 41 of the 49 hospitals which were the basis for the analysis in this study. The 8 hospitals with incomplete data comprised 4 from Oromia, 2 from Amhara and one each from Afar and Tigray. Confirmed malaria cases decreased from a mean of 78,325 during 2001–2005 to 30,780 cases in 2011 (Figure 4a), an observed decline of 61%, and a 66% decline (95% confidence interval [CI], 44–79%) from the number of cases predicted in 2011 if the trend during 2001–2005 had continued (Table 1). The number of confirmed cases at the midpoint of 2006–2011 was lower by 50% (CI 24–68%) than the values predicted. The SPR was 24% in 2001 and 11% in 2011 (Figure 4b); SPR decreased from a mean of 22% during 2001–2005 to 11% in 2011 (Table 1) and declined 37% (CI, 20%–51%) compared with the predicted value of 2011. Malaria inpatient cases and malaria deaths were highest in 2003, decreased during 2005–2008, and then rose slightly in 2009 but fell again in 2011 (Figure 4c, 4d). Overall, malaria inpatient cases in all ages were 54% lower and malaria deaths 68% lower in 2011 than that predicted by trends during 2001–2005, however, these declines were not statistically significant.

Concomitantly, non-malaria outpatient cases, inpatient cases, and deaths either increased or remained unchanged (Table 1, Figure 4a, 4c, 4d). The number of laboratory tests performed varied from a mean of 350,000 during 2001–2005 to 292,000 in 2011. The decrease in the number of microscopy tests performed is approximately similar to the decrease in the number of confirmed malaria cases (78,000 to 30,000) during the same time period.

A sensitivity analysis of the malaria cases for the 132 months covering the years 2001–2011 indicated that the month with the maximum change in the trendline was the 62nd month (January 2006) for confirmed malaria and the 66th month (June, 2006) for SPR, admissions and deaths 2006.

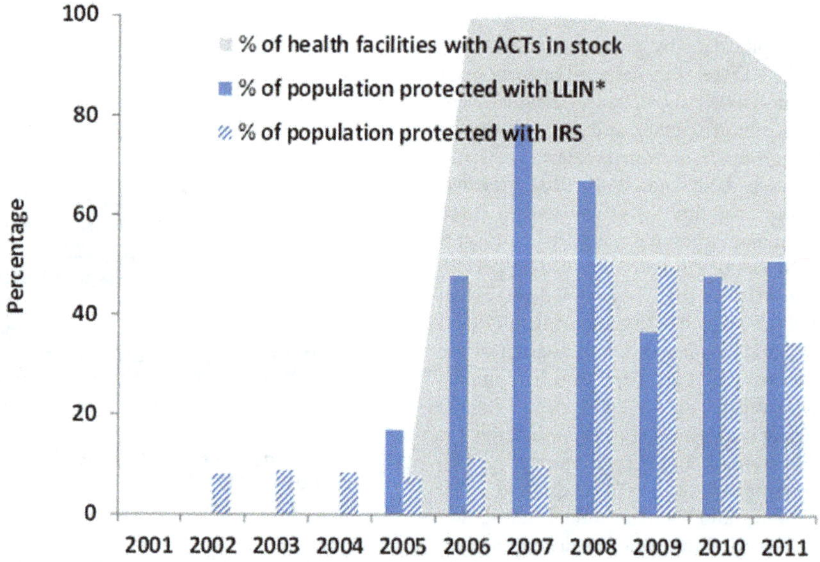

Figure 3. Percentage of population potentially protected with LLINs*, IRS and percentage of health facilities with stock of ACT available by year, 2001–2011, Ethiopia (*number of LLINs distributed during the 3 year period ×1.8/population).

Among children under 5 years of age, observed inpatient malaria cases were 41% lower in 2011 than the mean of the observed values during 2001–2005 (Table 1), and lower by 81% (CI, 47%–94%) than the level predicted for 2011. In this age-group, malaria deaths were 73% (CI, 48%–86%) lower in 2011 than predicted by previous trends. Among those 5 years and older, malaria inpatient cases and malaria deaths were lower in 2011 than predicted based on 2001–2005 trends, however these changes were not statistically significant. The proportions of inpatient cases due to malaria (of all-cause inpatient) in children under 5 years fell from 23% in 2001–2005 to 11% in 2011; and malaria deaths fell from 17% to 8% of all-cause deaths during the same period. The proportion of inpatient cases due to malaria in 5 years and above fell from 15% to 6% and the proportion of malaria deaths decreased from 19% to 5%.

The observed number of confirmed malaria cases in 2011 was lower than the mean number of confirmed cases during 2001–2005 in all 10 regions (Table 2). The decrease in confirmed cases varied among regions from 36 to 99%. Similarly, the SPR and the number of malaria deaths were lower in all regions, while malaria inpatient cases were higher in 2011 in one region, Gambella. Confirmed malaria cases were lower in 2011 compared with 2001–2005 in 33 of 41 hospitals; inpatient cases were lower in 34 hospitals and malaria deaths were lower in 37 hospitals.

Seasonality

Using the Hodrick-Prescott filter method to remove short-term (monthly) fluctuations and determine the long term time-series over multiple years, a decrease in all malaria indicators is seen (Figure 5). Confirmed malaria cases and SPR decreased through 2011, while malaria inpatient cases and malaria deaths decreased until 2008, followed by stability between 2008 and 2011. The spectral analysis showed that the fundamental frequency components of these series is one or annual.

Monthly mean confirmed malaria cases, SPR, malaria inpatient cases, and malaria deaths were lower for all months during 2006–2011 (post-intervention period) compared to 2001–2005 (pre-intervention period (Figure 6 a, b, c, d). Malaria inpatient cases and malaria deaths varied widely by month during 2001–2005, while little variation in monthly means was seen during 2006–2011.

Rainfall

Precipitation data of five regions and national aggregates made available by the International Research Institute for Climate and Society (IRI) were analysed. No significant difference in precipitation between pre- and post-intervention years was observed (Figure 7). Rainfall remained favourable for malaria transmission and peaked in 2006 and 2010 while it was lowest in 2009 across the regions. A linear regression of rainfall on national aggregates of confirmed cases and SPR showed no significant effect ($p>0.05$). Linear regression on confirmed cases and SPR by region showed no significant effect during the pre-intervention period in all regions except in SNNP region (where rainfall had significant increasing effect on both). During the post-intervention period, rainfall had a significant increasing effect on confirmed cases and SPR in all the regions except in Oromia, where rainfall had significant decreasing effect ($p<05$) and in Tigray with no significant effect.

Discussion

In this study reviewing data from hospitals in Ethiopia, malaria decreased between 2001 and 2011 by several measures. Among all age groups, the number of confirmed malaria cases, malaria inpatient cases and deaths declined by more than half, while malaria inpatient cases and malaria deaths among children under 5 years old decreased more than two-thirds from the numbers predicted if levels at the start of the decade had persisted. The observed declines in malaria cases and deaths were seen across all regions where malaria transmission occurs and could not be accounted for by changes in outpatient visits or by the number of diagnostic tests performed. During this time, measured rainfall was sufficient to support malaria transmission and levels of rainfall could not be consistently correlated with changes in malaria cases. Counts of cases and deaths were used in this analysis as the catchment population of each hospital was not known. Given the

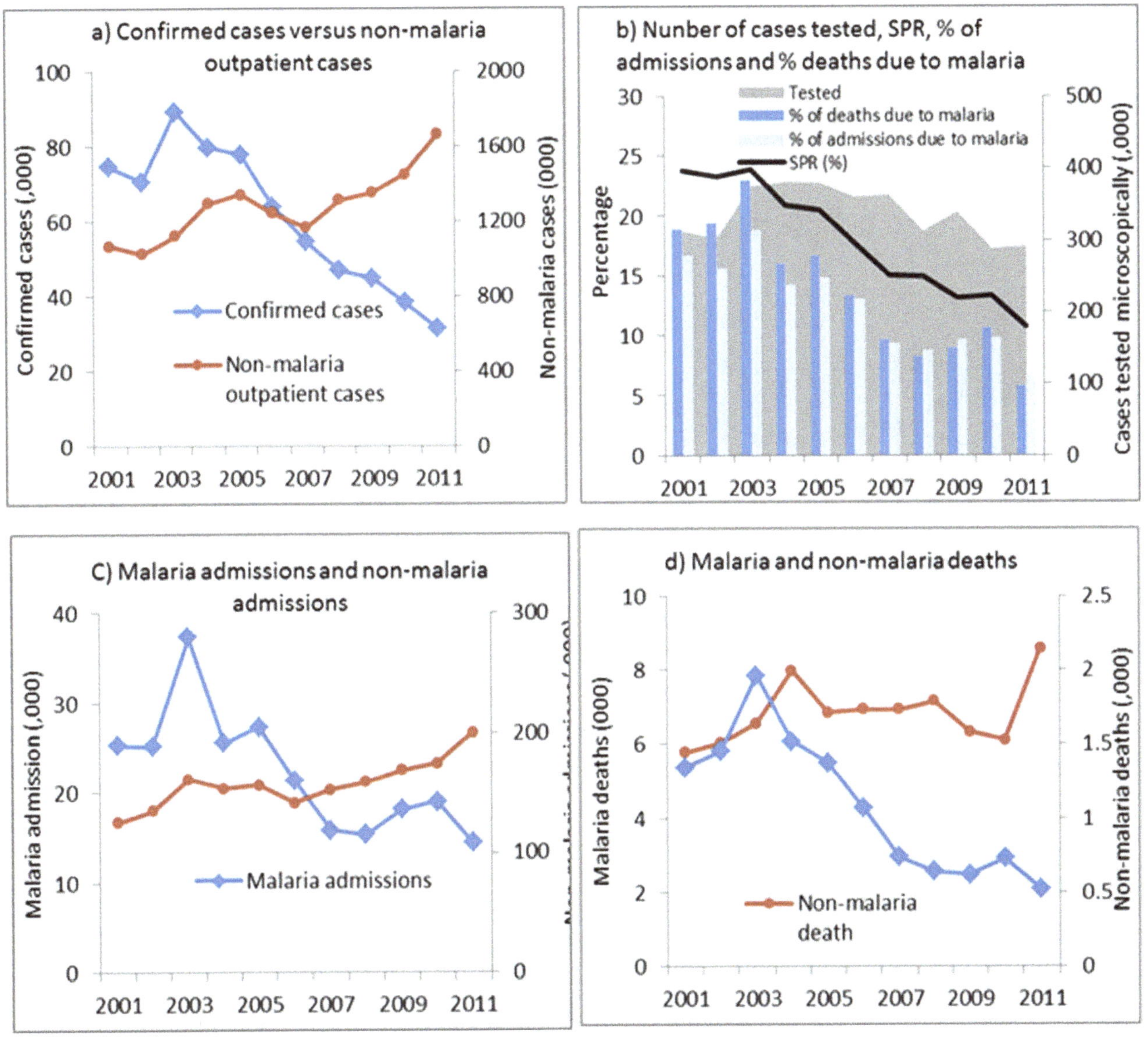

Figure 4. Trends of confirmed malaria cases and non-malaria outpatient visits (a); slide positivity rate and number of microscopic slides examined (b); malaria admissions and non-malaria admissions (c); malaria deaths and non-malaria deaths in all ages (d) in 41 hospitals, Ethiopia 2001–2011.

increase in population of Ethiopia during this time, the decline in malaria cases and deaths as rates per population may have been greater.

The downward trend in malaria cases and deaths was consistent across several approaches to the time series analysis. Comparing the observed number of cases in 2011 to the level predicted in 2011 by extrapolating trends from the first 5 years of the time period, 2001–2005, before full scale-up of malaria interventions, resulted in the largest measured decrease in cases and deaths. For confirmed cases, this can be explained in part by a slight increase in cases during the baseline period resulting in a higher predicted level in 2011 than the mean level during the 2001–2005. In contrast, for SPR, comparing the observed level in 2011 to the predicted level resulted in a smaller decrease due to an already decreasing trend of SPR in the baseline period. These examples demonstrate how characteristics of the baseline period chosen can affect the magnitude of measured changes over time [13]. Comparing the mid-point level of the regression line from 2006–2011 to the mean level 2001–2005 resulted in the smallest decrease for all primary indicators. Therefore this could be seen as the most conservative approach to this time series analysis. In addition to the decreasing trends seen in annual cases and deaths, lower numbers of malaria cases, admissions and deaths were seen when comparing the mean for each month during the post-intervention period to the same month in the pre-intervention period. Seasonal peaks also appeared lower in the post-intervention period compared to pre-intervention period.

The hospital data analysed for this study indicate that the decreases in cases and deaths coincided with the scale-up of malaria interventions. Analysis of the breakpoints in the time series of malaria cases and deaths were consistent with a change in the trend approximately when interventions were either introduced, or increasing during 2005 and 2006. The proportion of population potentially protected with LLINs increased from negligible levels

Table 1. Percentage change in malaria and non-malaria related indicators post-intervention years compared to pre-intervention period (2001–2005), by age, 41 hospitals < 2000 m elevation, Ethiopia, 2001–2011.

Age group	Indicator	Indicator	Observed values and changes			Change (%) in predicted versus observed (95% CI)	
			Observed values in 2011	Preintervention ave (2001–2005)	Observed change in 2011 (vs ave 2001–2005)	Midpoint 2006–2011	2011
Children <5 years	Malaria	Outpatient malaria cases	21,257	32,287	−34	−47% (−70%−−6%)†	−57% (−78%−−15%)†
		Malaria admissions	3,998	6,773	−41	−80% (−92%−−51%)†	−81% (−94%−−47%)†
		Malaria deaths	119	289	−59	−64% (−80% − −37%)†	−73% (−86%−−48%)†
	Nonmalaria	Nonmalaria outpatient cases	175,028	121,849	44	−20% (−57%-47%)	−22% (−62%-59%)
		Nonmalaria inpatient cases	32,242	22,366	44	−3% (−29%-34%)	−3% (−33%-41%)
		Nonmalaria deaths	1,396	1,388	1	−28% (−42%−−11%)†	−40% (−53%−−23%)†
5 years and above	Malaria	Outpatient malaria cases	77,863	113,158	−31	−54% (−65%−−41%)†	−63% (−73%−−50%)†
		Malaria admissions	10,423	21,374	−51	−43% (−77%-41%)	−52% (−83%-39%)
		Malaria deaths	406	1,240	−67	−58% (−88%-46%)	−66% (−92%-46%)
	Nonmalaria	Nonmalaria outpatient cases	1,488,596	1,048,716	42	−15% (−39%-20%)	−10% (−39%-34%)
		Nonmalaria inpatient cases	167,603	123,765	35	−13% (−44%-33%)	−9% (−45%-51%)
		Nonmalaria deaths	7,192	5,249	37	−20% (−56%-47%)	−8% (−56%-89%)
All ages	Malaria	Outpatient malaria cases	99,121	145,445	−32	−53% (−65%−−36%)†	−62% (−73%−−45%)†
		Malaria admissions	14,421	28,147	−49	−45% (−77%-30%)	−54% (−83%-27%)
		Malaria deaths	525	1,530	−66	−59% (−86%-22%)	−68% (−91%-17%)
		Laboratory examined cases	292,801	350,086	−16	−33% (−51%−−7%)†	−46% (−63%−−21%)†
		Laboratory confirmed cases	30,780	78,325	−61	−50% (−68%−−24%)†	−66% (−79%−−44%)†
		Slid positivity rate	11	22	−53	−28% (−41%−−11%)†	−37% (−51%−−20%)†
	Nonmalaria	Nonmalaria outpatient cases	1,663,624	1,170,565	42	−15% (−40%-21%)	−11% (−41%-34%)
		Nonmalaria inpatient cases	199,845	146,131	37	−12% (−41%-33%)	−8% (−43%-49%)
		Nonmalaria deaths	8,589	6,637	29	−22% (−52%-27%)	−16% (−53%-51%)

A negative percentage (ratio between observed and predicted indicators level multiplied by 100) indicates a decrease se in the indicator in the year compared to baseline period.
A positive percentage indicate an increase of the indicator or impact in the year compared to baseline.
†: 95% Confidence Interval (CI) does not include zero and change of trend (pre versus post-intervention) is statistically significant.

Table 2. Percentage change in inpatient malaria cases, malaria deaths and slide positivity rate in 2011 compared to pre-intervention period (2001–2005), by hospital and region, in 41 hospitals below 2000 m elevation, Ethiopia, 2001–2011.

Region	Hospital	Confirmed cases			SPR			Malaria admissions			Malaria deaths			% of population protected with LLIN	
		Mean (2001–2005)	2011	% Change in 2011	Mean (2001–2005)	2011	% Change in 2011	Mean (2001–2005)	2011	% Change in 2011	Mean (2001–2005)	2011	% Change in 2011	2005	2011
Afar	*Dubti*	*5089*	*2540*	*−50*	*39*	*26.8*	*−32*	*193*	*154*	*−20*	*27*	*8*	*−71*	*22*	*53*
Amhara	Dessie	975	89	−91	13	1.7	−87	254	11	−96	20	3	−86		
	Gondar Referal	483	399	−17	10	9.1	−8	286	313	9	34	25	−26		
	Woldia	455	77	−83	51	3.2	−94	134	45	−66	11	2	−83		
Total Amhara		*1914*	*565*	*−70*	*15*	*4.8*	*−68*	*674*	*369*	*−45*	*66*	*30*	*−55*	*10*	*48*
BGumuz	Asossa	5147	936	−82	41	41.5	2	559	334	−40	17	7	−58		
	Pawe	3341	1501	−55	28	28.0	0	2366	1382	−42	47	7	−85		
Total Bgumuz		***8489***	***2437***	***−71***	***35***	***32.0***	***−7***	***2924***	***1715***	***−41***	***64***	***14***	***−78***	***34***	***50***
Dire Dawa	***Dil Chora***	***742***	***24***	***−97***	***12***	***1.1***	***−91***	***1197***	***41***	***−97***	***87***	***4***	***−96***	***66***	***50***
Gambella	***Gambella***	***5167***	***3599***	***−30***	***31***	***21.4***	***−30***	***1045***	***2293***	***119***	***100***	***17***	***−83***	***95***	***100***
Harari	Hiwot Fana	624	6	−99	10	0.1	−99	497	22	−96	59	1	−99		
	Jegol	720	2	−100	13	0.2	−99	359	25	−93	38	3	−91		
Total Harari		***1343***	***8***	***−99***	***12***	***0.1***	***−99***	***855***	***47***	***−95***	***96***	***4***	***−96***	***62***	***70***
Oromia	Adama	NA	NA	NA	NA	NA	NA	120	121	0	13	4	−72		
	Ayira	1204	36	−97	9	0.6	−92	191	14	−93	18	2	−89		
	Bishoftu	NA	NA	NA	NA	NA	NA	221	52	−77	13	24	78		
	Bisidimo	686	0	−100	16	0.0	−100	169	0	−100	3	0	−100		
	Bule Hora	931	616	−34	46	8.4	−82	223	378	69	23	15	−36		
	Chiro	304	381	25	13	7.9	−40	272	95	−65	59	3	−95		
	Dembi Dolo	323	250	−23	13	3.6	−71	103	49	−53	15	5	−67		
	Gelemso	5195	6	−100	45	0.2	−100	4897	6	−100	86	0	−100		
	Gimbi Adventist	370	68	−82	10	1.6	−85	223	71	−68	10	0	−100		
	Ginnir	353	812	130	5	8.1	50	58	0	−100	3	0	−100		
	Jimma University	2820	1388	−51	19	8.9	−54	409	141	−66	58	19	−67		
	Mettu Karl	310	58	−81	5	0.9	−83	196	103	−48	25	7	−74		
	Mizan Aman	1740	503	−71	20	8.1	−60	581	309	−47	28	41	48		
	Nekemte	10363	298	−97	15	0.8	−95	1140	394	−65	63	15	−76		
	Shashemene	1076	90	−92	11	1.6	−86	361	92	−74	40	22	−45		
	St. Lukas Catholic	1287	667	−48	15	5.9	−60	443	571	29	30	46	53		
Total Oromia		***26963***	***5172***	***−81***	***17***	***4.1***	***−76***	***9608***	***2396***	***−75***	***488***	***201***	***−59***	***8***	***40***
SNNP	Arba Minch	5687	2962	−48	30	25.7	−15	3887	1952	−50	136	38	−72		

Table 2. Cont.

Region	Hospital	Confirmed cases			SPR			Malaria admissions			Malaria deaths			% of population protected with LLIN	
		Mean (2001–2005)	2011	% Change in 2011	Mean (2001–2005)	2011	% Change in 2011	Mean (2001–2005)	2011	% Change in 2011	Mean (2001–2005)	2011	% Change in 2011	2005	2011
	Atat	3355	2097	−37	27	17.6	−36	1225	957	−22	100	29	−71		
	Butajira HC	1376	1757	28	22	12.9	−40	267	167	−37	14	21	51		
	Dilla	2558	3428	34	31	47.8	56	1333	449	−66	43	12	−71		
	Gebretsadik Showa	3697	163	−96	27	5.4	−80	21	46	115	0	0	−100		
	Jinka Zonal	2316	2097	−9	28	16.0	−43	689	726	5	40	22	−47		
	Tarecha	741	722	−3	31	11.0	−64	138	512	270	14	8	−42		
	Wolayita	1188	652	−45	21	8.8	−58	861	732	−15	59	40	−32		
	Yirgalem	1974	810	−59	25	6.3	−74	716	429	−40	156	50	−68		
Total SNNP		*22893*	*14687*	*−36*	*28*	*16.9*	*−41*	*9137*	*5969*	*−35*	*562*	*219*	*−61*	*26*	*41*
Somali	Gode	1114	554	−50	44	16.5	−62	246	166	−33	7	3	−63		
	Karamara Regional	35	5	−85	4	0.4	−90	41	15	−62	5	0	−100		
Total Somalia		*1149*	*559*	*−51*	*33*	*12.1*	*−63*	*287*	*181*	*−37*	*11*	*3*	*−78*	*17*	*45*
Tigray	Abi Adi	388	302	−22	29	8.3	−71	284	261	−8	10	2	−80		
	Adwa	2756	452	−84	38	14.7	−61	345	153	−56	6	2	−67		
	Alamata	623	251	−60	19	4.6	−76	1122	625	−44	31	4	−89		
	Suhul	957	773	−19	19	13.1	−29	680	217	−68	19	18	−8		
Total Tigray		*4724*	*1778*	*−62*	*27*	*9.8*	*−63*	*2430*	*1256*	*−48*	*66*	*25*	*−62*	*15*	*44*
All hospital (regions)		*78472*	*31370*	*−60*	*23*	*10.7*	*−53*	*28351*	*14421*	*−49*	*1568*	*525*	*−67*	*21*	*51*

A negative percentage indicates a decrease of the indicator or impact in the year compared to baseline.

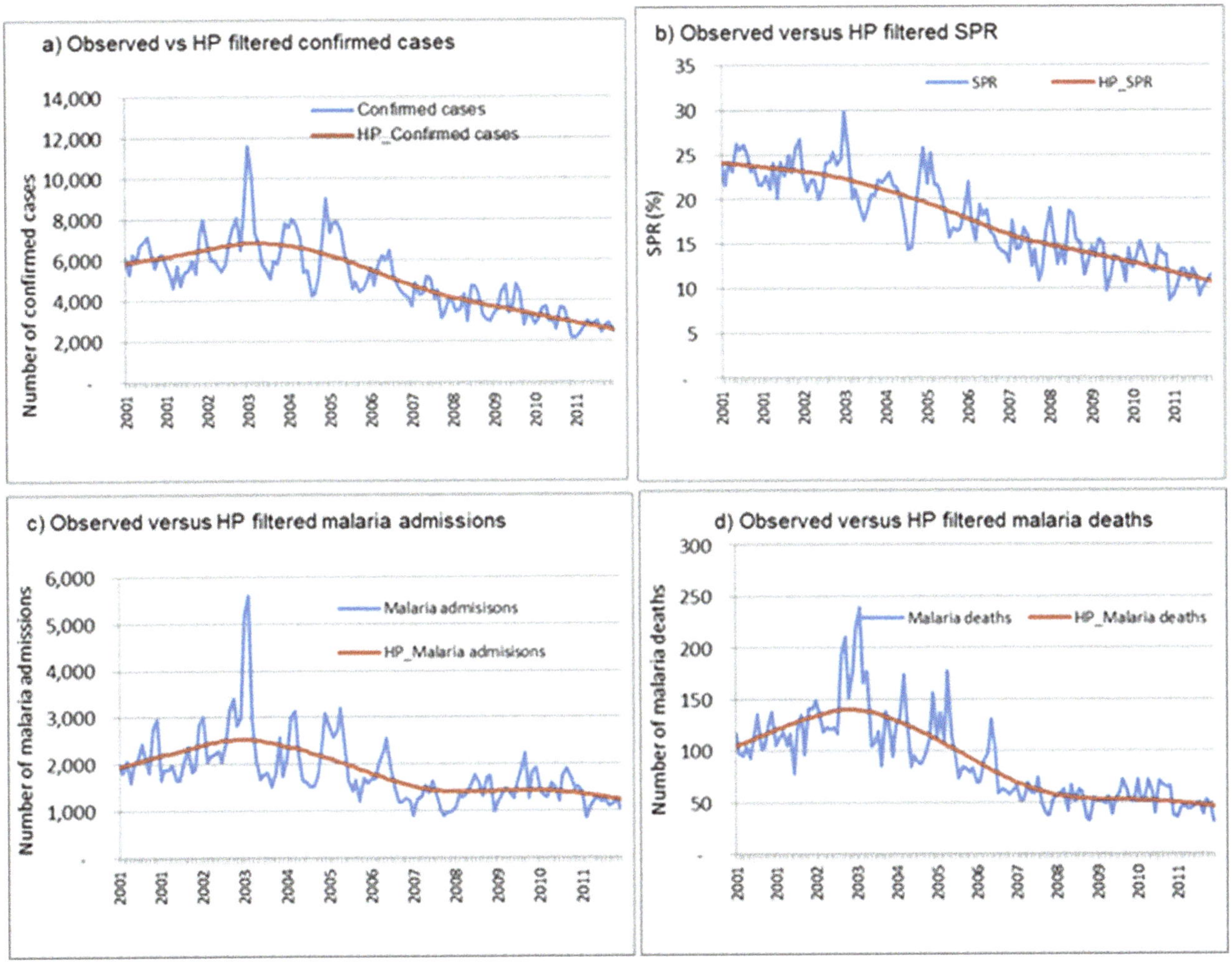

Figure 5. Time series of monthly confirmed malaria cases, slide positivity rate, admissions and deaths extracted by use of a Hodrick-Prescott filter with monthly smoothing parameter $\lambda = 14{,}400$ (HP = Hodrick-Prescott filter; MAl-IPDAll Ages = Inpatient malaria cases in all ages; Mal-DeathsAll Ages = Malaria deaths in all ages, SPRAll Ages = Slide positivity rate in all ages; PositiveAll ages = Number of confirmed cases).

prior to mass LLIN distribution starting in 2005 to levels 60% and above during 2006–2011. The proportion of the population protected by IRS also increased substantially during this time, reaching nearly 50% of the population at risk in 2008. By analysis of data on stock-outs at hospitals, ACTs were available in more than 90% of facilities after they were introduced in July 2004.

While confirmed malaria cases and the SPR decreased consistently until 2011, no additional decreases in malaria inpatient cases or malaria deaths were observed in recent years (during 2009–2011) compared to that of the early post-intervention period (2006–2008). This may be partly due to saturation of the protective effect of interventions following the attainment of the LLIN coverage and provision of ACTs by 2008. It may also be attributed to relatively slower changes in some of the major hospitals of high transmission areas in Oromia, SNNP and Gambella. A portion of LLIN distributed in 2006–2008 may also have been lost or rendered less effective during 2009–2011 due to reduced physical integrity and insecticidal waning after their estimated three-year effective lifespan. The measure of ACT availability used in this study, based on documentation of ACT stock-outs at facilities, does not provide a direct measure of what proportion of patients with malaria received adequate treatment, therefore it is unknown if changes in treatment patterns had an effect.

Assessment of trends in malaria cases and deaths and the effect of malaria control activities reported previously by Ethiopia, and other sub-Saharan African countries (Zanzibar [18,19], Rwanda [20], The Gambia [21] and Sao Tome and Principe [22]) have utilized both facility data and household survey results and have shown significant decrease following scale up of interventions. Compared to the 2008 study in Ethiopia [23], the present study benefits from three additional years of data and attempts to address concerns regarding analysis of trends given large variability in malaria transmission based on historical data in Ethiopia and a short, possibly spurious baseline in available facility data.

This study is subject to several limitations. A key challenge in assessing the trends in malaria in Ethiopia is the historically high variability in baseline malaria transmission. An attempt was made to account for this in the analysis; however, the time period reviewed may have been too short to reveal longer term trends in malaria transmission that may have been unrelated to malaria

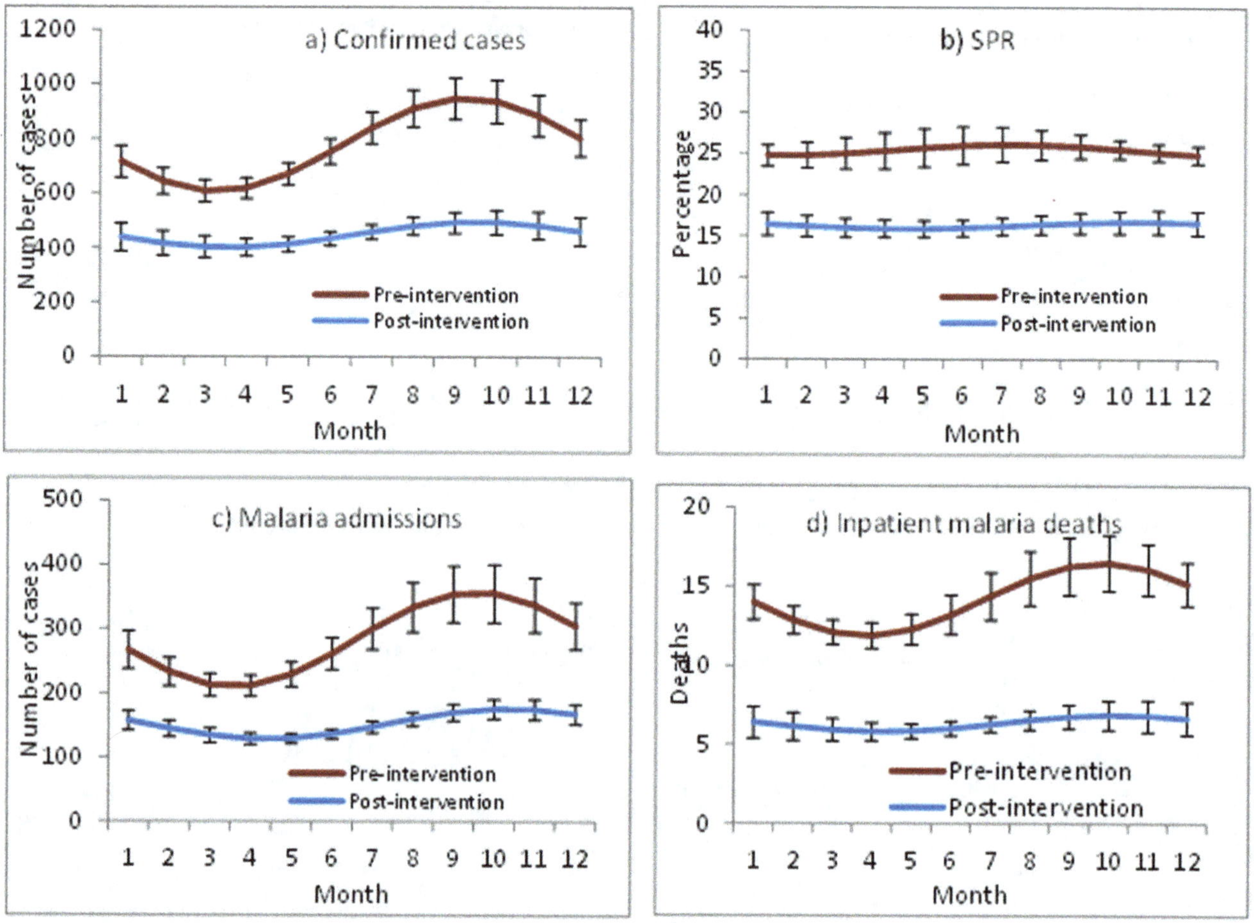

Figure 6. Monthly mean number of malaria confirmed cases, malaria inpatient cases, malaria deaths and slide positivity rate, 2001–2005 and 2006–2011, 41 hospitals, Ethiopia.

interventions. Visiting hospitals and reviewing data at hospitals helped in minimizing reporting bias present in routine surveillance. Even so, excluding visited hospitals with incomplete data introduces its own potential bias; this is likely to be small as the excluded hospitals represent a small fraction of the hospitals visited. The main reason for the incomplete data at the hospitals was disappearances of record books and monthly reports (for some months or years particularly the early years) and improper handing over of records during change of health staff. The study did not include lower level health facilities and it is unclear if trends there would be the same as those seen in the hospitals considered. There were no data on the volume of patients cared for or the number of malaria cases identified through community case management in the Health Extension Programme. The effect of this program on trends in hospital malaria cases appears to be limited as the decline in malaria cases and deaths occurred two years before the scale-up of community case management in 2009 and, given health care seeking patterns in Ethiopia, only a third of patients treated in the community were likely to have been seen at hospitals [24]. In addition, significant decrease in malaria cases and deaths were observed against the background of increased all-cause outpatient and all-cause inpatient cases and deaths in the hospitals. Information on testing practices at the district hospitals was limited. The number of suspected cases presenting to health facilities that should be tested for malaria was not recorded in standard reporting forms and therefore, it was difficult to assess whether the proportion of suspect patients tested changed over time. The measures of malaria control intervention coverage in this study were crude estimates of these interventions in the community however, they did reflect the time period during which interventions were available and were adequate to denote large changes in intervention coverage. More precise measures of LLIN coverage and ACT treatment would be needed to more closely relate changes in coverage to changes in malaria occurrence. Given the very high ecological variations within a region, annual average rainfall for the major regions may not be conclusive to accurately assess the climatic effect on trends of malaria cases and deaths. In a separate analysis of rainfall data by the International Research Institute for Climate and Society, Columbia University, New York, USA, using Enhancing National Climate Services (ENACTS) (not shown here), for most regions there was lower rainfall in the pre-intervention (baseline) period (2000–2005) relative to the post-intervention period (2006–2010). In addition, analysis of temperature indicate that the climate of Ethiopia has been getting warmer over the last 30 years –particularly in highland areas. Higher temperatures and rainfall in the intervention period suggest that the climate suitability for malaria from 2006–2010 was above that of the baseline period. Any large-scale declines in malaria cases and deaths during 2006–2010 are unlikely therefore to be as a result of a drier or cooler climate and an associated reduction in transmission suitability.

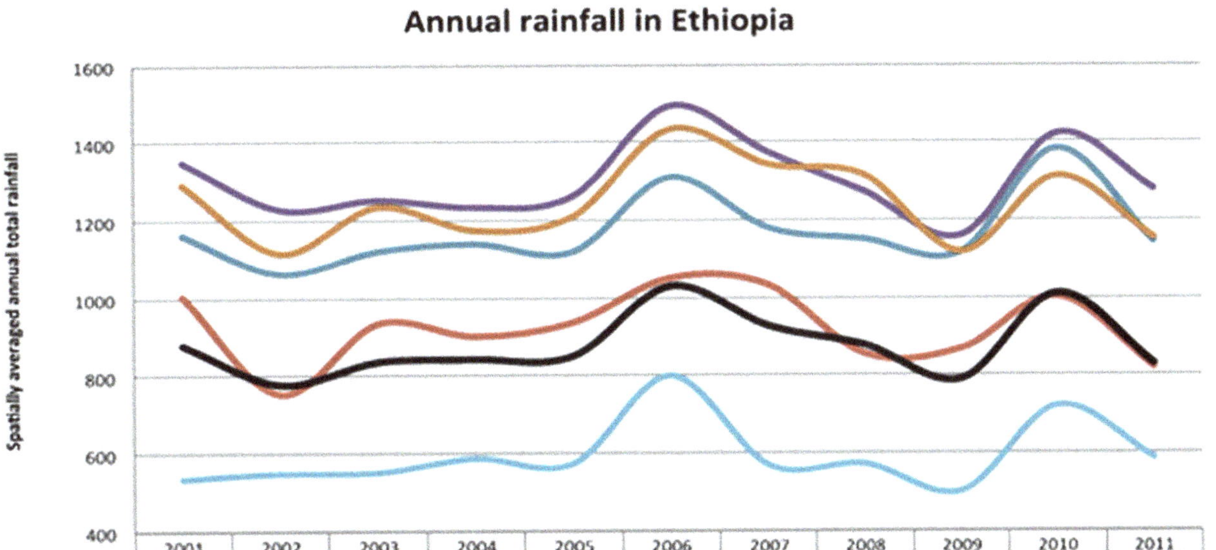

	2001	2002	2003	2004	2005	2006	2007	2008	2009	2010	2011
SNNPR	1349	1228	1252	1233	1261	1493	1373	1272	1159	1421	1278
Oromia	1160	1062	1120	1139	1119	1310	1179	1150	1117	1382	1143
Amhara	1290	1115	1234	1173	1209	1434	1342	1314	1118	1312	1153
Tigray	1005	752	934	901	936	1050	1031	854	867	1001	819
Somali	536	548	550	587	573	800	568	571	501	720	586
Country	879	778	836	843	850	1030	927	878	790	1010	830

Figure 7. Trends of annually averaged rainfall (mm) in the major regions, 2001–2011, Ethiopia.

The results of health facility-based changes in disease occurrences should be cautiously interpreted, as they may be influenced by changes in service utilization, testing rates, reporting, and other factors [25]. To the extent that these are addressed, review of hospital data from Ethiopia shows that malaria cases and deaths have decreased during the second half of the study period and these changes may be related to the increase in malaria control interventions. Given the history of malaria transmission in Ethiopia, strengthening of the surveillance system to allow regular monitoring of the disease trends is crucial to the success of the programme. Malaria in Ethiopia is highly heterogeneous and despite the recent reduction in malaria, the risk of resurgence and epidemics is still very real [5]. Intensive malaria control activities guided by epidemiological stratification with high resolution and adequate funding are therefore needed to reduce malaria transmission further and remove the risk of resurgence. In moderate-high transmission areas with considerable number of outpatient malaria cases, national malaria control programmes should consider surveillance on aggregates of outpatient cases and use line-listing of inpatient cases for assessing the use of interventions and causes of continued transmission in some areas. In low transmission areas where number of cases are manageable, line-listing of outpatient cases should be considered for in-depth geo-referencing and investigation of foci [26].

It has been difficult to discern trends in malaria cases and deaths from national aggregates reported in Ethiopia because of inconsistent and incomplete reporting [6]. This study was undertaken to attempt to account for reporting inconsistencies. Similar studies from sample hospitals will likely be required until the health information system becomes fully functional at national level to provide facility-level quality data to allow reliable assessment of trends of malaria cases and deaths; and other related indicators. Such studies would be stronger if complemented by trend analysis at levels of health centres and health posts to confirm if trends observed in hospitals are consistent with that of lower level facilities.

Acknowledgments

We thank Ministry of Health of the Federal Government of Ethiopia and the health staff who were involved in data collection and supervision. We also thank the Global Fund for availing resources for this study. We are grateful to the support provided by the International Research Institute for Climate and Society, Columbia University, New York, USA, in compiling and analysing spatial and temporal climate data for Ethiopia and to the National Meteorological Agency of Ethiopia for availing meteorological data mainly Enhanced National Climate Services (ENACTS) rainfall data aggregated for five major regions of the country. We thank Mehran Hosseini and John Aponte for their critical review and suggestion on the statistical methods. We thank Richard Cibulskis, Robert Newman, Umberto D'Alessandro and Christopher Dye for their critical review.

Author Contributions

Conceived and designed the experiments: MA. Performed the experiments: MA WB MY AL HK. Analyzed the data: MA. Contributed reagents/materials/analysis tools: MA RW. Wrote the paper: MA ML DJ HT MC. Provided precipitation data: MT. helped in strategic guidance, design of the study and reviewing of the manuscript: FNT KA TAG. Provided critical review and technical guidance: MC.

References

1. United Nations, UN Population Division New York (2013) World population prospects. Available: http://esa.un.org/wpp/Accessed 2014 May 6.
2. Zhou G, Minakawa N, Githeko AK, Yan G (2004) Association between climate variability and malaria epidemics in the East African highlands. Proc Natl Acad Sci U S A. 24; 101(8): 2375–80.
3. Fontaine RE, Najjar AE, Prince JS (1961) The 1958 malaria epidemic in Ethiopia. Am J Trop Med Hyg. 10: 795–803.
4. Checchi F, Cox J, Balkan S, Tamrat A, Priotto G, et al. (2006) Malaria Epidemics and Interventions, Kenya, Burundi, Southern Sudan, and Ethiopia, 1999–2004. Emerging Infectious Diseases. CDC. Volume 12.
5. Negash K, Kebede A, Medhin A, Argaw D, Babaniyi O, et al. (2006) Malaria epidemics in the highlands of Ethiopia. East Afr Med J 82(4): 186–92.
6. World Health organization (2013) World Malaria Report 2013. Geneva, Switzerland. ISBN 978 92 4 156469 4. Available: http://www.who.int/malaria/publications/world_malaria_report_2013/en/Accessed 2014 May 7.
7. Ministry of Health of the Federal Democratic Republic of Ethiopia (2004) Malaria Diagnosis and Treatment Guidelines for Health Workers in Ethiopia, 2nd Edition.
8. Teklehaimanot HD, Teklehaimanot A (2013) Human resource development for a community-based health extension program: a case study from Ethiopia. Hum Resour Health.20; 11(1): 39.
9. United Nations, United Nations Population Division New York (2011) World population prospects. Available: http://esa.un.org/wpp/unpp/panel_population.htm. Accessed 2014 Mar 25.
10. Dinku T, Hilemariam K, Grimes D, Kidane A, Connor S (2011) Improving availability, access and use of climate information. WMO Bulletin 60(2)
11. Thomson M, Indeje M, Connor S, Dilley M, Ward N (2003) Malaria early warning in Kenya and seasonal climate forecasts. Lancet. 362(9383): 580.
12. STATA website. Data Analysis and Statistical Software. Available: www.stata.com. Accessed 2014 Mar 25.
13. Wagner AK, Soumerai SB, Zhang F, Ross-Degnan D (2002) Segmented regression analysis of interrupted time series studies in medication use research. J Clin Pharm Ther. 27(4): 299–309
14. Box GEP, Jenkins G (1976) Time Series Analysis: Forecasting and Control, Holden-Day.
15. Ryan SE, Porth LS (2007) A tutorial on the piecewise regression approach applied to bedload transport data. Gen. Tech. Rep. RMRS-GTR-189. Fort Collins, CO: U.S. Department of Agriculture, Forest Service, Rocky Mountain Research Station. 41 p.
16. Hodrick RJ, Prescott E (1997) Postwar U.S Business Cycles: An Empirical Investigation. J Money, Credit, and Banking. 29 (1) pp. 1–16.
17. Thomson M, Indeje M, Connor S, Dilley M, Ward N (2003) Malaria early warning in Kenya and seasonal climate forecasts. Lancet 16; 362(9383): 580.
18. Aregawi MW, Ali AS, Al-mafazy A, Molteni F, Katikiti S, et al. (2011). Reductions in malaria and anaemia case and death burden at hospitals following scale-up of malaria control in Zanzibar, 1999–2008. Malaria J. 10: 46.
19. Bhattarai A, Ali AS, Kachur SP, Mårtensson A, Abbas AK, et al. (2007) Impact of artemisinin-based combination therapy and insecticide-treated nets on malaria burden in Zanzibar. PLoS Med 6; 4(11): e309.
20. Karema C, Aregawi MW, Rukundo A, Kabayiza A, Mulindahabi M, et al. (2012) Trends in malaria cases, hospital admissions and deaths following scale-up of anti-malarial interventions, 2000–2010, Rwanda. Malar J 11: 236.
21. Ceesay SJ, Casals-Pascual C, Erskine J, Anya SE, Duah NO, et al. (2008) Changes in malaria indices between 1999 and 2007 in The Gambia: a retrospective analysis. Lancet 1; 372(9649): 1545–54.
22. Teklehaimanot HD, Teklehaimanot A, Kiszewski A, Rampao HS, Sachs JD (2009). Malaria in São Tomé and Principe: on the brink of elimination after three years of effective antimalarial measures. Am J Trop Med Hyg. 80(1): 133–40.
23. Otten M, Aregawi MW, Were W, Karema C, Medhin A, et al. (2009) Initial evidence of reduction of malaria cases and deaths in Rwanda and Ethiopia due to rapid scale-up of malaria prevention and treatment. Malar J 14; 8: 14.
24. Central Statistical Agency [Ethiopia], ICF International (2012) Ethiopia Demographic and Health Survey 2011. Addis Ababa, Ethiopia and Calverton, Maryland, USA: Central Statistical Agency and ICF International.
25. Rowe AK, Kachur SP, Yoon SS, Lynch M, Slutsker L, et al. (2009) Caution is required when using health facility-based data to evaluate the health impact of malaria control efforts in Africa. Malar J 8: 209.
26. World Health Organization-Geneva, Switzerland (2012) Global Malaria Disease surveillance for malaria control. An operational manual. ISBN: 9789241503341.

2

Factors Affecting Family Satisfaction with Inpatient End-of-Life Care

Erin Sadler[1], Brigette Hales[2], Blair Henry[3], Wei Xiong[4], Jeff Myers[5], Lesia Wynnychuk[5], Ru Taggar[6], Daren Heyland[7], Robert Fowler[8]*

1 Department of General Surgery, University of Toronto, Toronto, Ontario, Canada, **2** Quality and Patient Safety, Sunnybrook Health Sciences Centre, Toronto, Ontario, Canada, **3** Bioethics, Sunnybrook Health Sciences Centre, Toronto, Ontario, Canada, **4** Trauma, Emergency and Critical Care Program, Sunnybrook Health Sciences Centre, Toronto, Ontario, Canada, **5** Palliative Care, Sunnybrook Health Sciences Centre, Toronto, Ontario, Canada, **6** Quality and Patient Safety, Chief Nursing and Health Professions Executive, Sunnybrook Health Sciences Centre, Toronto, Ontario, Canada, **7** Department of Critical Care Medicine, Queen's University, Kingston, Ontario, Canada, **8** Department of Critical Care Medicine, Sunnybrook Health Sciences Centre, Toronto, Ontario, Canada; Department of Medicine, University of Toronto, Toronto, Ontario Canada

Abstract

Background: Little data exists addressing satisfaction with end-of-life care among hospitalized patients, as they and their family members are systematically excluded from routine satisfaction surveys. It is imperative that we closely examine patient and institution factors associated with quality end-of-life care and determine high-priority target areas for quality improvement.

Methods: Between September 1, 2010 and January 1, 2012 the Canadian Health care Evaluation Project (CANHELP) Bereavement Questionnaire was mailed to the next-of-kin of recently deceased inpatients to seek factors associated with satisfaction with end-of-life care. The primary outcome was the global rating of satisfaction. Secondary outcomes included rates of actual versus preferred location of death, associations between demographic factors and global satisfaction, and identification of targets for quality improvement.

Results: Response rate was 33% among 275 valid addresses. Overall, 67.4% of respondents were very or completely satisfied with the overall quality of care their relative received. However, 71.4% of respondents who thought their relative did not die in their preferred location favoured an out-of-hospital location of death. A common location of death was the intensive care unit (45.7%); however, this was not the preferred location of death for 47.6% of such patients. Multivariate Poisson regression analysis showed respondents who believed their relative died in their preferred location were 1.7 times more likely to be satisfied with the end-of-life care that was provided ($p = 0.001$). Items identified as high-priority targets for improvement included: relationships with, and characteristics of health care professionals; illness management; communication; and end-of-life decision-making.

Interpretation: Nearly three-quarters of recently deceased inpatients would have preferred an out-of-hospital death. Intensive care units were a common, but not preferred, location of in-hospital deaths. Family satisfaction with end-of-life care was strongly associated with their relative dying in their preferred location. Improved communication regarding end-of-life care preferences should be a high-priority quality improvement target.

Editor: Yiru Fang, Shanghai Mental Health Center, Shanghai Jiao Tong University School of Medicine, China

Funding: The Heart and Stroke Foundation of Ontario, the University of Toronto Department of Medicine Integrating Challenge Grant, and the Technology Evaluation in the Elderly Network Center of Excellence have supported this body of work. The funders had no role in study design, data collection and analysis, decision to publish, or preparation of the manuscript.

Competing Interests: The authors have declared that no competing interests exist.

* Email: Rob.fowler@sunnybrook.ca

Introduction

Most elderly Canadians, when asked, would prefer to die at home. However in 1997, 73% of Canadians spent their final days in hospital and more recent reports estimate between 54–63% of all deaths continue to occur in hospital [1]. Despite most patients desiring a non-technologically assisted death, nearly one-fifth of all hospitalized patients were admitted to an intensive care unit (ICU) on their final hospitalization [2]. Therefore, it is imperative that our health care system evolve both a capacity to provide quality end-of-life (EOL) care in the location preferred by patients; and in parallel, that our health care system comprises clinicians who have the skills to provide compassionate, and high quality EOL care regardless of location of death.

Despite recognizing EOL care as an important area for quality improvement in hospitals, information related to its provision remains limited and insufficient [3]. Most hospitals systematically exclude the names of recently deceased patients and their family members from routine surveys intended to measure satisfaction with care. In 2000, the Canadian Senate recommended federal and provincial health care data custodians develop indicators for EOL care; however, this has yet to be achieved [4]. In Canada, we urgently require information about current practice and performance in order to guide quality improvement in EOL care. Preferences for care at the end of life vary among the population. Therefore, it is important to seek the perspective of patients and families in any assessment of performance. Prior work has demonstrated close patient proxies can reliably report on quality of services and observable symptoms for dying patients [5]. As the Canadian population is increasingly multicultural it is also important that hospitals understand how individual and cultural differences may influence patients' perception of the provision of EOL care.

The aim for this study was to evaluate the provision and quality of EOL care from the perspective of bereaved family members of recently deceased patients in a large academic tertiary care Canadian hospital. The specific objectives were: 1) assess family members' satisfaction with EOL care; 2) identify associations between level of satisfaction and patient factors (e.g. circumstances of death including location, preference of location and cultural factors); and 3) identify high-priority targets for quality improvement in the care of dying patients and their family members.

Methods

Study Design

The study received approval from Sunnybrook Health Sciences Centre's Research Ethics Board. Informed consent was obtained from all participants prior to entering the study. This study involved a non-incentivized routine mail-out questionnaire protocol. The Canadian Health care Evaluation Project (CANHELP) Bereavement Questionnaire, a letter of information, and return envelope were post-mailed to a random sample of 352 family member contacts of patients for whom death occurred between September 1, 2010 and January 1, 2012. Among those who had not responded after the first mail-out, a second mail-out was sent just over three weeks later. Although previous studies have demonstrated increased response rates using repeat mail-outs and reminders, the decision were made to limit the number of mail-outs to two in order to limit possible distress among family members [6]. Mail, email and phone contacts were provided in the letter of information to all potential respondents should they wish to contact the study investigators. Given the nature of the population, a sample size was not calculated as the number of participants would be determined by the total number of deaths occurring among admitted patients during the study period and for who contact information of their family member was available.

Survey Tool

The Canadian Health care Evaluation Project (CANHELP) Bereavement Questionnaire is a 40-item tool that has been previously validated for use in evaluating quality EOL care [7]. Each item has a 5-point Likert scale to rate level of satisfaction [1-not at all satisfied, 2-not very satisfied, 3-somewhat satisfied, 4-very satisfied, 5-completely satisfied]. The items collectively address eight domains of care including patient pain and symptom management; timely and clear communication; information to prepare the family for approaching death; compassionate care, comfort, dignity, and respect; patient-centred decision making; care of the family; family support; and caregiver satisfaction with hospital facilities and staff. At the end of the questionnaire additional optional items regarding ethnicity, language, and spiritual faith were added to explore their respective associations with EOL care satisfaction.

Data Analysis

The primary outcome variable was the CANHELP Bereavement Questionnaire's global rating of satisfaction which asked: "In general, how satisfied were you with the quality of care your relative received in the last month of life?" Secondary outcomes included: rates of actual versus preferred location of death; associations among demographic factors (patient ethnicity, primary language of patient, religion, and religiosity) and global satisfaction; and identification of targets for quality of care improvement.

Descriptive statistics of demographic data and Likert scale responses included counts and proportions, means (and standard deviations), and medians (and interquartile ranges). The distributions of all responses were assessed visually to determine appropriate parametric or non-parametric analyses. Univariate analysis included Pearson χ^2 and the Mann-Whitney U Test which examined associations between levels of satisfaction and particular characteristics of the respondents and their deceased relative. Levels of satisfaction were dichotomized into satisfied ("very satisfied or completely satisfied") vs. not satisfied ("not at all satisfied, not very satisfied, or somewhat satisfied"); ethnicity into Caucasian vs. non-Caucasian; religion into Christian vs. non-Christian; religiosity into religious vs. non-religious; and primary patient language into English speaking vs. other.

Given the high prevalence of the outcome variable "global rating of satisfaction," the statistic measure of prevalence ratio (relative risk) is preferable to odds ratio. A recent study has proposed a modified Poisson approach to analyze binary data for relative risk with robust error variance [8]. Six independent variables were pre-selected to build a multivariate Poisson regression model. These independent variables were selected *a priori* based on preliminary data exploration and clinical relevance based on the experimental question. A univariate Poisson regression model was applied to each independent variable to identify trending of satisfaction. Age factor was highly insignificant ($p = 0.999$) in the univariate Poisson regression and thus excluded from the multivariate Poisson regression. The other five independent variables were chosen for multivariate modeling due to significant trending ($p<0.2$) or clinical relevance. These variables included location of death (ICU vs. other), preferred location of death (yes vs. no), religiosity (religious vs. non-religious), patient language (English-speaking vs. other) and length of stay (7 to17 days vs. 1 to 6 days, or greater than 18 days vs. 1 to 6 days).

A respondent versus non-respondent analysis was performed to assess for significant differences between these population samples. Fisher's Exact test was used to determine significance when cell sizes were less than five. A Missing Value Analysis was performed to identify questions with a high proportion of unanswered values and estimate their potential impact on results [9].

Spearman Correlations were used to define the relative importance of the questionnaire's items by their association with the global rating of satisfaction. Importance-Satisfaction plots were constructed to identify areas that are of high-priority as targets for improvement by plotting the percent of "very" and "completely satisfied" responses (by their Spearman correlation coefficient) with the global rating of satisfaction [7,10,11]. Four quadrants were then established by plotting a vertical and horizontal line at the median values of the satisfied responses, and the correlation coefficients, respectively. Items in quadrant A (upper left) were considered to be areas of highest-priority for improvement because they were correlated strongly with global satisfaction, yet had lower ratings of satisfaction. A threshold significance level of $\alpha < 0.05$ was used for all analyses. All statistical analysis was completed

Table 1. Characteristics of Respondents and Non-Respondents.

	Respondents Mean (SD) or N (%)	Non-Respondents Mean (SD) or N (%)	χ^2	p
N	92 (33.5%)	183 (67%)	-	
Age (years)	75.7 (16.0)	74.2 (17.8)	-	0.500
Sex of patient			4.81	0.028
Male	58 (63.7%)	91 (49.7%)	-	
Female responses	45 (77.6%)			
Male responses	13 (22.4%)			
Female	33 (36.3%)	92 (50.3%)	-	
Female responses	11 (33.3%)			
Male responses	22 (66.7%)			
Length of stay (days)	15.5 (30.1)	16.9 (33.6)		0.742
Time since death (days)	41.8 (22.0)	46.4 (22.1)		0.112
Location of death				0.583
Intensive care unit	41 (45.1%)	77 (42.1%)		
Hospital ward	48 (52.7%)	95 (51.9%)		
Other	2 (2.2%)	11 (6.0%)		
Relationship to patient			2.11	0.715
Spouse	52 (57.1%)	98 (53.6%)		
Son/Daughter	29 (31.9%)	69 (37.7%)		
Sibling	3 (3.2%)	3 (1.6%)		
Parent	2 (2.2%)	6 (3.3%)		
Other	5 (5.5%)	7 (3.8%)		
Cause of death			11.19	0.263
Cancer	21 (23.1%	54 (39.5%)		
Cardiac	19 (20.8%)	28 (15.3%)		
Respiratory	16 (17.6%)	24 (13.1%)		
Neurological	14 (15.4%)	16 (8.7%)		
Trauma	7 (7.7%)	17 (9.3%)		
Sepsis	6 (6.6%)	10 (5.5%)		
Other	4 (4.4%)	12 (6.6%)		
Vascular	3 (3.3%)	8 (4.4%)		
Renal	0	5 (2.7%)		
GI	1 (1.1%)	9 (4.9%)		

Abbreviations: GI = gastrointestinal.

using SPSS 20.0 (IBM Corporation, Armonk, NY) or SAS 9.3 (SAS Institute, Cary NC).

Results

Response rate was 33% (92/275 valid addresses from an initial sample of 352 deceased patients) after two mail-outs (57 responses after the first, 35 after the second). The original sample of 352 was reduced to 275 valid addresses due to questionnaire packages that were returned to sender. Missing Value Analyses revealed that non-responses to items were missing randomly as opposed to systematically (Little MCAR test, p = 0.820). Only one respondent elected not to answer the optional demographic and cultural items. There were no significant differences among respondents and non-respondents according to age of the deceased, cause of death of the deceased, location of death, length of stay, duration of time since death, or relationship with the deceased; however family member contacts of deceased male patients were more likely to respond than family member contacts of deceased female patients (OR 1.77, p = 0.028) (Table 1).

Overall, 67.4% of respondents were *very* or *completely* satisfied with the overall quality of care their relative received in the last month of life. The most common location of death was the ICU (45.7%); however, this was not the preferred location of death for 47.6% of patients dying in the ICU (Table 2). Overall, 46.7% believed their relative did not die in the preferred location and of these, 71.4% believed their family member would have preferred an out-of-hospital ("home or retirement home") location. In Table 3, univariate Poisson regression analysis showed that, respondents who believed their relative died in their preferred location of death were 1.9 times more likely to be satisfied with the quality of EOL care (p<0.001).

The risk-adjusted multivariate Poisson regression model also indicated that patients' preferred location was a highly significant predictor for family global satisfaction (p = 0.001; Table 3). Families of patients who died in their preferred location were

1.7 times more likely to be satisfied with the quality of EOL care than families of patients who did not die in their preferred location using the multivariate model. The other four variables (location of death, religiosity, patient language and length of stay) did not demonstrate a significant relationship with family global satisfaction. The multivariate Poisson model fits the data well, since the ratio of deviance over degrees of freedom was less than 1.0, suggesting that there was no over-dispersion in the data. A Poisson model may be preferable over negative binomial model when the data is not over-dispersed.

Figure 1 outlines the Importance-Satisfaction Grid [7,10,11]. Quadrant A identifies survey items that are high-priority targets for improvement and include: relationships with the doctors; characteristics of the doctors and nurses; illness management; and communication and decision-making (Table 4). The survey items in quadrant D signify areas less correlated with global satisfaction, but are potentially worthwhile targets given the lower levels of satisfaction with current practice.

Discussion

Although family members of recently deceased patients were generally satisfied with the quality of EOL care, this study identified several important targets for quality improvement. First, nearly half of respondents believed that patients did not die in their preferred location, and most commonly would have preferred an out-of-hospital, at home death. Second, despite the population stating that they would like to avoid aggressive, technology-laden EOL care, the most common location of death in hospital was the ICU. Importantly, families of patients who died in their preferred location were nearly two times more likely to be satisfied with EOL care.

Although only one of many factors, dying in a preferred location has been shown in other studies to be strongly associated with satisfaction [12]. This indicates that our health care system should evolve mechanisms to provide such care outside of hospitals, in palliative homes or hospices; and, hospitals should reassess resources available to provide EOL care in alternative settings to the ICU. Our findings are consistent with the work of others who have found a mismatch in the care which patients and their families' desire, and the default institutionalized and aggressive EOL care which they often receive [2].

The discrepancy between preferred and actual location of death might also be due to ineffective advance care planning processes. In a recently performed study of 513 elderly inpatients at high risk of dying at 12 Canadian acute care hospitals, although 76% of patients had thought about EOL care, only 12% had preferred life-prolonging care, and fewer than half had completed an advance care plan. Of those who had discussed their wishes, 30% had done so with their family physician and only 55% with any member of the health care team [13]. Before hospitalization, only 20% of patients discussed prognosis with a physician.

The Importance-Satisfaction grid highlights the areas of EOL care that should be high-priority targets for quality of care improvement. Our results echo those of other investigators who surveyed both patients and families finding that emotional support for patients, relationships with doctors, and communication and decision-making are highly correlated with satisfaction yet often poorly performed [7,14]. Items most strongly correlated with global satisfaction included the level of trust in the doctor(s) and nurse(s), availability of the doctor(s) when their relative needed them, and compassionate and supportive care of their relative and themselves. One systematic review highlighted several similar areas of EOL care that were important to overall satisfaction, including accessibility and coordination, effective symptom management, comfort level with the dying process, education and communication, emotional support, care on the individual level, and support of patients' decision-making [15]. The similarity with other literature adds confidence to this study's findings and lends support to generalizability to other care settings. Our results suggest that levels of satisfaction with the quality of EOL care may be improved by targeting a select number of high-impact aspects of care, such as doctor availability, caring for patients in the absence of family members, the health care team working together as a cohesive team, and attentive listening to patients and families.

An overarching and important finding from this study is that the CANHELP Bereavement Questionnaire provides a feasible tool to evaluate care provided to patients at the end of life, to measure satisfaction, and to identify high-priority targets for quality improvement. This has been shown in other literature to be a reasonable method of obtaining accurate and representative views of the patients [5]. In addition, surveying family members can be a powerful vehicle for families to not only provide feedback, but to share their experiences, which may be an important element of the grieving process. A substantial number of returned surveys included narratives of the experience. Many requested an opportunity to communicate with study investigators directly, and this provided a subsequent mechanism to support families

Table 2. Actual and Preferred Location of Death.

Location of Death	N (%)
Intensive Care Unit	42 (45.7)
Palliative Care Unit	4 (4.3)
Hospital Ward	39 (42.4)
Other	3 (3.3)
No Answer	4 (4.3)
Patient's Preferred Location	
Yes	38 (41.3)
No	42 (45.7)
Prefer Home or Retirement Home	30 (71.4)
Prefer Other	12 (28.6)
No Answer	12 (13)

Table 3. Factors Associated with Satisfaction with End-of-Life Care.

Variables	Categories	Univariate Poisson regression		Multivariable Poisson regression	
		Prevalence ratio (95% CI)	p value	Prevalence ratio (95% CI)	p value
Preferred Location of Death	Yes vs No	1.9 (1.4–2.8)	<0.001	1.7 (1.2–2.4)	0.001
Location of Death	ICU vs Other	1.2 (0.9–1.6)	0.279	1.2 (0.9–1.6)	0.120
Religiosity	Very or Somewhat vs Other	1.5 (1.0–2.1)	0.020	1.2 (0.9–1.7)	0.191
Language	English vs Other	0.7 (0.5–0.9)	0.006	0.9 (0.7–1.1)	0.316
Age	>=80	1.0 (0.6–1.7)			
	71–79		0.999		
	<=70 (ref)	1.0 (0.7–1.4)			
Length of Stay	>=18	0.9 (0.7–1.2)		0.9 (0.7–1.2)	
	7–17		0.133		0.744
	<=6 (ref)	0.6 (0.4–1.0)		0.8 (0.5–1.4)	

Abbreviations: ref = reference; vs = versus.

through their loss, and, possibly an additional mechanism to improve their own satisfaction with care delivery.

This study is not without limitations. First, the response rate to the survey was modest. The response rate may have improved with subsequent mail-outs; however, we purposely limited such reminders in case families were not yet ready or willing to engage in discussion of their recent loss. As well, there has been a recent shift towards assessing survey response rate by the potential for non-respondent bias, and whether the response population is representative of the population of interest [16]. Importantly, we found very little difference in measured characteristics of respondents and non-respondents. However, this modest response rate does limit the external validity of the current study, and it is recommended that larger datasets be collected in order to determine reliability of the present results. Second, the respondent population was predominantly Caucasian, English-speaking and

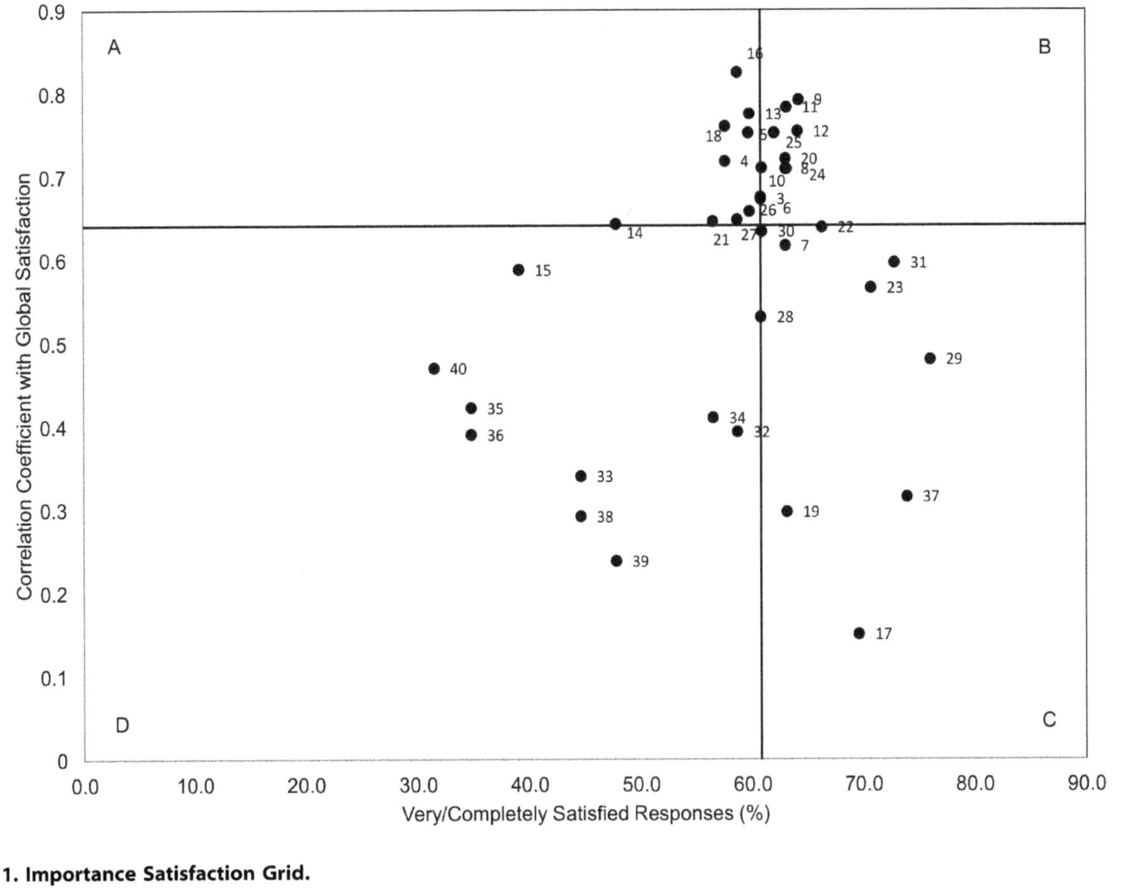

Figure 1. Importance Satisfaction Grid.

Table 4. High-Priority Areas for Quality Improvement.

Domain		Questionnaire Item
Relationship with Doctors	3.	How satisfied are you that you knew the doctor(s) in charge of your relative's care in the last month of life?
	4.	How satisfied are you that the doctor(s) took a personal interest in your relative in the last month of life?
	5.	How satisfied are you that the doctor(s) were available when you or your relative needed them (by phone or in person) in the last month of life?
	6.	How satisfied are you with the level of trust and confidence you had in the doctor(s) who looked after your relative in the last month of life?
Characteristics of the Doctors and Nurses	10.	How satisfied are you that the doctors and nurses looking after your relative in the last month of life were compassionate and supportive of you.
Illness Management	13.	How satisfied are you that physical symptoms (i.e. pain, shortness of breath, nausea, etc.) your relative had in the last month of life were adequately assessed and controlled?
	16.	How satisfied are you that, in the last month of life, your relative received good care when you were not able to be with him/her?
	18.	How satisfied are you that health care workers worked together as a team to look after your relative in the last month of life?
	21.	How satisfied are you that care and treatment your relative received in the last month of life was consistent with his/her wishes?
Communication and Decision Making	26.	How satisfied are you that the doctor(s) listened to what you had to say in the last month of your relative's life?
	27.	How satisfied are you with the discussions in the last month of life with the doctor(s) about where your relative would be cared for (in hospital, home, elsewhere)?

Christian. Ensuring delivery of culturally sensitive care should be an important goal for hospitals as we have previously shown that such factors often predict desires for different care at the end of life [17]. Although our respondent pool was of only modest size, it is important that we did not find evidence that specific aspects of culture – ethnicity, language, religion – were significantly associated with satisfaction with the quality of EOL care in this setting. It is possible that in more or less culturally diverse patient settings, such factors may have an even greater relationship with satisfaction. A related limitation is that our survey was administered only in English. The questionnaire is also available in French, and future work should explore further translations, especially among ethnic groups that have may have culturally unique EOL needs or practices. An additional limitation to the dataset is the anonymized nature of the survey responses. Analysis of the demographic data of the respondents and non-respondents was done on a pooled, gross level. However, respective survey responses were anonymized from their demographic data in order to fulfill the Research Ethics requirements of the study's institution. This meant that analysis at the individual respondent level was unable to be completed. Finally, although the results of our study represent the views of families at a single tertiary academic centre, we suspect the emerging of importance of communication, relationships and location of death are broadly generalizable to other hospitals and we encourage other centres to undertake a similar exercise towards understanding how to better improve quality of EOL care.

Conclusion

Administration of the CANHELP bereavement questionnaire to family members of recently deceased inpatients is feasible and associated with a high degree of internal consistency. Many patients die in a location other than is preferred and dying in the preferred location is highly associated with family satisfaction with EOL care. This represents an urgent health care system and hospital target for quality improvement. Additionally, this questionnaire allows construction of a hospital-specific Importance-Satisfaction grid that can help hospitals identify unique quality improvement targets. We recommend that hospitals and health care systems adopt a common instrument to measure and improve EOL care that allows for local quality of care improvement and comparisons across institutions en route to addressing the needs of patients and families at the end of life.

Author Contributions

Conceived and designed the experiments: ES RF B. Hales B. Henry JM. Performed the experiments: ES RF B. Hales. Analyzed the data: ES RF WX. Contributed reagents/materials/analysis tools: ES RF B. Hales B. Henry JM LW RT DH WX. Wrote the paper: ES RF B. Hales B. Henry JM LW RT DH WX.

References

1. Heyland DK, Lavery JV, Tranmer JE, Shortt SED, Taylor SJ (2000) Dying in Canada: Is it an institutionalized, technologically supported experience? J Palliat Care 16: s10–s16.
2. Canadian Institute for Health Information (2007) Health Care Use at the End of Life in Western Canada (Ottawa: CIHI).
3. Singer PA, Bowman KW (2002) Quality care at the end of life: Should be recognised as a global problem for public health and health systems. BMJ 324(7349): 1291–1292.
4. Standing Senate Committee on Social Affairs, Science and Technology (2000) Recommendation 11. In: Quality end-of-life care: the right of every Canadian: final report of the subcommittee to update Of Life and Death. Ottawa: Senate of Canada.
5. McPherson CJ, Addington-Hall JM (2003) Judging the quality of care at the end of life: Can proxies provide reliable information? Soc Sci Med 56: 95–109.
6. Burns K, Duffett M, Kho ME, Meade MO, Adhikari N, et al. (2008) A guide for the design and conduct of self-administered surveys of clinicians. CMAJ 179(3): 245–252.
7. Heyland DK, Cook DJ, Rocker GM, Dodek PM, Kutsogiannis DJ, et al. (2010) The development and validation of a novel questionnaire to measure patient and family satisfaction with end-of-life care: the Canadian Health Care Evaluation Project (CANHELP) Questionnaire. Palliat Med 24(7): 682–695.

8. Zou G (2004) A modified Poisson regression approach to prospective studies with binary data. Am J Epidemiol 159(7): 702–6.
9. SPSS Missing Value Analysis. Available http://priede.bf.lu.lv/grozs/Datorlietas/SPSS/SPSS%20Missing%20Value%20Analysis%207.5.pdf. Accessed: Mar 15 2013.
10. Dodek PM, Heyland DK, Rocker GM, Cook DJ (2004) Translating family satisfaction data into quality improvement. Crit Care Med (9): 1922–1927.
11. Soberman LR, Murray M, Norton PG, van Maris B, Tasa K (1997) Satisfaction of residents and families in longterm care: III. Dissemination of results. Qual Manag Health Care 5: 63–71.
12. Teno JM, Clarridge BR, Casey V, Welch LC, Wetle T, et al. (2004) Family perspectives on end-of-life care at the last place of care. JAMA 291(1): 88–93.
13. Heyland DK, Barwich DB, Pichora D, Dodek P, Lamontagne F, et al. (2013) Failure to engage hospitalized elderly patients and their families in advance care planning. JAMA Intern Med l: 1–10.
14. Heyland DK, Cook DJ, Rocker GM, Dodek PM, Kutsogiannis DJ, et al. (2010) Defining priorities for improving end of life care in Canada. CMAJ 182(16): 747–752.
15. Dy SM, Shugarman LR, Lorenz KA, Mularski RA, Lynn J (2008) A systematic review of satisfaction with care at the end of life. J Am Geriatr Soc 56: 124–129.
16. Johnson TP, Wislar JS (2012). Response rates and nonresponse errors in surveys. JAMA 307(17): 1805–1806.
17. Frost DW, Cook DJ, Heyland DK, Fowler RA (2011) Patient and health care professional factors influencing end-of-life decision-making during critical illness: A systematic review. Crit Care Med 39(5): 1174–1189.

3

Treatment Results in the Different Surgery of Intradural Extramedullary Tumor of 122 Cases

Shaohui Zong[1], Gaofeng Zeng[2], Li Du[1], Ye Fang[1], Taihang Gao[1], Jingmin Zhao[3]*

1 Department of Spine Osteopathia, the First Affiliated Hospital of Guangxi Medical University, Nanning, Guangxi, P.R. China, 2 College of Public Hygiene of Guangxi Medical University, Nanning, Guangxi, P.R. China, 3 Department of Orthopaedics Trauma and Hand Surgery, the First Affiliated Hospital of Guangxi Medical University, Nanning, Guangxi, P.R. China

Abstract

Study Design: A retrospective study of intradural extramedullary tumor.

Objective: To compare the treatment results in the different surgeries of spinal intradural extramedullary tumor.

Methods: The study retrospectively reviewed 122 patients. The minimally invasive surgery (MIS) group was divided into Group A (hemilaminectomy + tumor microscopic excision) and Group B (laminectomy + tumor microscopic excision + pedicle screw fixation). Meanwhile, the non-MIS group was divided into Group C (hemilaminectomy + tumor excision), Group D (laminectomy + tumor excision), and Group E (laminectomy + tumor excision + pedicle screw fixation). In order to study postoperative spinal stability, we simultaneously divided all of the subjects into three categories, namely Group HE: hemilaminectomy + tumor excision; Group LE: laminectomy + tumor excision; and Group LEPSF: laminectomy + tumor excision + pedicle screw fixation.

Results: The MIS group exhibited fewer postoperative complications ($p<0.05$), better short-term clinical efficacy ($p<0.05$) and less non-surgical cost ($p<0.05$) than in non-MIS group. The rate of postoperative spinal instability in hemilaminectomy was lower than in laminectomy in a single spinal segment ($p<0.05$). The rate of postoperative spinal instability in laminectomy + pedicle screw fixation was lower than in hemilaminectomy and laminectomy in two or more spinal segments ($p<0.05$).

Conclusion: In the case of appropriate surgical indications, minimally invasive surgery for intradural extramedullary tumor is a useful method that can successfully produce good clinical results and reduce non-surgical cost. In addition, pedicle screw fixation helps avoid spinal postoperative instability.

Editor: Zachary A. Smith, Northwestern University, United States of America

Funding: The authors acknowledge support from the Guangxi Science and Technology Plan Fund, Gui Ke Gong 1298003-5-1. The funders had no role in study design, data collection and analysis, decision to publish, or preparation of the manuscript.

Competing Interests: The authors have declared that no competing interests exist.

* Email: zhaojingmin3008@sina.com

Introduction

Intradural extramedullary tumors are very common in the osteopathic departments, accounting for approximately two-thirds of all primary intraspinal neoplasms [1]. As the tumors grow larger, the main outcome may be the compression of the spinal cord, which can cause back pain and worsening sensory and motor loss. The analyses of data from 25 cases revealed that the remaining spinal canal area was decreased to 20–30% of the normal spinal canal [2]. Therefore, the primary goal of the therapy for spinal intradural tumors is to decompress the spinal cord and remove it thoroughly without recurrence.

Nowadays, surgery is the effective approach for benign intradural extramedullary tumors [3]. For older people, minimally invasive surgery for benign intradural extramedullary tumor removal still represents the best therapeutic option [4,5]. Although a conventional approach without a microscope can have a good curative effect, several drawbacks still exist, including greater intraoperative blood loss and a higher risk of injury to the spinal cord or nerve roots. With the development of technology, manipulation with a microscope could avoid these problems as far as possible. When removing spinal intradural extramedullary tumors by MIS or non-MIS, the damage to the anatomical structure of the posterior column of the spine will affects postoperative spinal stability.

This study reviewed a series of 53 consecutive patients with spinal intradural extramedullary tumors who underwent MIS and 69 consecutive patients with spinal intradural extramedullary tumors who underwent non-MIS. The purpose of this retrospective study is to compare the treatment results between MIS and non-MIS in these cases of spinal intradural extramedullary tumor and to analyze the postoperative spinal stability and health economics arising from the different surgical techniques.

Table 1. Summary of baseline characteristics of intradural extramedullary tumor patients.

Groups	N	Age (year)	Male/Female	Course of disease (mouth)
MIS group	53	41.15±14.73	29/24	32.45±6.81
Non-MIS group	69	43.25±16.42	37/32	30.67±5.28
Group A	19	42.84±11.25	11/8	28.25±8.14
Group B	34	41.42±13.47	16/18	29.53±8.75
Group C	24	40.26±15.08	14/10	33.67±7.99
Group D	18	43.71±12.23	10/8	30.73±7.43
Group E	27	43.54±14.67	15/12	31.84±6.58
Group HE	43	40.87±12.54	21/22	29.72±4.73
Group LE	18	41.62±13.75	10/8	34.91±7.54
Group LESPF	61	43.92±15.68	35/26	33.14±9.36

There was no significant difference between the MIS group and Non-MIS group ($p>0.05$). This was the same among the five groups (Group A, Group B, Group C, Group D, Group E; $p>0.05$) and among the three groups (Group HE, Group LE, Group LESPF; $p>0.05$). Data are expressed as the mean ± standard deviation.

Materials and Methods

Ethical statement

All study procedures were reviewed and approved by the Institutional Ethics Review Board at the First Affiliated Hospital of Guangxi Medical University and conducted according to the principles expressed in the Declaration of Helsinki. Informed consent was exempted by the board due to the retrospective nature of this research.

Patient characteristics

122 patients who underwent surgical resection of intradural extramedullary tumors were retrospectively analyzed from January 2010 to June 2012. Data were obtained from the departments of surgery of six hospitals in the south of China. The ages of patients ranged from 15 to 82 years, with a mean age of 42 years. Symptom duration before surgery ranged from 2 months to 9 years, with a mean symptom duration of 31.2 months. The following inclusion criteria were used: 1) all of the subjects had intradural extramedullary tumor; 2) all of the subjects exhibited integrity of the spine and spinal stability before surgery; 3) clinical diagnosis was determined by physical examination, magnetic resonance imaging (MRI), and pathology; and 4) clinical and radiological follow-up was carried out for 12–60 months (average 28 months). Patients who underwent surgery again because of the recurrence of intraspinal tumor were excluded. The spinal levels of intradural extramedullary tumor were cervical vertebrae in 36 cases, cervicothoracic vertebrae in 2 cases, thoracic vertebrae in 39 cases, thoracolumbar vertebrae in 3 cases, and lumbosacral vertebrae in 42 cases.

Surgical methods

All the patients were placed in the prone position under general anesthesia and a posterior median approach was chosen. The choice of surgical procedure depended on the location and size of the tumor. Hemilaminectomy was adopted when the tumor was small or located laterally or dorsolaterally to the spinal cord. Laminectomy was adopted when the tumor was large or located ventrally to the spinal cord. Pedicle screw fixation was required after multilevel laminectomy. Based on the spinal level of tumor, we inserted the pedicle screws in above 1-below 1. The subjects were divided into two groups according to the type of differential surgery, namely the MIS group (53 cases) and the non-MIS group (69 cases). The MIS group was subdivided into two groups, as follows:

- Group A: hemilaminectomy + tumor microscopic excision, 19 cases; and
- Group B: laminectomy + tumor microscopic excision + pedicle screw fixation, 34 cases.

Table 2. Summary of the results for operating time, intraoperative blood loss, resection rate, duration of hospital stay, and complications.

Groups	N	Operating time (min)	Intraoperative blood loss (ml)	Resection rate (%)	Duration of hospital stay (d)	Complications
MIS group	53	270.00±147.99★	307.14±185.13★	77.36▲	21.88±10.15★	2★
Non-MIS group	69	173.26±81.36	540.08±282.15	72.46	26.42±11.60	12

This table shows the results for operating time, intraoperative blood loss, resection rate, duration of hospital stay, and complications in the MIS and Non-MIS group. "Resection rate" means the percentage of the cases of total resection of tumor. Data are expressed as the mean ± standard deviation.
★$p<0.05$ vs. MIS group;
▲$p>0.05$ vs. Non-MIS group.

Table 3. Analysis of short-term and long-term clinical efficacy.

Groups	N	Short-term clinical efficacy			Long-term clinical efficacy		
		Effectivity	Nullity	Rate of effectivity (%)	Effectivity	Nullity	Rate of effectivity (%)
MIS group	53	52	1	98.11*	51	2	96.22▲
Non-MIS group	69	59	10	85.50	64	5	92.75

This table shows the results for short-term and long-term clinical efficacy in the MIS and Non-MIS groups.
*$p<0.05$ vs. Non-MIS group;
▲$p>0.05$ vs. Non-MIS group.

Meanwhile, the non-MIS group was subdivided into the following three groups:

- Group C: hemilaminectomy + tumor excision, 24 cases;
- Group D: laminectomy + tumor excision, 18 cases;
- Group E: laminectomy + tumor excision + pedicle screw fixation, 27 cases.

In order to study postoperative spinal stability, 122 patients were simultaneously divided into three categories, as follows:

- Group HE: hemilaminectomy + tumor excision, 43 cases;
- Group LE: laminectomy + tumor excision, 18 cases; and
- Group LEPSF: laminectomy + tumor excision + pedicle screw fixation, 61 cases.

Clinical outcome evaluation

The preoperative neurological status and neurological status at the time of discharge were evaluated in terms of back pain, dysesthesia, dyskinesia, and sphincter disturbance. Each category was divided into three grades, namely improved, unchanged, and deteriorative. In the postoperative evaluation of recent clinical efficacy, improvement and no change in neurological status were regarded as effectivity and deterioration of neurological status was regarded as nullity.

The evaluation of the long-term clinical efficacy was carried out using the American Spinal Injury Association classification (ASIA) [6]. In the evaluation of long-term clinical efficacy at the time of final follow-up (12–60 months, average 28 months), improvement was regarded as effectivity, while no change and deterioration were regarded as nullity.

All of the patients underwent examination of lateral roentgenograms during follow-up every 6 months. A spinal instability was diagnosed when either of the following conditions was observed [7]: 1. Abnormal mobility: abnormal segmental motion of a vertebral body of more than 15°; and 2. abnormal slide: anterior or posterior slide of a vertebral body of more than 3 mm.

Health economics analysis

The total costs of hospitalization included surgical and non-surgical costs. Internal fixation device cost was included in surgical cost. Non-surgical cost included drug cost and hospital bed cost. Because the patients were from different socioeconomic backgrounds, an accurate estimation of work loss-related costs was not possible and this item was excluded from the cost analysis.

Statistical analysis

All data are presented as the mean ± standard error of the mean (SEM). The statistical analysis was performed using SPSS 16.0 (SPSS, Inc., Chicago, IL, USA). Enumeration data were tested by the chi-squared test. Measurement data were tested by analysis of variance and t tests. A value of $p<0.05$ (two-tailed) was considered statistically significant.

Results

There was no significant difference in age, gender or the course of disease between the MIS group and non-MIS group ($p>0.05$; Table 1). This was the same among the five groups (Group A, Group B, Group C, Group D, Group E; $p>0.05$; Table 1) and among the three groups (Group HE, Group LE, Group LESPF; $p>0.05$; Table 1).

Table 4. Summary of results of duration of hospital stay, recovery time, loss of working time.

Groups	N	Duration of hospital stay (d)	Recovery time (d)	Loss of working time (d)
A	19	21.42±10.36	19.29±8.92	50.13±15.76
B	34	22.35±9.83	31.12±7.79	59.98±12.83
C	24	24.76±7.81★	22.31±6.78★	52.69±10.33★
D	18	25.29±11.92•	42.72±7.25▲	75.38±15.22▲
E	27	28.73±13.47▲	34.18±9.6•	71.81±17.19▲

This table shows the results for the duration of hospital stay, recovery times, and loss of working time in five groups (Group A, Group B, Group C, Group D, Group E). "Recovery time" means the postoperative activity time. "Duration of hospital stay" means the postoperative days in hospital. "Loss of working time" represents the duration from admission to the start of work after hospital discharge. Data are expressed as the mean ± standard deviation.

★$p>0.05$ vs. Group A;

▲$p<0.05$ vs. Group B;

•$p>0.05$ vs. Group B.

Clinical results

In the MIS group (53 cases), postoperative pathologies showed schwannoma in 26 cases, meningioma in 12, dermoid cyst in 4, hemangioma in 3, and lipoma in 2. Among these, 41 tumors were totally removed, 10 were subtotally removed, and 2 were partially removed. Two complications were observed in the MIS group, including one case of infection and one case of myasthenia. Meanwhile, in the non-MIS group (69 cases), postoperative

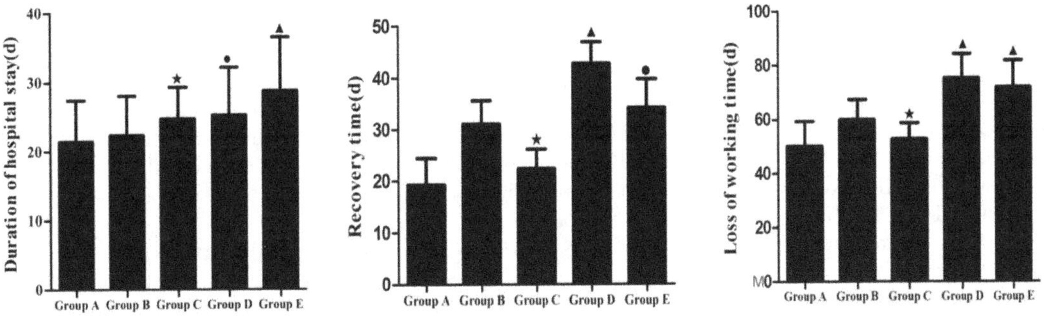

Group A: hemilaminectomy + tumor microscopic excision

Group B: laminectomy + tumor microscopic excision + pedicle screw fixation

Group C: hemilaminectomy + tumor excision

Group D: laminectomy + tumor excision

Group E: laminectomy +tumor excision + pedicle screw fixation

Duration of hospital stay: the postoperative days in hospital

Recovery time: the postoperative activity time

Loss of working time: the duration from admission to the start of work after hospital discharge

Fig 1: This table shows the results for the duration of hospital stay, recovery times, and loss of working time in five groups (Group A, Group B, Group C, Group D, Group E). Data are expressed as the mean ± standard deviation. ★ $p > 0.05$ vs. Group A; ▲$p < 0.05$ vs. Group B; •$p>0.05$ vs. Group B.

Figure 1. This table shows the results for the duration of hospital stay, recovery times, and loss of working time in five groups (Group A, Group B, Group C, Group D, Group E). Data are expressed as the mean ± standard deviation. ★p>0.05 vs. Group A; ▲p<0.05 vs. Group B; ●p>0.05 vs. Group B. Group A: hemilaminectomy + tumor microscopic excision. Group B: laminectomy + tumor microscopic excision + pedicle screw fixation. Group C: hemilaminectomy + tumor excision. Group D: laminectomy + tumor excision. Group E: laminectomy + tumor excision + pedicle screw fixation. Duration of hospital stay: the postoperative days in hospital. Recovery time: the postoperative activity time. Loss of working time: the duration from admission to the start of work after hospital discharge.

Table 5. Summary of various expenses.

Groups	N	Surgical cost (CNY)	Non-surgical cost (CNY)	Cost of hospitalization (CNY)
A	19	13467±7682	7782±3129	20971±12318
B	34	29314±12854	6459±2743	34354±13214
C	24	10525±9078★	10974±5607▲	21509±8842★
D	18	11628±7216*	11691±8329*	22319±11327*
E	27	27612±10722■	9621±6031*	37234±11999■

This table shows the analysis of health economics for the five surgical approaches. Data are expressed as the mean ± standard deviation.
★$p>0.05$ vs. Group A;
▲$p<0.05$ vs. Group A;
*$p<0.05$ vs. Group B;
■$p>0.05$ vs. Group B.

pathologies showed schwannoma in 29 cases, meningioma in 15, dermoid cyst in 12, arachnoid cyst in 9, enterogenous cyst in 3, and hemangioma in 1. Among these, 50 tumors were totally removed, 15 were subtotally removed, and 4 were partially removed. Twelve complications were observed in the non-MIS group, including six cases of leakage of cerebrospinal fluid, three cases of infection, two cases of myasthenia, and one case of localized pain.

There was no significant difference in the rate of tumor resection between the MIS group and non-MIS group (p>0.05). The estimated blood loss and hospital stay durations observed in the MIS group were significantly less than in the non-MIS group (p<0.05). The operating time observed in the MIS group was significantly longer than in the non-MIS (p<0.05). The rate of postoperative complication in the MIS group was lower than in the non-MIS group (p<0.05) (Table 2).

As the neurological status was reevaluated at the time of discharge, the results were as follows: In the MIS group, postoperative neurological status improved or remained unchanged in 52 cases and worsened in 1 case (dysesthesia). In the non-MIS group, postoperative neurological status improved or remained unchanged in 59 cases and worsened in 10 cases (4 cases of back pain, 3 cases of dysesthesia, 2 cases of dyskinesia, 1 case of sphincter disturbance). Based on the results above, the short-term clinical efficacy in the MIS group was superior to that in the non-MIS group (p<0.05; Table 3).

According to ASIA, the results of the long-term clinical efficacy were observed as follows: In the MIS group, as the neurological status was reevaluated at the time of the final follow-up (12–60 months, average 28 months), neurological status improved in 51 cases and remained unchanged in 2 cases. In the non-MIS group, as the neurological status was reevaluated at the time of the final follow-up (12–60 months, average 28 months), neurological status improved in 65 cases, remained unchanged in 4 cases, and worsened in 1 case. Based on the results, there was no statistically significant difference between the MIS group and non-MIS group in terms of long-term clinical efficacy (p>0.05; Table 3).

Health economics analysis

There were no significant differences in the hospital stay durations, recovery times, or loss of working time between Group A and Group C (p>0.05). The hospital stay durations and loss of working time observed in Group B were significantly less than in Group E (p<0.05). There was no significant difference in recovery times between Group B and Group E (p>0.05). The recovery times and loss of working time in Group B were significantly less than in Group D (p<0.05). There was no significant difference in hospital stay durations between Group B and Group D (p>0.05; Table 4; Figure 1).

In terms of the costs of surgery, there is no significant difference between Group A and Group C (p>0.05), which was same between Group B and Group E (p>0.05). Group B was significantly higher than Group D (p<0.05). Meanwhile, in relation to non-surgical costs, those in Group A were significantly less than those in Group C (p<0.05). In addition, those of Group B were significantly less than those of Group E (p<0.05), while those of Group B were significantly less than those of Group D (p<0.05). Regarding the total costs of hospitalization, the total costs of hospitalization between Group A and Group C showed no significant difference (p>0.05), which was same between Group B and Group E (p>0.05). On the other hand, those of Group D were significantly less than those of Group B (p<0.05) (Table 5).

Study of postoperative spinal stability

The rate of postoperative spinal instability in Group HE and Group LEPSF were significantly lower than that in Group LE in a single spinal segment (p<0.05). The rate of postoperative spinal instability between Group HE and Group LEPSF showed no significant difference in a single operative segment. The rate of postoperative spinal instability in Group LEPSF was significantly lower than those in Group HE and Group LE in two or more spinal operative segments (p<0.05). The rate of postoperative spinal instability between Group HE and Group LE showed no significant difference in two or more operative segments (p>0.05; Table 6).

Discussion

Intradural extramedullary tumors account for two-thirds of primary spinal tumors [8]. Most intradural extramedullary tumors are benign, and they exhibit no specific symptoms. Radicular pain and worsening sensory and motor loss are common manifestations. Therefore, most of the patients are wrongly diagnosed with cervical spondylopathy or intervertebral disk herniation. MRI is very crucial to confirm the diagnosis of intradural extramedullary tumors. Once the diagnosis is confirmed, the best treatment for nonmalignant intradural extramedullary tumor is surgery. The goal of surgery is complete surgical resection while preserving spinal stability, without worsening the preoperative neurological status.

All the processes of conventional surgical tumor resection are carried out without using microscope, which may lead to a greater likelihood of incomplete tumor resection, as well as more damage to the spinal cord and vessels surrounding the spinal canal. With

Table 6. Summary of postoperative spinal stability in different segments.

Groups	1 segment			2 segments			>2 segments		
	stable	instable	Rate of stability (%)	stable	instable	Rate of stability (%)	stable	instable	Rate of stability (%)
HE	21	0	100.00	8	5	61.54	3	6	33.33
LE	4	2	66.67★	3	3	50.00'	1	5	16.67'
LEPSF	22	1	95.65▲'	26	2	92.86★▲	9	1	90.00★▲

This table shows the results of postoperative spinal stability of various surgical approaches in different segments. Abbreviations: HE: hemilaminectomy + tumor excision; LE: laminectomy + tumor excision; LEPSF: laminectomy + tumor excision + pedicle screw fixation.

★$p<0.05$ vs. Group HE;

▲$p<0.05$ vs. Group LE;

'$p>0.05$ vs. Group HE.

the improvement of medical devices, surgeons are increasingly using microscopy to perform surgical tumor resection. MIS can provide a clearer visual operative field and more delicate operative maneuvers, which can avoid the damage to the spinal cord and peripheral nerves as far as possible, reduce intraoperative blood loss and postoperative complications, and increase the rate of complete removal of tumors. It was reported that MIS allowed removal of the tumor with minimal impairment from cutting of nerve fibers at the nerve root [9]. Regarding intramedullary tumors, MIS made it possible to reduce postoperative mortality from 38.5 to 4.5%, exclude various complications (postoperative liquorrhea, meningitis), restore the disturbed functions of the spinal cord fully, and prolong postoperative remission and the patient's survival [10]. After total resection, restoration of full spinal cord function can happen in limited numbers of cases.

In our present study, the MIS group had the advantages of less estimated blood loss, shorter hospital stays, and fewer postoperative complications than those were observed in the non-MIS group ($p<0.05$). The short-term clinical efficacy of the MIS group was superior to that of the non-MIS group ($p<0.05$). However, there was no significant difference in the resection rates of tumors or long-term clinical efficacy between the MIS group and non-MIS group ($p>0.05$). Micromanipulation achieved less intraoperative blood loss than in the non-MIS group through avoiding accidental injury of epidural and spinal cord vessels as much as possible and precisely intercepting arteries supplying the tumor. In the MIS group, micromanipulation prevented as many complications as possible, such as postoperative infection and cerebrospinal leakage; this is because micromanipulation could reduce intraoperative blood loss and trauma to tissues around surgical site. What's more, a small mount of intraoperative blood loss has modesty impact on patient's body immunity and the duration before functional exercises on limb function, which is helpful to reduce postoperative infection effectively. Although non-MIS manipulation did not directly damage the anatomical structure of the spinal cord, it increased the damage to the vessels supplying the spinal cord than in the MIS group, which could lead to less-than-ideal postoperative spinal function recovery and short-term clinical efficacy.

Although we cannot use health economics analysis to determine the best treatment for any particular disease, we can get some useful references for surgical options. In this study, the non-surgical cost in MIS is less than in non-MIS ($p<0.05$), this is because MIS can result in the less intraoperative blood loss, lower postoperative complications, shorter durations of hospital stay and better short-term clinical efficiency. As surgical cost takes a great proportion in the total cost of hospitalization, the total costs of hospitalization between Group A (hemilaminectomy + tumor microscopic excision) and Group C (hemilaminectomy + tumor excision) showed no significant difference, which was same between Group B (laminectomy + tumor microscopic excision + pedicle screw fixation) and Group E (laminectomy + tumor excision + pedicle screw fixation). Because the costs of the internal fixation device must be taken into consideration, the total cost of hospitalization in Group B (laminectomy + tumor microscopic excision + pedicle screw fixation) is not less than in Group D (laminectomy + tumor excision). The health economics analysis was based on data from six hospitals, and therefore, may not be representative of costs at other hospitals.

In our study, we found that hemilaminectomy for intradural extramedullary tumor had better postoperative spinal stability than laminectomy with a single spinal segment. However, conventional laminectomy is still widely used for the surgical removal of spinal intradural extramedullary tumor, which can offer more familiar exposure and a wider view of the surgical field to surgeons than in hemilaminectomy. In contrast, some serious drawbacks of laminectomy still exist, such as spinal instability, epidural fibrosis, the absence of osseous protection for the spinal cord, and postoperative dorsal pain [11,12].

The removal of the posterior lamina, spinous process, paravertebral muscles, supraspinous ligament, interspinous ligament, and ligamentum flavum is needed in the surgical corridor of laminectomy, which causes great damage to the posterior column of the spine, in turn jeopardizing spinal stability [13,14,15,16]. In an effort to maintain spinal stability, hemilaminectomy avoids damage to the posterior structure of the vertebral column by preserving the supraspinous ligament, interspinous ligament, and paravertebral muscle of the opposite side. Therefore, hemilaminectomy has less impact on spinal biomechanics [17,18]. On the other hand, the disadvantage of hemilaminectomy is the narrow surgical corridor, which increases the risk of injury to spinal cord [19]. In our study, there was no statistical difference about spinal stability between hemilaminectomy and laminectomy in two or more operative segments of spine. Another result was that laminectomy + pedicle screw fixation showed better postoperative spinal stability than hemilaminectomy and laminectomy in two or more spinal operative segments. It is generally known that pedicle screw fixation offers a significant biomechanical advantage [20], and is superior to other techniques regarding the promotion of mechanical strength [21,22]. As a result, great internal stability is observed.

In this study, we have found that MIS is advantageous in the removal of intradural extramedullary tumor, this is because MIS can reduce intraoperative blood loss, duration of hospital stay, postoperative complications, non-surgical cost and have better short-term clinical efficacy compared with non-MIS. In addition, in two or more spinal operative segments, pedicle screw fixation helps avoid spinal postoperative instability. However, we have not investigated if the MIS is helpful to postoperative stability in this study. Besides that, the follow-up time and preoperative radiographic assessment of spinal stability need to be further improved in our future study. In summary, the study provides some insight to help surgeons choose the appropriate surgical method for intradural extramedullary tumor.

Author Contributions

Conceived and designed the experiments: JZ SZ. Performed the experiments: GZ LD. Analyzed the data: YF TG. Contributed to the writing of the manuscript: LD SZ GZ.

References

1. Albanese V, Platania N (2002) Spinal intradural extramedullary tumors. Personal experience. Journal of neurosurgical sciences. 46(1): 18–24.
2. Yeo DK, Im SB, Park KW, Shin DS, Kim BT, et al. (2011) Profiles of spinal cord tumors removed through a unilateral hemilaminectomy. Journal of Korean Neurosurgical Society. 50(3): 195–200.
3. Sachdev S, Dodd RL, Chang SD, Soltys SG, Adler JR, et al. (2011) Stereotactic radiosurgery yields long-term control for benign intradural, extramedullary spinal tumors. Neurosurgery. 69(3): 533–539.
4. Postalci L, Tugcu B, Gungor A, Guclu G (2010) Spinal meningiomas: recurrence in ventrally located individuals on long-term follow-up; a review of 46 operated cases. Turkish neurosurgery. 21(4): 449–453.
5. Sun Z, Sun L, Li T, Ma X, Zhang Z (2011) Intraosseous trigeminal schwannoma of mandible with intracranial extension. The Journal of Laryngology & Otology. 125(04): 418–422.
6. Kirshblum SC, Memmo P, Kim N, Campagnolo D, Millis S, et al. (2002) Comparison of the revised 2000 American Spinal Injury Association classification standards with the 1996 guidelines. American journal of physical medicine & rehabilitation. 81(7): 502–505.
7. Lida Y, Kataoka O, Sho T, Sumi M, Hirose T, et al. (1990) Postoperative lumbar spinal instability occurring or progressing secondary to laminectomy. Spine. 15(11): 1186–1189.
8. Helseth A, Mørk SJ (1989) Primary intraspinal neoplasms in Norway, 1955 to 1986: a population-based survey of 467 patients. Journal of neurosurgery. 71(6): 842–845.
9. Kobayashi S, Uchida K, Kokubo Y, Yayama T, Nakajima H, et al. (2007) A schwannoma of the S1 dural sleeve was resected while the intact nerve fibers were preserved using a microscope. Report of a case with early MRI findings. Minimal Invasive Neurosurgery. 50(2): 120–123.
10. Starodubtsev AI (1984) Surgical treatment of intramedullary tumors. Zhurnal voprosy neirokhirurgii imeni NN Burdenko. (4): 22–25.
11. Mayfield FH (1976) Complications of laminectomy. Clinical neurosurgery. 23: 435–439.
12. Yasuoka S, Peterson HA, MacCarty CS (1982) Incidence of spinal column deformity after multilevel laminectomy in children and adults. Journal of neurosurgery. 57(4): 441–445.
13. Smith ZA, Vastardis GA, Carandang G, Havey RM, Hannon S, et al. (2014) Biomechanical Effects of a Unilateral Approach to Minimally Invasive Lumbar Decompression. PloS one. 9(3): e92611.
14. Canbay S, Hasturk AE, Basmaci M, Erten F, Harman F (2012) Management of thoracal and lumbar schwannomas using a unilateral approach without instability: an analysis of 15 cases. Asian spine journal. 6(1): 43–49.
15. Iacoangeli M, Gladi M, Di Rienzo A, Dobran M, Alvaro L, et al. (2012) Minimally invasive surgery for benign intradural extramedullary spinal meningiomas: experience of a single institution in a cohort of elderly patients and review of the literature. Clinical interventions in aging. 7: 557–564.
16. Zong S, Zeng G, Xiong C, Wei B (2013) Treatment Results in the Differential Surgery of Intradural Extramedullary Schwannoma of 110 Cases. PloS one. 8(5): e63867.
17. Panjabi MM, White AA 3rd (1980) Basic biomechanics of the spine. Neurosurgery. 7(1): 76–93.
18. Ogden AT, Bresnahan L, Smith JS, Natarajan R, Fessler RG (2009) Biomechanical comparison of traditional and minimally invasive intradural tumor exposures using finite element analysis. Clinical Biomechanics. 24(2): 143–147.
19. Guidetti B (1974) Removal of extramedullary benign spinal cord tumours. In: Advances and technical standards in neurosurgery. Springer Vienna. 173–197.
20. Mazel C, Hoffmann E, Antonietti P, Grunenwald D, Henry M, et al. (2004) Posterior cervicothoracic instrumentation in spine tumors. Spine. 29(11): 1246–1253.
21. Kotani Y, Cunningham BW, Abumi K, McAfee PC (1994) Biomechanical analysis of cervical stabilization systems: an assessment of transpedicular screw fixation in the cervical spine[J]. Spine. 19(22): 2529–2539.
22. Kothe R, Rüther W, Schneider E, Linke B (2004) Biomechanical analysis of transpedicular screw fixation in the subaxial cervical spine. Spine. 29(17): 1869–1875.

4

Adding More Junior Residents May Worsen Emergency Department Crowding

Takahisa Kawano[1]*, Kei Nishiyama[2], Hiroyuki Hayashi[3]

1 Department of Emergency Medicine, University of Fukui Hospital, Yoshida county, Fukui Prefecture, Japan, 2 Department of Primary Care and Emergency Medicine, Kyoto University Graduate School of Medicine, Kyoto city, Kyoto Prefecture, Japan, 3 Department of General Medicine, University of Fukui Hospital, Yoshida county, Fukui Prefecture, Japan

Abstract

Background: Although increasing staff numbers during shifts when emergency department (ED) crowding is severe can help meet patient demand, it remains unclear how different types of added staff, particularly junior residents, may affect crowding.

Methods: To identify associations between types of staff and ED crowding, we conducted a cross-sectional, single-center study in the ED of a large, teaching hospital in Japan between January and December 2012. Patients who visited the ED during the study period were enrolled. We excluded (1) patients previously scheduled to visit the ED, and (2) neonates transferred from other hospitals. During the study period, 27,970 patients were enrolled. Types of staff analyzed were junior (first and second year) residents, senior (third to fifth year) residents, attending (board-certified) physicians, and nurses. A generalized linear model was applied to length of ED stay for all patients as well as admitted and discharged patients to quantify an association with the additional staff.

Results: In the model, addition of one attending physician or senior resident was associated with decreased length of ED stay for total patients by 3.88 or 1.64 minutes, respectively (95% CI, 2.20–5.56 and 0.81–2.48 minutes); while additional nursing staff had no association. Surprisingly, however, one additional junior resident was associated with prolonged length of ED stay for total patients by 0.97 minutes (95% CI 0.37–1.57 minutes) and for discharged patients by 1.01 minutes (95% CI 0.45–1.59 minutes).

Conclusion: Staffing adjustments aimed at alleviating ED crowding should focus on adding more senior staff during peak-volume shifts.

Editor: Robert Lane Schmidt, University of Utah School of Medicine, United States of America

Funding: Financial incentives were provided to the authors by the Emergency Promotion Foundation (http://www.fasd.or.jp/). The funders had no role in study design, data collection and analysis, decision to publish, or preparation of the manuscript.

Competing Interests: The authors have declared that no competing interests exist.

* Email: maketenakunarakattenake@hotmail.com

Introduction

Emergency department (ED) crowding, in which patient care cannot be provided within a reasonable time due to excess demand for emergency services, is a serious and challenging problem [1,2]. In Japan, 13,100 patients in critical condition experienced an ambulance diversion more than four times during one ambulance transportation; about 21% of these ambulance diversions were caused by ED crowding [3]. While ED crowding decreases an ED's capacity to accept patients who are transported by ambulance service, it can also have serious consequences: the mortality of patients admitted from the ED has been shown to increase when ED crowding is severe [4,5]. Additionally, ED crowding decreases ED physician productivity and satisfaction [6]. Importantly, a study of the association between hospital resources and ED crowding demonstrated that an increased ratio of ED staff to patient volume shortened patient treatment time in the ED [7].

When ED crowding is severe, adding more staff, e.g., board-certificated ED physicians, residents, and nurses, can be an effective countermeasure [2]. In Japan, however, hospitals commonly add only junior (first and second year) residents on shifts with high patient volumes. This practice arose from a shortage of board-certified ED physicians; the current number of these physicians is just 3,400 [8]. Meanwhile, the number of hospitals with EDs was 39,00 in 2008, and the total number of patients visited at ED in Japan was 0.57 million per day in 2011 [9,10]. Although the additional allowance was paid to emergency physicians by government to increase number of them, the shortage is widespread in Japan. It creates staffing difficulties; adding more junior residents on shift instead of adding more board-certificated emergency physicians when ED crowding is severe. However, the contribution of junior residents to alleviating ED crowding has been questioned [11]. Thus, although the prevailing ED staffing plan in Japan might exacerbate ED crowding, this hypothesis has not yet been proven.

In this study, we used a generalized linear model to investigate the association of staff type—junior or senior resident, nurse, and attending (board-certified) physician—on the length of ED stay. The findings will provide basic information that supports the need for an increase the number of board-certificated ED physicians in Japan.

Methods

Study design and setting

A cross-sectional, single-center study was conducted in the ED of the Fukui Prefectural Hospital in Fukui, Japan. The Fukui Prefectural Hospital, a large teaching hospital in an urban setting, has the largest ED in Fukui Prefecture, where approximately 380,000 residents live. The area is also served by a second ED in a large academic hospital. These hospitals serve both urban and rural communities in an area of 830 km^2. The population density of this area is 450 persons per km^2. Seven fire departments and 7 emergency dispatch centers are located in this area. Fukui Prefectural Hospital has about 1,080 beds and 14 intensive care unit beds. The main treatment location in our ED has four beds for serious cases or patients being resuscitated. There are also four examination rooms for low-acuity patients and four beds for observation. Almost all patients who visited this ED were self-referred. The ED accepts all patients regardless of their age, including pediatric patients. In our department, nursing staff triages the new arrival patients like at other institutions. Residents are responsible for the first encounter to evaluate new arrival patients after this triage. However, nursing staff can skip this evaluation; nursing staff chooses patients with high acuity and allocates them to ED beds where senior residents and attending physicians treat and evaluate patients. All other specialist consultants are available when necessary.

Selection of participants

Patients who visited the ED of Fukui Prefectural Hospital from 08:00 January 1, 2012 to 07:59 December 31, 2012 were enrolled in our study. We excluded (1) patients who were scheduled for admission or pharmaceutical prescription, and (2) neonates requiring intensive care who were transferred from other hospitals. The regular reception desks at our hospital are closed on weekends, therefore patients for scheduled admission or pharmaceutical prescription visit the reception desk at the ED. Patients who need pharmaceutical prescription mainly receive daily intravenous antibiotic administration at outpatient clinics. These patients quickly depart the ED without any evaluation or treatment, so the length of ED stay of these patients is quiet small. Neonates requiring intensive care transferred from another hospital typically stay in the ED during registration only, so their length of ED stay is also small. Because these patients rarely consume any ED resources beyond registration, we excluded them from this study.

Study outcome

Study outcome was the length of ED stay, which is one of the most common proxy measures of ED overcrowding [12]. The length of ED stay was defined as the time, in minutes, from registration in ED to ED departure.

Definitions

To assess the association of staffing types with ED crowding, we chose the number of staff (junior resident, senior resident, attending physician, and nurse) and common covariates of ED crowding in our analysis (number of walk-in patients, number of ambulance arrivals, mode of arrival, bed occupancy, ED boarding, patient age, arrival time, percentage of admission).

Junior residents were defined as first- and second-year residents. Senior residents were defined as third- to fifth-year residents. Attending physicians were defined as board-certified in Emergency Medicine and working at the ED for over six years. Junior residents determine the disposition of the patient after consulting with senior residents or attending physicians; senior residents and attending physicians determine the disposition of patients by themselves. Number of walk-ins was defined as the number of walk-in patients arriving in the ED each hour [4]. The number of ambulance arrivals was determined hourly. Mode of arrival was defined as the method of patient entry to the ED, by ambulance or walk-in [13]. Bed occupancy was defined as the percentage of hospital beds occupied per day [14]. ED boarding was defined as the number of patients at each hour who remained in the ED for more than 1 hour after admission by an ED physician [14]. Arrival time was classified into periods (08:00–15:59, 16:00–23:59, and 00:00–07:59). The percentage of admissions represented the percentage of total hospital admissions generated from the ED per day [15].

Measurement

The number of junior and senior residents, attending physicians, and nurses was obtained from recorded work schedules. We obtained the data from the electronic medical record system (EMR) and the electronic hospital administrative data system of our hospital. Patient age, arrival time, time of decision to admit, departure time, disposition of patient, mode of arrival, and execution of any diagnostic tests were obtained from EMR. This record is considered to be accurate because every patient account is generated from it. When a patient needs to be admitted, the physician orders admission through EMR. Nurses follow the necessary procedures after this order and transfer patients to hospital wards. If patients have to wait in the ED for the arrangement of a hospital bed, nurses record these patients and provide care to them appropriately. We obtained this nursing record to calculate ED boarding. ED clerks obtained the number of available hospital beds at 09:00 each day from the electronic hospital administrative data system and calculated hospital bed occupancy. We could not obtain hourly hospital bed occupancy information.

Statistical analysis

Descriptive analyses were conducted with the use of frequency tabulations. We described the medians and interquartile ranges (IQR) for all variables.

Primary analysis

We defined 280 minutes, which was the upper 5% of length of ED stay for total patients when no junior resident was on shift, as a clinically significant delay. To assess the contribution of junior residents to ED crowding, we classified total patients according to the number of junior residents on shift and described the proportion of the number of patients who stayed at the ED for more than the clinically significant delay in each category. We conducted the Cochran-Armitage test to assess the presence of an association between the proportion of patients with significant delay in each category and the number of junior residents.

Secondary analysis

To assess the association of staff types in the ED with length of ED stay, a generalized linear model (GLM) with a log-link function and gamma distribution was conducted. In this study, length of ED stay was not normally distributed (absolute skew value 2.3, absolute kurtosis 10.0) and corresponded to findings of previous studies [14,16,17]. GLM is commonly used to analyze length of ED stay to fit skewedness and can report the results in the original time units as opposed to a log-transformed outcome [14,16]. The distribution of this model was determined by result of modified park test [18]. This model can determine the range of change in length of ED stay when each variable changes per its original unit and other variables are fixed to their mean.

We constructed the GLM to assess the association of each staff type with length of ED stay in the total patient group with other covariates. Next, patients were stratified into discharged and admitted groups. The model was then constructed in each group to investigate the association of each staff type with ED stay in the different acuity groups.

All analyses were conducted with STATA version 12.1 (STATA Corp LP, College Station, TX). The authors had full access to the data and take responsibility for its integrity. All authors have read and agreed to the content of the manuscript.

Ethical statement

The study protocol was based on the guidelines for epidemiologic studies issued by the Ministry of Health, Labor and Welfare of Japan. [19] Fukui Prefectural Hospital ethics committees approved the research protocol. All data was collected retrospectively. All patient data was anonymous when researchers accessed it. Our study didn't include any personally identifiable information, so the requirement of oral or written informed consent was allowed to be waived by the ethics committees [19,20]. So, we didn't obtain oral or written informed consent from participants. We posted the poster about our study protocol on the bulletin board at the gate of ED instead of informed consent.

Results

Characteristics of study participants

During the study period, 28,611 patients visited the ED. Of these, 619 patients who were scheduled to visit the ED for admission or pharmaceutical prescription as well as 22 newborn babies who were transferred from other hospitals were excluded. The study therefore included 27,970 (97.8%) of the total patients who visited the ED. Of the included patients, 4,024 (14.4%) were admitted to the hospital, and 23,946 (85.6%) were discharged (Figure 1).

Patient demographics and primary outcomes

The median (quartiles) age of participants was 38 years [interquartile range (IQR), 17–74 years] (Table 1). The median daily number of ambulances was 10 cars (IQR, 8–13 cars). Of included patients, 13.5% were transported by ambulance. The median daily number of walk-in patients was 56 (IQR, 48–76). The number of walk-in patients peaked between 16:00 to 23:59 (37: IQR, 31–44). The median length of ED stay for total patients was 88 minutes (IQR, 53–147 minutes). The median length of ED stay for admitted and discharged patients were 170 and 70 minutes, respectively (IQR, 117–233, and 50–128 minutes).

Staffing in the ED

The median hourly numbers of junior residents, senior residents, attending physicians, and nurses on shift were four, two, one, and three, respectively (IQR: 2–5, 1–3, 1–2, and 2–3)(Table 2). The median hourly number of junior residents, senior residents, and nurses peaked between 16:00 to 23:59 (4: IQR, 4–5; 2: IQR, 1–3; and 3: IQR, 3–3; respectively). This peak in the number of staff was consistent with the peak in number of walk-in patients.

Primary analysis

The proportion of patients with a clinically significant delay is described in Figure 2. A statistically significant association between the proportion of patients with a significant delay in each category and the number of junior residents was not detected ($P = 0.054$).

Secondary analysis

The GLM was applied to estimate the associations of changes in ED staffing on length of stay in ED. In our model, adding one attending physician was associated with decreased length of ED stay for total patients (3.9 minutes, 95% CI, 2.2–5.5 minutes)(Table 3). Adding one senior resident was associated with decreased length of ED stay (1.6 minutes, 95% CI, 0.8–2.5 minutes). However, the range of decrease in length of ED stay when adding a senior resident was smaller than for an attending physician (−1.6 vs. −3.9 minutes). In contrast, adding one junior resident was associated with prolonged length of ED stay for total patients (1.0 minutes, 95% CI, 0.4–1.6). Adding one nurse did not have a statistical association on length of ED stay for total patients.

The model was then applied to patients grouped by admitted and discharged status. Adding one attending physician was associated with decreased length of ED stay for both admitted (−6.5 minutes, 95% CI, −1.2–−11.8 minutes) and discharged patients (−4.0 minutes, 95% CI, −2.4–−5.6 minutes)(Table 4). The range of change in length of ED stay was wider in admitted patients than in discharged patients. Similarly, adding one senior resident was associated with decreased length of ED stay for discharged patients (−1.9 minutes, 95% CI, −1.1–−2.7 minutes). However, adding a senior resident did not have a statistical association with the length of ED stay for admitted patients. Interestingly, adding one junior resident on shift was associated with prolonged length of ED stay for discharged patients (1.0 minutes, 95% CI 0.5–1.6 minutes) but had no statistical association with length of ED stay for admitted patients. An additional nurse had no statistical association with length of ED stay for either patient group.

Discussion

Using actual ED data to supply our model, we demonstrated the contribution of each type of ED staff to the length of ED stay. Our model is consistent with previous studies, in that the addition of an attending physician was associated with reduced length of ED stay for both admitted (by ~6.5 minutes) and discharged (by ~4 minutes) patients [11]. The addition of one senior resident in the model was associated with reduced length of ED stay, but only for discharged patients (by ~2 minutes). Interestingly, in contrast, an additional junior resident was associated with prolonged length of ED stay for total patients and discharged patients (by ~1.0 minute each). The addition of one nurse had no statistical association with the length of ED stay for any patient group. These findings indicate that the addition of senior physicians can improve ED crowding, but the addition of junior physicians might worsen ED crowding.

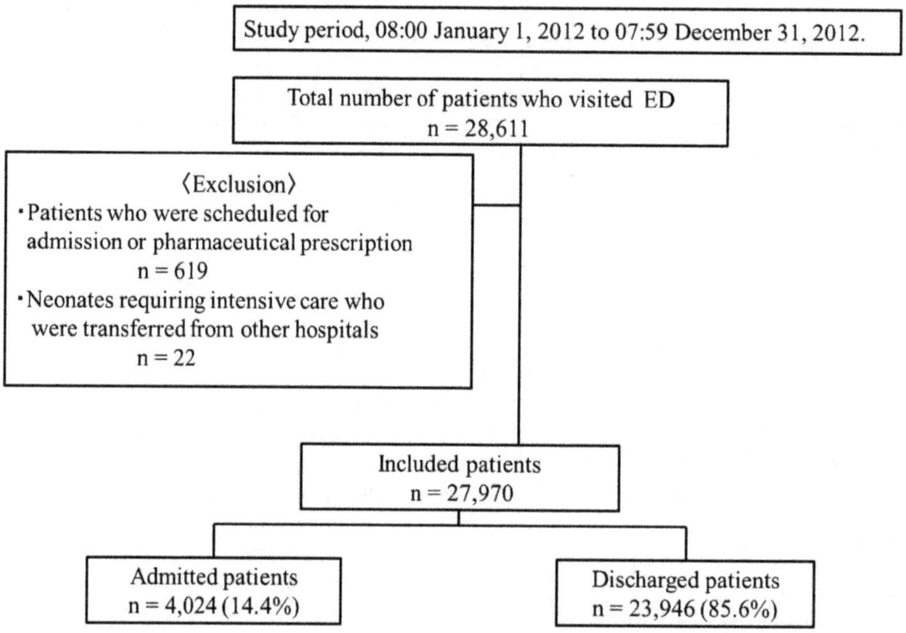

Figure 1. Patient recruitment diagram. ED, emergency department.

Table 1. Patient demographics and primary outcomes.

	n = 27,970
Median age, years (IQR)	38 (17–64)
Walk-in patients, n	24,186
per day, n (IQR)	56 (48–76)
08:00 to 15:59, n (IQR)	19 (15–34)
16:00 to 23:59, n (IQR)	37 (31–44)
0:00 to 07:59, n (IQR)	11 (8–14)
Ambulance, n	3784
per day, n (IQR)	10 (8–13)
08:00 to 15:59, n (IQR)	6 (3–6)
16:00 to 23:59, n (IQR)	4 (3–6)
0:00 to 07:59, n (IQR)	2 (1–3)
Admissions, n	7,843
per day, n (IQR)	11 (8.3–13)
Percentage of admission, % (IQR)	13.7 (9.8–18.0)
Hospital occupancy	
per day, % (IQR)	68.5 (66.3–70.7)
ED boarding	
per day, n (IQR)	2 (1–3)
Deaths, n (%)	96 (0.3)
Median Length of ED stay	
Total patients, min (IQR)	88 (53–147)
Admitted patients, min (IQR)	170 (117–233)
Discharged patients, min (IQR)	70 (50–128)

IQR, interquartile range; ED, emergency department.

Table 2. Staffing in ED.

	Median (IQR)
Junior resident	
per hour, n	4 (2–5)
08:00 to 15:59, n	2 (1–4)
16:00 to 23:59, n	4 (4–5)
0:00 to 07:59, n	3 (3–4)
Senior resident	
per hour, n	2 (1–3)
08:00 to 15:59, n	1 (1–2)
16:00 to 23:59, n	2 (1–3)
0:00 to 07:59, n	1 (1–1)
Attending physician	
per hour, n	1 (1–2)
08:00 to 15:59, n	1 (1–2)
16:00 to 23:59, n	1 (1–2)
0:00 to 07:59, n	1 (1–1)
Nurse	
per hour, n	3 (2–3)
08:00 to 15:59, n	2 (2–2)
16:00 to 23:59, n	3 (3–3)
0:00 to 07:59, n	2 (2–2)

IQR, interquartile range; ED, emergency department.

To provide quality care within an appropriate timeframe when ED crowding is severe, adding staff helps meet patient volume [2]. However, the contribution of residents to the alleviation of ED crowding has been debated. For example, during a resident strike in Australia, ED shifts were comprised of board-certified physicians, and the total number of physicians on shift was lower than before the strike; however, the length of ED stay was lower during the strike [11]. Our findings support and extend this previous study; we estimated the associations of each type of medical staff with length of ED stay directly. The results suggest that, when demand is estimated to be high in the ED, staffing managers should consider adding senior residents or attending physicians to shifts rather than junior residents.

Our study emphasizes the role of board-certificated ED physicians in alleviating ED crowding; only this type of staff was associated with reduced length of ED stay of both admitted and

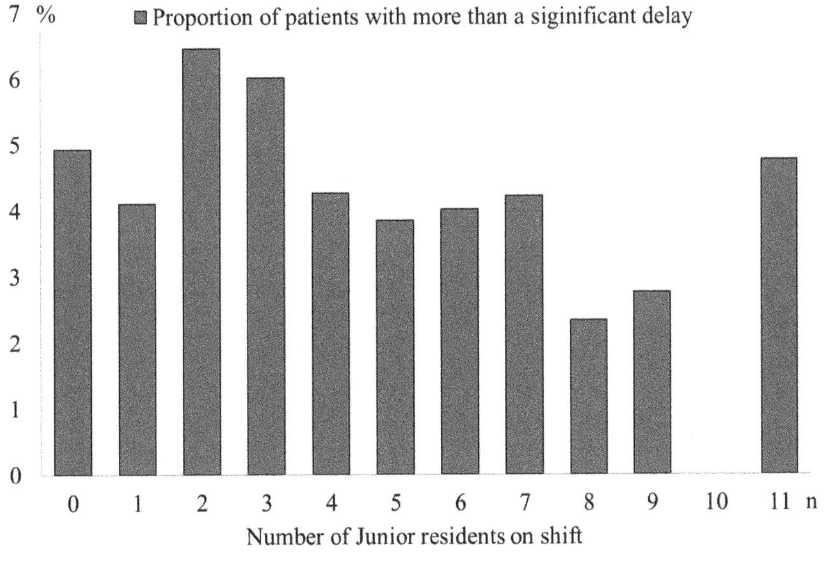

Figure 2. Proportion of patients with a significant delay in each category classified by the number of junior residents on shift.

Table 3. The range of change in length of ED stay for total patients when each variable changed per its original unit.

	Total patients (n = 27,970)	
Characteristic	**Length of stay, minutes (Unstandardized slope coefficient)**	**95% CI**
Mode of arrival		
Walk-in	Reference	
Ambulance	30.4*	27.1–33.6
Number of walk-in patients	0.4	-<0.1–0.7
Number of ambulance arrivals	3.6*	2.3–4.9
Staff in ED		
Junior resident	1.0*	0.4–1.6
Senior resident	−1.6*	−2.5–−0.8
Attending physician	−3.9*	−5.6–−2.2
Nurse	−0.6	−2.4–1.2
Bed occupancy	0.4*	0.7–0.7
ED boarding	−0.4	−3.3–1.3
Patient age	0.8*	0.8–0.9
Arrival		
08:00–15:59	Reference	
16:00–23:59	−4.2*	−7.0–−1.4
0:00–07:59	2.5	−0.9–5.9
Percentage of admissions	0.9*	0.8–1.1

*, P<0.05; 95% CI, 95% confidence intervals; ED, emergency department

Table 4. The range of change in length of ED stay for admitted and discharged patients when each variable changed per its original unit.

	Admitted patients (n = 4,024)		Discharged patients (n = 23,946)	
Characteristic	**Length of stay, minutes (Unstandardized slope coefficient)**	**95% CI**	**Length of stay, minutes (Unstandardized slope coefficient)**	**95% CI**
Mode of arrival				
Walk-in	Reference		Reference	
Ambulance	−41.6*	−49.4–−33.8	39.3*	25.7–42.9
Number of walk-in patients	1.6*	0.3–2.9	0.4*	0.6–0.8
Number of ambulance arrivals	0.3	−4.0–4.6	3.4*	2.2–4.7
Staff in ED				
Junior resident	0.4	−1.5–2.4	1.0*	0.5–1.6
Senior resident	−1.0	−3.7–1.7	−1.9*	−2.7–−1.1
Attending physician	−6.5*	−11.8–−1.2	−4.0*	−5.6–−2.4
Nurse	0.4	−6.0–6.9	0.2	−1.5–2.0
Bed occupancy	0.1	−0.9–1.1	0.6*	0.3–0.9
ED boarding	6.1	−1.4–13.7	−0.9	−3.1–1.3
Patient age	0.5*	0.4–0.6	0.7*	0.7–0.7
Arrival				
08:00–15:59	Reference		Reference	
16:00–23:59	−13.6*	−22.8–−4.4	−1.8	−4.4–0.9
0:00–07:59	37.2*	26.3–48.0	2.3	−0.9–5.5
Percentage of admissions	0.4	−0.1–1.0	0.4*	0.3–0.6

*, P<0.05; 95% CI, 95% confidence intervals; ED, emergency department.

discharged patients. To improve ED efficacy, hospital administrators and Japanese government officials should increase efforts to end the shortage of ED physicians. In Japan, medical students have a right of free selection of their specialties, and their selections are influenced by the advice of senior doctors [21]. However, 32% of senior residents who studied emergency medicine were reportedly not satisfied with their specialty [22]. In particular, the stress of working in the ED was the primary factor contributing to their dissatisfaction compared to other factors including their working conditions, and training and teaching systems at ED [22]. To increase the number of board-certificated ED physicians, measures should focus on relieving stressful conditions for ED residents, thereby encouraging medical students to select Emergency Medicine as their specialty. Such measures will be increasingly important, as ED crowding in Japan is estimated to become more severe due to the advancing age of the population [23].

Patient volume in the ED is considered to be relatively predictable [2]. The National Hospital Ambulatory Medical Care Survey indicated that patient volume in EDs in the U.S. is highest in the evening and on Mondays, Tuesdays, and Sundays than on other days of the week [16]. Additionally, the percentage of admissions from the ED on weekdays was higher than that on weekends [24]. Thus, ED crowding is likely severe on Monday and Tuesday evenings, with a high percentage of admissions from ED, and on Sundays, with a low percentage of admissions. From our findings, one could propose that adding another attending physician to the usual shift staff on Monday and Tuesday evenings would be the best action, as attending physicians can reduce length of ED stay for admitted patients. When ED crowding is severe on Sundays, adding an attending physician or senior resident could reduce the length of stay (for discharged patients only, in the case of senior residents). Further, analysis of patient arrival patterns and admission rates for particular times could allow even more effective shift scheduling to meet patient demand.

In this study, the peak in number of staff on shift was consistent with the peak in number of walk-in patients. However, the additional staff on shift comprised junior and senior residents and nurses. According to our model, this staffing plan in our hospital may be, in part, responsible for exacerbated ED crowding. The addition of five junior residents on a shift when ED crowding is severe would add another five minutes to the length of ED stay for each patient during the shift; thus, the additional residents will not alleviate ED crowding. This approach to ED staffing is common in Japan; however, our study demonstrates that this prevalent staffing plan is not successful for reducing ED crowding.

Two phenomena may explain why the addition of a junior resident contributed to increased length of ED stay. First, junior residents likely require more time to evaluate patients. One study found that when an ED patient was initially assessed by an attending physician, compared to a resident, the length of ED stay was shorter. [1]. Second, teaching hospitals typically require that a senior resident or attending physician evaluates and treats a patient after initial evaluation by a junior resident. This additional step introduces a delay that may prolong ED stay [25]. However, high-acuity patients are typically not evaluated by a junior resident first, as attending physicians or senior residents will begin evaluation and treatment immediately. In our study, the addition of a junior resident was associated with a prolonged length of ED stay only for discharged patients. Thus, the time required for resident evaluation and follow-up by senior physicians in lower-acuity patients may have led to the lengthened stay identified in our study.

Patient volume in this study might have a smaller association with length of ED stay than it would in large EDs. However, large EDs having annual patients volumes of over 60,000 are less common, accounting for only 11% of total EDs in U.S. [26]. Although our ED volume is smaller, matching the annual ED volume of 20,000–40,000 in mid-sized U.S. EDs, these smaller EDs are more common, accounting for 25% of total EDs in the U.S. [26]. The trend of increasing associations of input factors on ED stay when patient volume is higher is observed even at smaller EDs with annual patient volumes of 20,000 [26]. Thus, our findings may be beneficial for mid- and smaller-sized EDs.

Limitations

Several limitations existed in our study. First, this study is a model-based analysis; our findings need to be validated in experimental situations. Second, the data were obtained from a single institution over just one year in Japan, which might reduce the generalizability of the conclusions. Our approach corresponds to that of previous studies of ED crowding in a single site [14]. Our findings may have limited generalizability due to the differences in health care systems between Japan and other nations, but are considered to be generalizable within Japan, especially for other teaching hospitals. Third, although ambulance diversion and patients leaving before evaluation are common proxy measures of ED crowding, we did not include them in this study because we did not measure them. Fourth, we could not obtain triage results, so patients were not classified according to level of disease severity. Patients who were considered as high acuity at triage but were eventually discharged from the ED might have a different time of assessment by senior residents because of difficulty of case management. Additionally, the range of decrease in length of ED stay of discharged patients by senior residents may be shortened due to these complex patients. Fifth, a lack of hourly bed occupancy counts in our data system precluded analysis of hourly hospital bed occupancy. Since bed occupancy changes each hour, an ideal analysis would be performed according to the precise hospital bed occupancy at a particular time. Despite this limitation, our findings are supported by previous studies that found an association between length of ED stay and daily bed occupancy [15,27]. Finally, we cannot exclude possible bias from unmeasured and unavailable factors such as the time involved in awaiting laboratory or radiology results and consultation from other specialists.

Conclusions

Our statistical model indicates that different types of ED staff make different contributions to length of patient stay in the ED. In particular, the addition of attending physicians and senior residents is associated with reduced ED stays. In contrast, adding a junior resident may prolong ED stays, which may worsen ED crowding. To improve efficacy at EDs in Japan, government and health care authorities should place on emphasis on addressing the shortage of board-certificated ED physicians.

Acknowledgments

The authors would like to thank Miho Tamamura and Kyoko Kawano for research assistance.

Author Contributions

Conceived and designed the experiments: TK KN. Analyzed the data: HH TK. Wrote the paper: TK.

References

1. Holroyd BR, Bullard MJ, Latoszek K, Gordon D, Allen S, et al. (2007) Impact of a triage liaison physician on emergency department overcrowding and throughput: a randomized controlled trial. Acad Emerg Med 14: 702–708.
2. Affleck A, Parks P, Drummond A, Rowe BH, Ovens HJ (2013) Emergency department overcrowding and access block. CJEM 15: 359–370.
3. Ministry of Internal Affairs and Communications (2010) Reserch of the acceptance of ambulance in the medical institution in 2009 (Japanese). Available: http://www.fdma.go.jp/neuter/topics/houdou/h22/2203/220318_6houdou.pdf. Accessed 2014 Aug 10.
4. Kennebeck SS, Timm NL, Kurowski EM, Byczkowski TL, Reeves SD (2011) The association of emergency department crowding and time to antibiotics in febrile neonates. Acad Emerg Med 18: 1380–1385.
5. Sun BC, Hsia RY, Weiss RE, Zingmond D, Liang LJ, et al. (2013) Effect of emergency department crowding on outcomes of admitted patients. Ann Emerg Med 61: 605–611 e606.
6. Derlet RW, Richards JR (2000) Overcrowding in the nation's emergency departments: complex causes and disturbing effects. Ann Emerg Med 35: 63–68.
7. Harris A, Sharma A (2010) Access block and overcrowding in emergency departments: an empirical analysis. Emerg Med J 27: 508–511.
8. Japanese Association for Acute Medicine (2012) The number of board certificated ED physicians in Japan (Japanese). Available: http://www.jaam.jp/index.htm. Accessed 2014 Aug 10.
9. Ministry of Health, Labour and Welfare (2009) The basic statistics of the regional health care in 2009 (Japanese) Available: http://www.mhlw.go.jp/toukei/saikin/hw/hoken/kiso/21.html. Accessed 2014 Aug 18.
10. Ministry of Health, Labour and Welfare (2011) The patient survey (Japanese). Available: http://www.mhlw.go.jp/toukei/saikin/hw/kanja/11/index.html. Accessed 2014 Aug 28.
11. Thornton V, Hazell W (2008) Junior doctor strike model of care: Reduced access block and predominant Fellow of the Australasian College for Emergency Medicine staffing improve emergency department performance. Emerg Med Australas 20: 425–430.
12. Timm NL, Ho ML, Luria JW (2008) Pediatric emergency department overcrowding and impact on patient flow outcomes. Acad Emerg Med 15: 832–837.
13. McCarthy ML, Zeger SL, Ding R, Levin SR, Desmond JS, et al. (2009) Crowding delays treatment and lengthens emergency department length of stay, even among high-acuity patients. Ann Emerg Med 54: 492–503 e494.
14. Hillier DF, Parry GJ, Shannon MW, Stack AM (2009) The effect of hospital bed occupancy on throughput in the pediatric emergency department. Ann Emerg Med 53: 767–776 e763.
15. Asaro PV, Lewis LM, Boxerman SB (2007) The impact of input and output factors on emergency department throughput. Acad Emerg Med 14: 235–242.
16. Kocher KE, Meurer WJ, Desmond JS, Nallamothu BK (2012) Effect of testing and treatment on emergency department length of stay using a national database. Acad Emerg Med 19: 525–534.
17. Gardner RL, Sarkar U, Maselli JH, Gonzales R (2007) Factors associated with longer ED lengths of stay. Am J Emerg Med 25: 643–650.
18. Buntin MB, Zaslavsky AM (2004) Too much ado about two-part models and transformation? Comparing methods of modeling Medicare expenditures. J Health Econ 23: 525–542.
19. Nakayama T, Sakai M, Slingsby BT (2005) Japan's ethical guidelines for epidemiologic research: a history of their development. J Epidemiol 15: 107–112.
20. Halperin H, Paradis N, Mosesso V Jr, Nichol G, Sayre M, et al. (2007) Recommendations for implementation of community consultation and public disclosure under the Food and Drug Administration's "Exception from informed consent requirements for emergency research": a special report from the American Heart Association Emergency Cardiovascular Care Committee and Council on Cardiopulmonary, Perioperative and Critical Care: endorsed by the American College of Emergency Physicians and the Society for Academic Emergency Medicine. Circulation 116: 1855–1863.
21. Tsukasa OJ, Takeda Y, Takahashi M, Housei M, Takada S (2010) Factors affecting future specialty choice and practice site among Japanese medical students and graduates - a nationwide survey (Japanese). Japanese Iji Shinpou 4471: 101–107.
22. Hagiwara Y, Hasegawa K, Watase H, Chiba T (2010) Residency and career satisfaction among ER-style emergency medicine residents in Japan. Nihon Kyukyu Igakukai Zasshi 21: 889–898.
23. Kawano T, Nishiyama K, Anan H, Tujimura Y (2014) Direct relationship between aging and overcrowding in the ED, and a calculation formula for demand projection: a cross-sectional study. Emerg Med J 31: 19–23.
24. Wiler JL, Handel DA, Ginde AA, Aronsky D, Genes NG, et al. (2012) Predictors of patient length of stay in 9 emergency departments. Am J Emerg Med 30: 1860–1864.
25. Chin L, Fleisher G (1998) Planning model of resource utilization in an academic pediatric emergency department. Pediatr Emerg Care 14: 4–9.
26. Pines JM, Decker SL, Hu T (2012) Exogenous predictors of national performance measures for emergency department crowding. Ann Emerg Med 60: 293–298.
27. Asaro PV, Lewis LM, Boxerman SB (2007) Emergency department overcrowding: analysis of the factors of renege rate. Acad Emerg Med 14: 157–162.

5

All-Cause Pneumonia Hospitalizations in Children <2 Years Old in Sweden, 1998 to 2012: Impact of Pneumococcal Conjugate Vaccine Introduction

Anders Berglund[1]*, Mats Ekelund[1], Mark A. Fletcher[2], Lars Nyman[1]

1 Pfizer Inc., Sollentuna, Sweden, **2** Pfizer Inc., Paris, France

Abstract

Background: In late 2007, some Swedish County Councils started 7-valent pneumococcal conjugate vaccine (PCV7) implementation for children, and PCV7 was included in the national immunization program in 2009. By 2010, both PCV10 and PCV13 were licensed, and the selection of vaccine was subject to County Councils tenders. This study investigated the impact of the order of PCV introduction into vaccination programs on the incidence of all-cause pneumonia hospitalizations in children <2 years-old.

Methods: Using population-based data from the publicly available National Inpatient Registry, the incidence of inpatient pneumonia (ICD-10 J12-J18) hospitalizations by County Councils among children <2 years old was identified between 1998 and 2012. Incidence rate ratios (IRR; 95% CI) were calculated during the nationwide implementation of PCV7 and then between County Councils, as based on the higher-valent vaccine chosen for a program.

Results: There was a lower risk of all-cause pneumonia hospitalization among <2 year-old children following the introduction of PCV7, as compared to the pre-PCV7 period (0.77; 0.63–0.93). A decreased risk of all-cause pneumonia was also observed in the County Councils that followed the order PCV7 then PCV13 (0.82; 0.66–1.01), while no trend was observed in County Councils with a program in the order PCV7 then PCV10 (1.03; 0.82–1.30). When comparing the higher-valent vaccines, there was a 21% (0.79; 0.66–0.96) lower risk for childhood pneumonia hospitalization in County Councils finally using PCV13 as compared to the experience in County Councils that ultimately adopted PCV10.

Conclusions: Among children <2 years-old, all-cause pneumonia hospitalizations were significantly reduced by 23% one to two years after introduction of PCV7 vaccination in Sweden. In those County Councils that next introduced PCV13, a further decline in all-cause pneumonia hospitalization was observed, in contrast to those County Councils that followed with PCV10; this 21% lower risk for childhood pneumonia hospitalization was statistically significant.

Editor: Bernard Beall, Centers for Disease Control & Prevention, United States of America

Funding: The present study was performed and funded in full by Pfizer Inc.

Competing Interests: The present study was performed and funded in full by Pfizer Inc.

* Email: anders.berglund@pfizer.com

Introduction

All-cause pneumonia remains a common cause of hospitalizations among infants throughout the world [1–3]. Since the introduction of the pneumococcal conjugate vaccines into the childhood national immunization programs (NIPs) of many countries, large reductions in all-cause pneumonia admissions have been observed, as based on experience with the 7-valent pneumococcal conjugate vaccine (PCV7) [4–14], which targets seven serotypes (4, 6B, 9V, 14, 18C, 19F and 23F) [15].

Recently, two higher-valent pneumococcal conjugate vaccines have become available for routine immunization of children: the 10-valent pneumococcal conjugate vaccine (PCV10), which includes three additional serotypes, 1, 5, and 7F [16], not covered by the PCV7, and the 13-valent pneumococcal conjugate vaccine (PCV13) that includes an additional six serotypes (1, 3, 5, 6A, 7F and 19A) [17].

In Sweden, PCV7 was included in the NIP for infants in 2009, although some County Councils already began implementation of PCV7 in late 2007. In 2010, both PCV10 and PCV13 were registered with a 3-dose schedule, and the selection of a higher-valent PCV was subject to County Council tenders that resulted in different choices between County Councils. The aim of the present study was to evaluate the impact of diverse PCV programs (i.e., pre-PV7 to PCV7, then either PCV7 to PCV10 or PCV7 to PCV13) on the rate of hospitalization due to all-cause pneumonia in children <2 years of age in Sweden.

In a review of the effect of PCV dosing schedules on the prevention of pneumonia, which included 37 studies of PCV7 and one study of PCV10, evidence for a reduction was found with each schedule [18]. Investigators in Nicaragua (3+0 schedule) recently observed lower rates of all-cause pneumonia hospitalizations among children after the introduction of PCV13 immunization through the GAVI Alliance [19]. Furthermore, two recent studies from Uruguay and France (both 2+1 schedules) reported a significant reduction among children <2 years old of consolidated pneumonia and community-acquired pneumonia when transitioning from PCV7 to PCV13 [20,21].

Material and Methods

Data sources

The present study is a retrospective analysis of aggregated data from the publicly available National Inpatient Registry administrated by the National Board of Health and Welfare that includes nationwide information on hospital admissions and discharges since 1987 in Sweden [22,23]. The proportion of data not properly registered in the National Inpatient Registry has been estimated to be <1% [22]. Each inpatient discharge record includes date of hospital admission, the age and sex of the patient, and discharge diagnosis coded according to the International Classification of Diseases (ICD). In the analysis, hospitalization for all-cause pneumonia was defined in accordance with the codes in the ICD-10 (J12–J18): J12 (viral pneumonia), J13 (pneumonia due to *Streptococcus pneumoniae*), J14 (pneumonia due to *Haemophilus influenzae*), J15 (bacterial pneumonia), J16 (pneumonia due to other infectious organisms), J17 (pneumonia in diseases classified elsewhere), and J18 (pneumonia, unspecified organism) (**Figure 1**). For the present study, all-cause pneumonia admission, irrespective of the causative agent, was used, as etiology is mostly unknown in children. The current standard for making the diagnosis of pneumonia is an X-ray-confirmed infiltrate in a child with acute respiratory disease, which would include cases with a viral cause also. We have used the hospital discharge diagnosis, and although the absolute majority of these are X-ray confirmed, there is no obligate requirement to have an X-ray-confirmed infiltrate to make the diagnosis, and thus a small minority may not be confirmed.

In addition, the total number of hospital admissions for any cause of disease (i.e., all ICD-10 codes together) was identified by calendar year and County Council.

Demographic characteristics for each County Council were assembled using public information from the government agency, Statistics Sweden [24], while information on health care characteristics was retrieved from a public statistical database of the Swedish Association of Local Authorities and Regions [25].

Study population

The number of in-patient hospital admissions for patients aged <1 year old and 1-<2 years old with one of the selected diagnosis codes (ICD-10 J12-J18) as primary diagnosis was retrieved per County Council or cluster of County Councils for each quarter in the years between 1 January 1998 and 31 December 2012. (Note that County Councils that introduced the same PCV simultaneously were clustered together.)

The Swedish health care system and vaccine coverage

In Sweden, the 21 *Landsting* are each responsible for financing and managing the delivery of their own health care. ("County Council" is the official translation of the word for this geographical division in Sweden.)

The central government is responsible for legislation about the main principles for health care delivery, as well as guidelines for care and the monitoring of quality, and it provides additional funding to financially disadvantaged County Councils in order to ensure equitable health care for all residents in Sweden.

PCV7 was included in the Swedish NIP in January 2009 in a 2+1 infant schedule (vaccinated at 3, 5 and 12 months of age) with no catch-up, although the first County Council had already started vaccination with PCV7 in October 2007. PCV coverage for children in Sweden born in 2010 was 97.6% (range 96.4–98.6% between County Councils) [26].

Each County Council tenders PCVs independently or together with other County Councils, leading to different tender criteria and evaluation algorithms between County Councils. In 2010, the County Councils introduced either PCV10 or PCV13, although one cluster of County Councils implemented PCV7, changed to PCV13, and then changed again to PCV10. Four County Councils had PCV introduction dates that differed from all other County Councils; the populations of these County Councils are small, representing about 10% of the source population, and available data did not allow a separate analysis for each one of them. They were each clustered into pairs with the County Council that had the closest introduction date (**Table 1**).

The fraction of infants belonging to each age group (<1 year or 1-<2 years old) exposed to at least one dose of vaccine in a given quarter was estimated on the simplifying assumptions that the number of births is equally distributed over the calendar year and that vaccine coverage was 100%. Consequently, if a vaccination scheme began the first day of January in a given year, the fraction of infants <1 year old that has been exposed to at least one dose of vaccine will increase from 0% in the beginning of the first quarter to 25% by the end of the first quarter; consequently, 12.5% of infants on average will have been exposed to at least one dose of vaccine during this first quarter. For each additional quarter, the fraction of vaccinated infants <1 year old will increase until the maximum is reached (i.e., 75% of infants <1 years of age exposed to at least one dose of vaccine). As the first dose is given at the age of 3 months after birth, no more than 75% of <1 year-olds are exposed to at least one dose of vaccine. By the same logic, the fraction of vaccinated 1-year-old infants starts to increase one year after the introduction of a vaccine and will eventually reach 100%.

Statistical Analyses

An additive time-series model was used to determine the trend, with seasonal and random components, by using moving averages. Trend is the long-term increase or decrease; the seasonal component relates to short-term, regular, wave-like patterns, while the random component describes the unpredictable residual fluctuations [27].

A pooled analysis combining time-series for several cross sections of clusters was applied, based on a generalized linear model for rates of hospitalization for all-cause pneumonia, using the negative binomial distribution (given that data were over dispersed) with a logarithmic link function and an offset equal to the log of the population divided by 100,000 [28,29]. A sandwich variance estimator was used to account for possible multiple hospitalizations. Residual analyses showed no substantial deviations from model assumptions. Using negative binomial regression models, hospitalization rates per 100,000 person-years and incidence rate ratios (IRR) with corresponding 95% confidence interval (95% CI) for each explanatory variable were estimated.

The crude regression models included only the particular PCV (PCV7, PCV10 or PCV13) that was being administered at each time point, whereas the adjusted regression models also accounted for seasonal effects, calendar year, clustered County Councils, and a covariate of "mixed exposure of PCV13 and PCV10". The variable *type of vaccine* was categorized as follows: pre-PCV7,

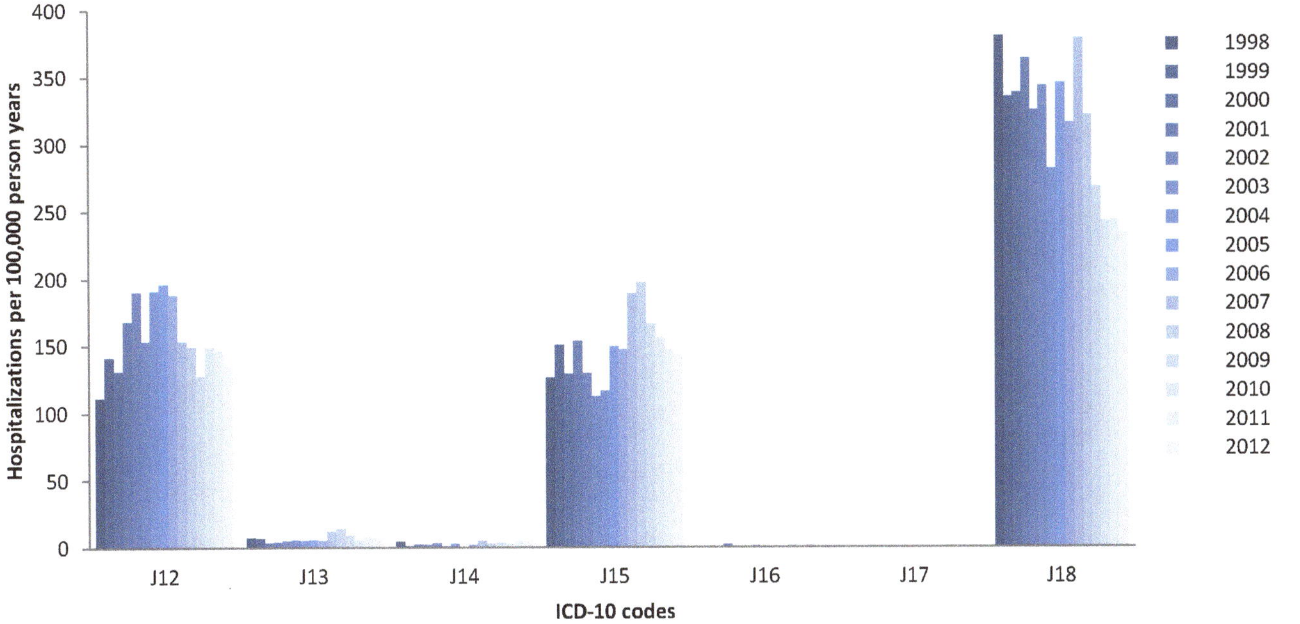

Figure 1. Distribution of ICD-10 code hospitalization rates by calendar year among children <2 years old: J12 (viral pneumonia), J13 (pneumonia due to Streptococcus pneumoniae), J14 (pneumonia due to Haemophilus influenzae), J15 (bacterial pneumonia), J16 (pneumonia due to other infectious organisms), J17 (pneumonia in diseases classified elsewhere), and J18 (pneumonia, unspecified organism).

PCV7, PCV10, or PCV13. The fundamental transition periods (e.g. pre-PCV7 to PCV7, PCV7 to PCV10, or PCV7 to PCV13) were excluded from the regression models. In a cluster of two paired County Councils, together representing 5.7% of the source population, there was a period (first quarter, 2011 to fourth quarter, 2012) with overlap where children in one of the County Councils were vaccinated with PCV10 and children in the other were vaccinated with PCV13. In the sensitivity analyses, the regression models were restricted to the same duration of time of use for PCV10 or PCV13.

All p-values were two-sided, and statistical significance was considered at $p<0.05$; R version 2.10.1 and STATA version 12 (STATA, College Station, Texas, USA) were used for all statistical analyses.

Results

In 2012, 15 of 21 County Councils were vaccinating with PCV10 and 6 of 21 with PCV13. The County Councils vaccinating with PCV13 correspond to 51% of the source population (**Figure 2**). There were no major differences between County Councils vaccinating with PCV10 or PCV13 with regard to key demographic or health care characteristics (**Table 2**).

A total of 37,553 hospitalizations for all-cause pneumonia among 6,013,445 person-years in children <2 years old was identified during the study period, 1998–2012. In 1998, the incidence rate per 100,000 person-years (95% CI) of all-cause pneumonia hospitalization was 615 (578–651). There was no particular trend between 1998 and 2007. A decrease commenced in 2008 and a further decrease was observed after 2009 (**Figure 3**).

In the County Councils that followed the order PCV7 then PCV13 (i.e., PCV7//PCV13), a pronounced decrease in the incidence rate was observed through 2012 (**Figure 3**); whereas for PCV7//PCV10 County Councils that introduced a program of PCV7 then PCV10, a further decrease following PCV10 was not apparent (**Figure 3**).

The crude rates of all-cause pneumonia hospitalizations per 100,000 person-years were greatest in the pre-PCV7 era (598; 568–622) and they were lowest among PCV7//PCV13 County Councils (464; 411–518) (**Table 3**). When adjustments were made for seasonal effects, calendar year, and clustered County Councils, the incidence rates for pre-PCV7, PCV7, PCV7//PCV10 County Councils and PCV7//PCV13 County Councils were 655 (619–691), 504 (414–595), 520 (440–599) and 413 (358–468), respectively.

In the pre-PCV7 period, the incidence rate was 584 per 100,000 person-years among County Councils that later chose PCV10 and 724 per 100,000 person-years among those that transitioned to PCV13. There was no difference in the PCV7 impact between the County Councils that eventually used PCV10 or PCV13; in particular, during the PCV7 era, the incidence decreased to 480 per 100,000 person-years in the County Councils ultimately using PCV10 and to 576 per 100,000 person-years in the PCV13 final County Councils, which was not a statistically significant difference ($p = 0.233$) between these groups of County Councils.

Compared with the pre-PCV7 period, there was a 23% reduced risk (0.77; 0.63–0.93) for all-cause pneumonia hospitalization in children <2 years old after PCV7 was introduced, based on a median time of follow-up of 14 months (**Table 3**). When comparing the post-PCV7 period incidence with the PCV13 period incidence, a further 18% decrease (0.82; 0.66–1.01) in the risk of hospitalizations due to all-cause pneumonia was observed in the PCV7//PCV13 County Councils, while no further decrease was observed in the PCV7//PCV10 County Councils that moved from PCV7 to a PCV10 program (1.03; 0.82–1.30).

When evaluating the rates of hospitalizations due to all-cause pneumonia among children <2 years of age in the pre-PCV7 period compared to the rates in the County Councils post-PCV10 or post-PCV13, the reduction in risk was 21% (0.79; 0.68–0.93) in

Table 1. Month of implementation (in parenthesis) and vaccine, PCV7, PCV10, or PCV13, in the implementation of vaccination programs by County Council or clustered County Council and by Calendar Year.

Clustered County Councils	% of the source population	Calendar Year						
		1998–2006	2007	2008	2009	2010	2011	2012
Stockholm	25.4		(Oct) PCV7	PCV7	PCV7	(Jan) PCV13	PCV13	PCV13
Halland, VGR, Kronoberg, Gotland	22.2				(Jan) PCV7	(Jan) PCV13	PCV13	PCV13
Jönköping[1]	3.5			(April) PCV7	PCV7	(Jan) PCV13	PCV13	PCV13
Västernorrland[1]	2.2			(July) PCV7	PCV7	(Jan) PCV13	(Mar) PCV10	PCV10
Östergötland, Jämtland, Västerbotten, Norrbotten	10.2				(Jan) PCV7	(Jan) PCV13	(Mar) PCV10	PCV10
Uppsala, Västmanland, Dalarna, Gävleborg	11.2				(Jan) PCV7	(Mar) PCV10	PCV10	PCV10
Värmland, Södermanland[2]	5.1				(Jan/Oct) PCV7	PCV10	PCV10	PCV10
Skåne, Kalmar	15.9				(Jan) PCV7	(May) PCV10	PCV10	PCV10
Blekinge[3]	1.4			(Oct) PCV7	PCV7	(May) PCV10	PCV10	PCV10
Örebro[3]	2.9			(Mar) PCV7	(Oct) PCV10	PCV10	PCV10	PCV10

[1]Jönköping and Västernorrland were clustered by the National Board of Health and Welfare in order to ensure confidentiality of records.
[2]PCV7 was introduced in January 2009. In October 2009 the present region switched to PCV10.
[3]Blekinge and Örebro were clustered by the National Board of Health and Welfare in order to ensure confidentiality of records.

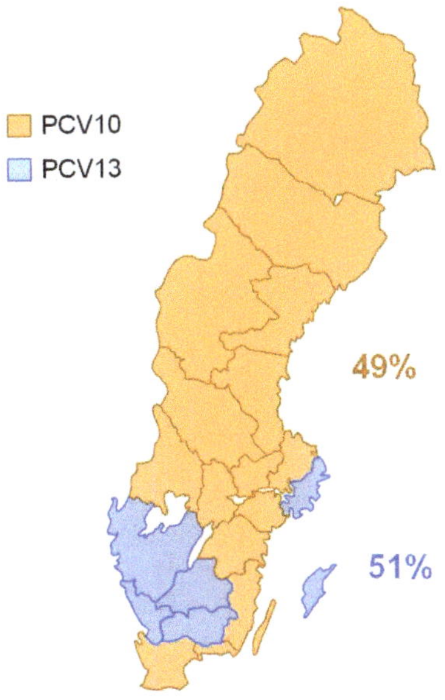

Figure 2. PCV use in 2012 in Sweden by County Council.

the PCV7//PCV10 County Councils and 37% (0.63; 0.54–0.74) in the PCV7//PCV13 County Councils.

When contrasting the two higher-valent vaccines, a 21% (0.79; 0.66–0.96) decreased risk was observed in County Councils finally using PCV13 rather than PCV10 (**Table 3**). In analyses restricted to the same duration of time exposed to either of the higher-valent vaccines, the results remained virtually unchanged (0.78; 0.63–0.97).

Discussion

For children <2 years of age, hospitalizations due to all-cause pneumonia were significantly reduced by 23% following the PCV7 vaccination program implemented in Sweden. In County Councils that then next chose PCV13, a trend to a further 18% decrease was observed; however, the PCV10 program that 15 County Councils followed was not associated with a further decline as compared to that already demonstrated with PCV7. In an analysis of all-cause inpatient pneumonia among <2-year-old children, there was a statistically significant 21% decreased risk among County Councils that vaccinated with PCV7 then PCV13 (PCV7//PCV13) as compared to those that followed the order PCV7//PCV10.

The introduction of PCV7 in Sweden decreased the likelihood of all-cause pneumonia hospitalizations by 23% among children < 2 years old. These reductions are within the range of results from previous observational studies, where the decline in all-cause pneumonia hospitalizations in children ranged from 13–65% after implementation of PCV7 [4–14]. The observed reduction for Sweden is at the lower end of this spectrum, and it might be that the duration of the immunization program had been too brief to allow for the full impact of PCV7 to be observed. For instance, in the present study, for the single County Council that implemented PCV7 in 2007, ahead of the NIP, the observed reduction was 41% compared to the pre-PCV7 period ($p<0.001$).

A recent study in Brazil after the introduction of PCV10 as the initial pneumococcal conjugate vaccine observed a 23–29% decline of pneumonia hospitalizations (ICD-10 J12-J18) in children in 3 of 5 cities one year after implementation of PCV10, compared to an earlier period with no use of vaccines [30]. Within the first two years of a PCV13 immunization program in Nicaragua, provided as the only PCV, investigators observed statistically significant lower risks of pneumonia hospitalizations, compared to the pre-vaccination period: 33% reduction in infants <1 year-old (0.67; 0.59–0.75) and 26% in children 1-<2 years-old (0.74; 0.67–0.81) [19].

An indication of a further effect following the switch from PCV7 to PCV13 was noted on the incidence of consolidated pneumonia in Uruguay [20]. The same pattern was observed in France, where an additional 32% reduction in community-acquired pneumonia was observed after the transition from PCV7 to PCV13 among children <2 years old [21]. But to our knowledge, no other investigators have compared the rates in all-cause pneumonia based on the order of introduction of different higher-valent vaccines, PCV7 then PCV10 or PCV7 then PCV13.

The observed difference in changes of hospitalization rates attributed to the higher-valent vaccines in the present study does not seem to be related to key demographic or health care characteristics between those County Councils vaccinating with

Table 2. Demographic and Health Care Characteristics Between County Councils Utilizing PCV13 and PCV10 in 2012.

	County Councils in 2012			
	Using PCV13		Using PCV10	
No. of County Councils (%)	6	(29%)	15	(71%)
No. of children <2 years (%)	115,958	(51%)	110,981	(49%)
Total population (%)	4,613,813	(48%)	4,942,080	(52%)
Share of the pop. with higher education (range)	26%	(18–30%)	21%	(17–27%)
Mean net income (>20 years) (range)[1,2]	€ 27,830	(€ 22,081–€ 29,648)	€ 23,211	(€ 21,792–€ 25,117)
Share of the pop. in urban areas (range) [3]	88%	(58–96%)	82%	(66–89%)
Share of the pop. born in Sweden (range)	82%	(78–95%)	87%	(82–95%)
Mean net health care spend per inhab. (range) [1]	€ 2,400	(€ 2,326–€ 2,650)	€ 2,382	(€ 2,257–€ 2,599)
Mean of hospital admissions per 1,000 (range)	166	(163–190)	170	(153–197)

[1]Swedish prices converted to euros (€) by using the exchange rate of August 12, 2014 (1 Swedish kronor [SEK] = 0.10891 euro [€]).
[2]Only available in 2011.
[3]Only available in 2010.

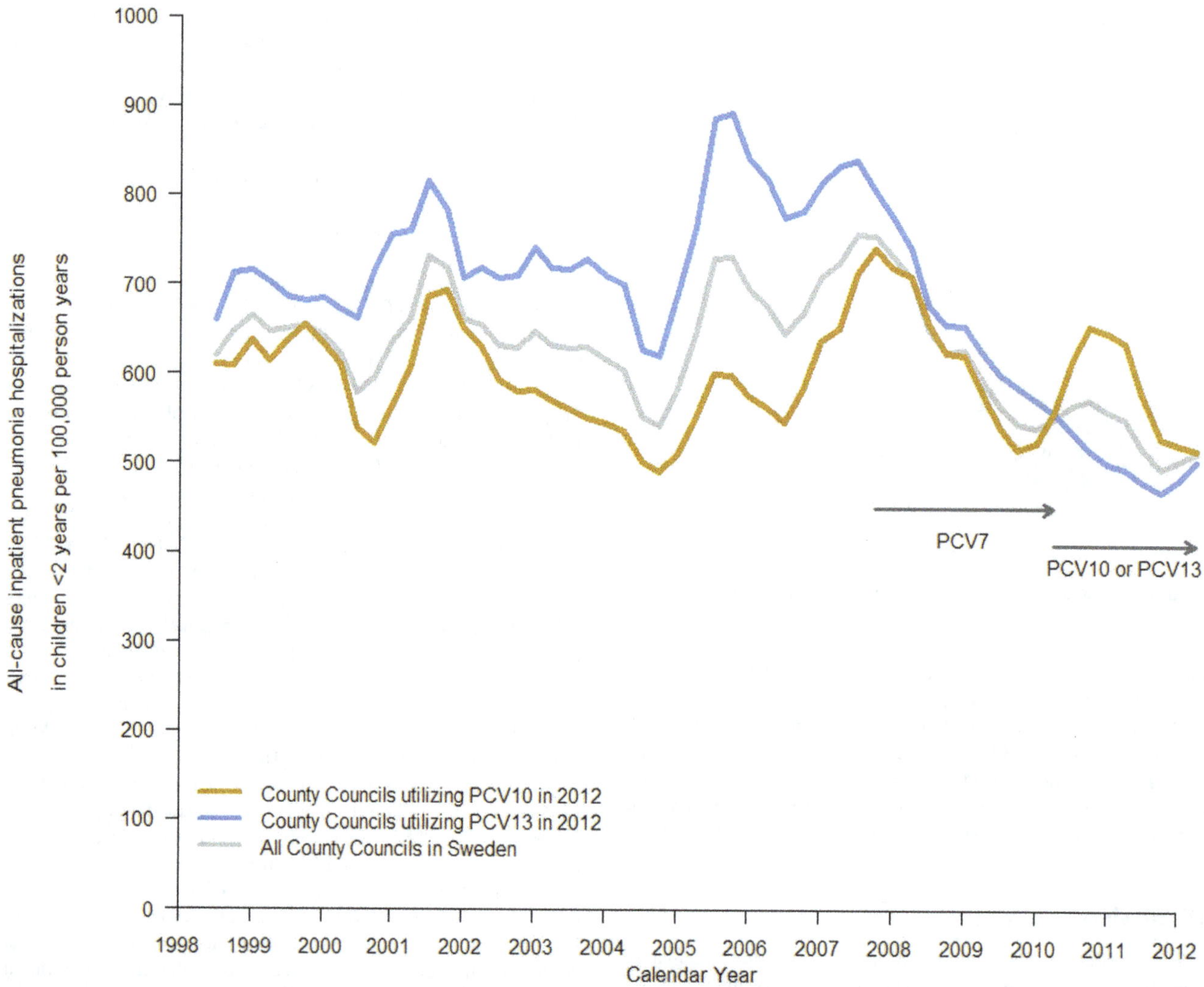

Figure 3. All−cause pneumonia hospitalizations per 100,000 person-years by all County Councils and by County Councils utilizing PCV10 only or PCV13 only in 2012.

PCV10 or PCV13 (**Table 2**). The median period of time from vaccine implementation at a County Council level was 14 months for PCV7; it was 34 and 36 months for PCV10 and PCV13, respectively. In separate analyses, restricted to the same duration of time of vaccination with PCV10 or PCV13, results remained virtually unchanged with regards to a lower risk of all-cause pneumonia hospitalizations among children <2 years old in the PCV7//PCV13 County Councils. Although the start date was adjusted for in the analyses, the indirect impact of the initial PCV7 program might enlarge the impact seen in later years. Another possible reason for the observed differences in all-cause pneumonia admissions may include modifications in the criteria for pneumonia hospitalizations or the introduction of new diagnostic methods, but neither seems to have changed in recent years.

A limitation of the present study is that the data were not on an individual level. The large numbers attained using the entire Swedish population provide adequate statistical power, and the fact that the population is divided in two equally sized geographically distinct groups from different parts of the country is likely to reduce potential biases induced by regional differences, such as any variations in the annual incidence of influenza and respiratory syncytial virus hospitalizations. Nonetheless, even with two equally sized populations, we are not able to account for all residual confounding, and the observed differences between the higher-valent vaccines in the reductions of all-cause pneumonia hospitalizations may be associated with regional differences in the serotypes most frequently causing pneumococcal pneumonia or differences in the etiology of pneumonia [31].

The uptake of PCV7, PCV10 or PCV13 in the County Councils did not show any meaningful differences, and the general vaccine uptake has been very high (total 97.6%, range 96.4–98.6%). By utilizing information from the National Inpatient Registry, we were able to include all registered inpatient pneumonia hospitalizations among children aged <2 years in Sweden during the study period. Moreover, the total number of hospital admissions for all causes of disease stayed the same during the study period, suggesting a similar access to hospital beds.

A factor underlying the differences in impact between the sequence PCV7//PCV10 and PCV7//PCV13 could be the serotype coverage. Sweden has mandatory reporting for invasive pneumococcal disease (IPD) and all isolates are serotyped by the Disease Control Agency [26]. As in other countries that have introduced a pediatric vaccination program against pneumococcal disease, Sweden has noted a clear decrease in IPD among

Table 3. Crude and Adjusted Incidence Rates and Incidence Rate Ratios (IRR) with Corresponding 95% Confidence Intervals (CI) during the pre-PCV7 and PCV7 period, and for County Councils utilizing by 2012 PCV10 and PCV13, among children <2 years old in Sweden.

	Crude				Adjusted[1]			
Exposure variables	**Rates**	**(95% CI)**	**IRR**	**(95% CI)**	**Rates**	**(95% CI)**	**IRR**	**(95% CI)**
Pre-PCV7	597.7	(567.8–621.6)	1.00	(ref.)	654.7	(618.5–690.8)	1.00	(ref.)
PCV7	508.5	(428.8–588.2)	0.86	(0.73–1.00)	504.4	(414.1–594.6)	0.77	(0.63–0.93)
Pre-PCV7	597.7	(567.8–621.6)	1.00	(ref.)	654.7	(618.5–690.8)	1.00	(ref.)
PCV10	510.7	(444.1–577.4)	0.86	(0.75–0.98)	519.9	(440.4–599.3)	0.79	(0.68–0.93)
Pre-PCV7	597.7	(567.8–621.6)	1.00	(ref.)	654.7	(618.5–690.8)	1.00	(ref.)
PCV13	464.4	(410.9–517.9)	0.78	(0.69–0.88)	412.6	(357.5–467.6)	0.63	(0.54–0.74)
PCV7	508.5	(428.8–588.2)	1.00	(ref.)	504.4	(414.1–594.6)	1.00	(ref.)
PCV10	510.7	(444.1–577.4)	1.00	(0.82–1.23)	519.9	(440.4–599.3)	1.03	(0.82–1.30)
PCV7	508.5	(428.8–588.2)	1.00	(ref.)	504.4	(414.1–594.6)	1.00	(ref.)
PCV13	464.4	(410.9–517.9)	0.91	(0.75–1.11)	412.6	(357.5–467.6)	0.82	(0.66–1.01)
PCV10	510.7	(444.1–577.4)	1.00	(ref.)	519.9	(440.4–599.3)	1.00	(ref.)
PCV13	464.4	(410.9–517.9)	0.91	(0.77–1.08)	412.6	(357.5–467.6)	0.79	(0.66–0.96)

ref. = reference group.

[1]The regression models were adjusted for County Councils, Seasonal effects, and Calendar Year.

vaccinated children. For children <2 years of age, the total number of IPD cases had fallen by 75% in 2012, as compared to the average number in the years before vaccination began. In particular, the total number of IPD cases in children <2 years in all of Sweden decreased between 2010 and 2012: 26 cases in 2010, 27 cases in 2011, and 18 cases in 2012 (for which results from serotyping of 17 of 18 cases are available) [26]. The Disease Control Agency calculated the serotype coverage in children <2 years of age for the different available pneumococcal vaccines, which had remained similar between 2010 and 2012: PCV7, 12%; PCV10, 18%; PCV13, 47%. The most prevalent IPD serotypes in Sweden in 2012 for all ages were 22F (13%), 3 (13%), 7F (9%), 19A (7%), 33F (5%) and 11A (4%); data for children <2 years only are not available. The serotypes 3 and 19A are particularly interesting in this aspect because these two serotypes covered by PCV13, but not by PCV10, constitute 20% of the remaining all-age IPD burden in Sweden. It might be estimated that these serotypes also constitute an important part of the remaining IPD for children <2 years, as exemplified by the 47% coverage for PCV13, as compared to 18% for PCV10 in this same age group. This suggests that the serotypes 3 and 19A constitute a substantial part of remaining IPD burden, and should the same serotypes play a similar role in pneumonia, it may serve as an explanation for differences noted between PCV10 and PCV13 on hospitalizations due to all-cause pneumonia.

Another possible explanation may come from the transition period between different PCV programs. All children in Sweden were primed by the PCV7 with a CRM197 carrier protein conjugate against the seven targeted serotypes. Although no catch-up schedules were implemented in Sweden, County Councils used different approaches for the transitions: one County Council continued with PCV7 for all children initiated on PCV7 and in parallel started with PCV10 for new infants; others made a direct switch from PCV7 to PCV10 individually within the 2+1 schedule of the NIP [15,16,32]. These latter County Councils subsequently introduced PCV10 vaccine to PCV7-primed but incompletely vaccinated infants, in spite of the fact that the PCV10 has carrier proteins that are different from PCV7 for the seven serotypes in common. Other County Councils subsequently introduced PCV13 to PCV7-primed infants, where PCV13 uses the same carrier protein as PCV7 and the switch is indicated at any dose [17,21].

Conclusions

In conclusion, our study provides additional findings of a decreased risk of all-cause pneumonia hospitalizations among children <2 years old since implementation of the PCV7 program, as compared to the period before the pediatric NIP in Sweden. Furthermore, comparing County Councils that subsequently introduced PCV10 or PCV13, there was an additional trend of reduction of all-cause inpatient pneumonia among children <2 years old only in County Councils transitioning to PCV13. In a comparison between County Council programs that followed the order PCV7 then PCV13 or the programs that followed the order PCV7 then PCV10, there was a statistically significant 21% lower risk of all-cause inpatient pneumonia among children <2 years old in County Councils that finally vaccinated with PCV13. It is important to continue observations to understand the evolution of all-cause pneumonia hospitalizations and further document the impact of the County Council pneumococcal disease childhood immunization programs.

Acknowledgments

The authors wish to thank their Pfizer colleagues, Alejandro Cane, Raymond A. Farkouh, Myint Tin Tin Htar, and Rogier Klok, for their expert guidance in the preparation of this manuscript.

Author Contributions

Conceived and designed the experiments: AB ME LN. Performed the experiments: AB ME LN. Analyzed the data: AB. Contributed reagents/materials/analysis tools: AB ME. Wrote the paper: AB ME MF LN.

References

1. World Health Organization (2013) Immunization surveillance, assessment and monitoring. Accessed 2013 Nov 5.
2. Wardlaw T, Salama P, Johansson EW, Mason E (2006) Pneumonia: the leading killer of children. Lancet 368(9541): 1048–50.
3. McIntosh K (2002) Community-acquired pneumonia in children. N Engl J Med 346(6): 429–37.
4. Grijalva CG, Nuorti JP, Arboqast PG, Martin SW, Edwards KM, et al (2007) Decline in pneumonia admissions after routine childhood immunisation with pneumococcal conjugate vaccine in the USA: a time-series analysis. Lancet 369(9568): 1179–86.
5. Griffin MR, Zhu Y, Moore MR, Whitney CG, Grijalva CG (2013) U.S. hospitalizations for pneumonia after a decade of pneumococcal vaccination. N Engl J Med 369(2): 155–63.
6. Jardine A, Menzies RI, McIntyre PB (2010) Reduction in hospitalizations for pneumonia associated with the introduction of a pneumococcal conjugate vaccination schedule without a booster dose in Australia. Pediatr Infect Dis J 29(7): 607–12.
7. Koshy E, Murray J, Bottle A, Sharland M, Saxena S (2010) Impact of the seven-valent pneumococcal conjugate vaccination (PCV7) programme on childhood hospital admissions for bacterial pneumonia and empyema in England: national time-trends study, 1997–2008. Thorax 65(9): 770–4.
8. Zhou F, Kyaw MH, Shefer A, Winston CA, Nuorti JP (2007) Health care utilization for pneumonia in young children after routine pneumococcal conjugate vaccine use in the United States. Arch Pediatr Adolesc Med 161(12): 1162–8.
9. Simonsen L, Taylor RJ, Young-Xu Y, Haber M, May L, et al (2011) Impact of pneumococcal conjugate vaccination of infants on pneumonia and influenza hospitalization and mortality in all age groups in the United States. MBio 2(1): e00309–10.
10. Durando P, Crovari P, Ansaldi F, Sticchi L, Sticchi C, et al (2009) Universal childhood immunisation against Streptococcus pneumoniae: the five-year experience of Liguria Region, Italy. Vaccine 27(25–26): 3459–62.
11. Lee GE, Lorch SA, Sheffler-Collins S, Kronman MP, Shah SS (2010) National hospitalization trends for pediatric pneumonia and associated complications. Pediatrics 126(2): 204–13.
12. Patrzalek M, Albrecht P, Sobczynski M (2010) Significant decline in pneumonia admission rate after the introduction of routine 2+1 dose schedule heptavalent pneumococcal conjugate vaccine (PCV7) in children under 5 years of age in Kielce, Poland. Eur J Clin Microbiol Infect Dis 29(7): 787–92.
13. Miller E, Andrews NJ, Waight PA, Slack MP, Gergoe RC (2011) Herd immunity and serotype replacement 4 years after seven-valent pneumococcal conjugate vaccination in England and Wales: an observational cohort study. Lancet Infect Dis 11(10): 760–8.
14. Rozenbaum MH, Boersma C, Postma MJ, Hak E (2011) Observed differences in invasive pneumococcal disease epidemiology after routine infant vaccination. Expert Rev Vaccines 10(2): 187–99.
15. European Medicines Agency (2013) European Public Assessment Report, Prevenar pneumococcal saccharide conjugated vaccine (adsorbed). Accessed 2013 Dec 5.
16. European Medicines Agency (2013) European Public Assessment Report, Synflorix pneumococcal polysaccharide conjugated vaccine (adsorbed). Accessed 2013 Dec 5.
17. European Medicines Agency (2013) European Public Assessment Report, Prevenar 13 pneumococcal polysaccharide conjugated vaccine (13-valent, adsorbed). Accessed 2013 Dec 5.
18. Loo JD, Conklin L, Fleming-Dutra KE, Deloria Knoll M, Park DE, et al (2014) Systematic review of the effect of pneumococcal conjugate vaccine dosing schedules on prevention of pneumonia. Pediatr Infect Dis J 33 Suppl 2: S140–51.
19. Becker-Dreps S, Amaya E, Liu L, Moreno G, Rocha J, et al (2014) Changes in childhood pneumonia and infant mortality rates following introduction of the 13-valent pneumococcal conjugate vaccine in Nicaragua. Pediatr Infect Dis J 33(8): 637–42.

20. Hortal M, Estevan M, Laurani H, Iraola I, Meny M (2012) Hospitalized children with pneumonia in Uruguay: pre and post introduction of 7 and 13-valent pneumococcal conjugated vaccines into the National Immunization Program. Vaccine 30(33): 4934–8.
21. Angoulvant F, Levy C, Grimprel E, Varon E, Lorrot M, et al (2014) Early impact of 13-valent pneumococcal conjugate vaccine on community-acquired pneumonia in children. Clin Infect Dis 58(7): 918–24.
22. Ludvigsson JF, Andersson E, Ekbom A, Feychting M, Kim JL, et al (2011) External review and validation of the Swedish national inpatient register. BMC Public Health 11: 450.
23. The National Board of Health and Welfare (2012) The statistical database on diagnosis in in-patient care. http://www.socialstyrelsen.se/statistik/statistikdatabas/diagnoserislutenvard. Accessed 3 December 2013.
24. Statistics Sweden (2012) The statistical database for demographic characteristics in Sweden. http://scb.se/sv_/Hitta-statistik/Statistik-efter-amne. Accessed 2013 Dec 3.
25. Swedish Association of Local Authorities and Regions (2012) The statistical database for municipalities and county councils. http://www.kolada.se. Accessed 2013 Dec 3.
26. Swedish Institute for Communicable Disease Control (2013) Annual epidemiological report in 2012. Stockholm.
27. Cleveland RB, Cleveland WS, McRae JE, Terpenning I (1990) STL: A seasonal-trend decomposition procedure based on loess. Journal of Official Statistics 6: 3–73.
28. Hilbe JM (2011) Negative Binomial Regression. Cambridge: Cambridge University Press. 570 p.
29. Frees EW (2004) Longitudinal and Panel Data. Cambridge: Cambridge University Press. 484 p.
30. Afonso ET, Minamisava R, Bierrenbach AL, Escalante JJ, Alencar AP, et al (2013) Effect of 10-valent pneumococcal vaccine on pneumonia among children, Brazil. Emerg Infect Dis 19(4): 589–97.
31. Fitzwater SP, Chandran A, Santosham M, Johnson HL (2012) The worldwide impact of the seven-valent pneumococcal conjugate vaccine. Pediatr Infect Dis J 31(5): 501–8.
32. World Health Organization (2012) Pneumococcal vaccines WHO position paper – 2012 – recommendations. Vaccine 30(32): 4717–4718.

6

A Meta-Analysis of Unilateral versus Bilateral Pedicle Screw Fixation in Minimally Invasive Lumbar Interbody Fusion

Zheng Liu[1], Qi Fei[2]*, Bingqiang Wang[2], Pengfei Lv[1], Cheng Chi[1], Yong Yang[2], Fan Zhao[2], Jisheng Lin[2], Zhao Ma[2]

1 Department of Orthopaedics, Peking University Shougang Hospital, Beijing, China, **2** Department of Orthopaedics, Beijing Friendship Hospital, Capital Medical University, Beijing, China

Abstract

Study Design: Meta-analysis.

Background: Bilateral pedicle screw fixation (PS) after lumbar interbody fusion is a widely accepted method of managing various spinal diseases. Recently, unilateral PS fixation has been reported as effective as bilateral PS fixation. This meta-analysis aimed to comparatively assess the efficacy and safety of unilateral PS fixation and bilateral PS fixation in the minimally invasive (MIS) lumbar interbody fusion for one-level degenerative lumbar spine disease.

Methods: MEDLINE/PubMed, EMBASE, BIOSIS Previews, and Cochrane Library were searched through March 30, 2014. Randomized controlled trials (RCTs) and controlled clinical trials (CCTs) on unilateral versus bilateral PS fixation in MIS lumbar interbody fusion that met the inclusion criteria and the methodological quality standard were retrieved and reviewed. Data on participant characteristics, interventions, follow-up period, and outcomes were extracted from the included studies and analyzed by Review Manager 5.2.

Results: Six studies (5 RCTs and 1 CCT) involving 298 patients were selected. There were no significant differences between unilateral and bilateral PS fixation procedures in fusion rate, complications, visual analogue score (VAS) for leg pain, VAS for back pain, Oswestry disability index (ODI). Both fixation procedures had similar length of hospital stay (MD = 0.38, 95% CI = −0.83 to 1.58; P = 0.54). In contrast, bilateral PS fixation was associated with significantly more intra-operative blood loss (P = 0.002) and significantly longer operation time (P = 0.02) as compared with unilateral PS fixation.

Conclusions: Unilateral PS fixation appears as effective and safe as bilateral PS fixation in MIS lumbar interbody fusion but requires less operative time and causes less blood loss, thus offering a simple alternative approach for one-level lumbar degenerative disease.

Editor: Mohammed Shamji, Toronto Western Hospital, Canada

Funding: The study was funded by Basic-Clinical Cooperation Project in Capital Medical University (NO. 13JL37) and Beijing Outstanding Talent Training Project (NO. 2013D003034000005). The funders had no role in study design, data collection and analysis, decision to publish, or preparation of the manuscript.

Competing Interests: The authors have declared that no competing interests exist.

* Email: spinefei@126.com

Introduction

Minimally invasive (MIS) lumbar interbody fusion is a popular technique used to treat various lumbar degenerative disorders. Over the traditional open surgery, MIS surgery offers multiple advantages; it not only reduces the approach-related muscle damage, blood loss, postoperative pain, length of hospital stay, and postoperative narcotic usage but also allows for early ambulation. Accordingly, MIS is popularized by most of the spine surgeons, especially when it is used with percutaneous pedicle screws [1].

Generally, bilateral pedicle screw (PS) fixation is accepted as a standard procedure in lumbar interbody fusion. Providing rigid fixation, bilateral PS have a great biomechanical stability and several clinical advantages [2]. Recently, unilateral PS fixation has been suggested as an effective approach as bilateral PS fixation in spinal fusion requiring significantly shorter operating time and hospital stay [3–5]. Ding et al. evaluated outcomes of patients with degenerative disc disease following unilateral and bilateral PS fixation procedures respectively and validated the efficacy and safety of unilateral PS fixation in traditional open lumbar interbody fusion. However, this meta-analysis included samples of patients with both one- and two-level degenerative lumbar spine diseases, which might increase the statistical heterogeneity [5]. No similar meta-analyses on unilateral versus bilateral PS fixation in MIS lumbar interbody fusion particularly for one-level degenerative lumbar spine disease are available in the current literature. The objective of this meta-analysis was to examine the effects of unilateral PS fixation and bilateral PS fixation in MIS lumbar interbody fusion for one-level degenerative lumbar spine disease by contrasting and combining results from previously reported relevant randomized controlled trials (RCTs) and controlled clinical trials (CCTs).

Methods

Literature search

The MEDLINE (through PubMed), EMBASE, Ovid (BIOSIS Previews included), and Cochrane databases were searched through March 18, 2014 using combinations of such key terms as 'lumbar interbody fusion', 'pedicle screw fixation', 'minimally invasive', 'unilateral', and 'bilateral' with the Boolean operators 'AND', 'NOT', and 'OR'. Studies cited in the identified articles were also searched manually. The included studies were published in a peer-reviewed journal as a full article, excluding the gray literature and conference proceedings.

Inclusion and exclusion criteria

RCTs and CCTs were included if the following criteria were met: (1) they were published in full-text in English in peer-reviewed journals but not in the gray literature and conference proceedings; (2) subjects were diagnosed with one-level lumbar degenerative disease; (3) bilateral and unilateral pedicle screw fixation procedures were comparatively evaluated; and (4) RCTs and comparative observational studies (CCTs). The exclusion criteria were: (1) combined anterior and posterior surgery; (2) lumbar tumors; (3) conditions such as severe osteoporosis, active infection, metabolic disease or symptomatic vascular disease; (4) previous lumbar surgery; and (5) an average follow-up time of <6 months.

Data extraction

Two reviewers independently screened the titles and abstracts of the retrieved articles to ensure that both inclusion and exclusion criteria were met. Disagreements, if any, were resolved by a third reviewer. Data on the primary outcome measures including visual analogue leg pain score (VAS), Oswestry disability index (ODI), fusion rate and complications and the secondary outcome measures including intra-operative blood loss, operating time and hospital stay were extracted from the included studies and are presented in Table 1.

Study quality

The methodological quality of the included studies was assessed by two independent authors based on the physiotherapy evidence database (PEDro) scale [6]. This scale is based on a list of 11 criteria, each conferring 1 point to the total score. One criterion was excluded from our calculation of the total PEDro score, and, subsequently there was a potentially maximum total score of 10 points for each of the individual studies included in this meta-analysis. Two reviewers performed the assessment independently. The agreement between the 2 reviewers was evaluated with both the correlation coefficient (r) for interrater agreement and the intraclass correlation coefficient.

Statistical analysis

The summary statistic was calculated for each individual study using the meta-analysis program of the Cochrane Collaboration (Review Manager 5.2). Binary data (e.g., fusion rate, incidence rate of screw complications) were presented as odds ratio (OR) and 95% confidence intervals (CIs). Continuous outcomes (VAS, ODI, intra-operative blood loss, operative time, and hospital stay) were summarized using the mean difference (MD) and respective 95% CI. Data on the primary and secondary outcome measures were analyzed as continuous or dichotomized variables using random effect model or fixed effect model. When there was no difference between the findings derived with the 2 models, the results were reported using the fixed-effect model, indicating the absence of significant statistical heterogeneity. Random-effects model was used as a more conservative estimate, less likely to reveal a difference between 2 treatment approaches as compared with the fixed-effects model. When any difference between treatment approaches really existed, both models were used. The possibility of publication bias was assessed by funnel plots, showing the intervention effect from each study against the corresponding standard error. Symmetrical and any asymmetry plots would suggest absence and presence of publication bias respectively. The strength and robustness of the pooled results by sequential omission of individual studies were tested by the sensitivity analysis.

Results

Eligible studies

A total of 1070 relevant titles were identified through electronic and manual searches. After review of the abstracts and titles, 802 studies were excluded in that they were irrelevant, not on human

Table 1. Outcome measurements in the studies included in this meta-analysis.

Clinical outcome	Choi Y 2013	Dahdaleh N 2013	Dong J 2014	Lin B 2013	Shen X 2013	Sonmez E 2013
VAS	Yes	Yes	Yes	Yes	Yes	Yes
ODI	Yes	Yes	Yes	Yes	Yes	Yes
JOA	NR	NR	Yes	NR	NR	NR
SF-36	NR	Yes	NR	NR	NR	NR
mProlo scores	NR	NR	NR	NR	Yes	NR
Fusion rate	Yes	Yes	Yes	Yes	Yes	Yes
Complication rate	Yes	Yes	Yes	Yes	Yes	Yes
Operation time	Yes	NR	Yes	Yes	NR	Yes
Blood loss	Yes	Yes	Yes	Yes	NR	Yes
Hospital stay	NR	Yes	Yes	NR	NR	Yes

subjects, not comparative studies or other forms of investigation. Forty articles on bilateral and unilateral PS fixation procedures were retrieved from the databases, and six studies (5 RCTs and 1 CCT) met the inclusion criteria (Figure 1). The characteristics of these six studies [7–12] are summarized in Table 2, and no significant differences were found in the baseline characteristics between the two groups. The six studies included a total of 298 participants with 146 adults treated with unilateral PS fixation and 152 adults treated with bilateral unilateral PS fixation.

Methodological quality

The total scores for all included studies assessed by PEDro quality criteria ranged from 5 to 7 (Table 3). Five studies were considered as being high quality (PEDro score ≥6), and one study was of low quality (PEDro score <6). The two independent reviewers reached consensuses on the scoring of all items without any disagreement.

Postoperative functional performance (VAS and ODI)

VAS and ODI are the most frequently used variables to assess the postoperative function performance of patients. Five studies assessed VAS for back pain, which was not significantly different between bilateral and unilateral groups (MD = −0.02, 95% CI = −0.17 to 0.13; P = 0.77) (Figure 2a). Three studies assessed VAS for leg pain, which was not different between the two groups either (MD = −0.10, 95% CI = −0.20 to 0.01; P = 0.06) (Figure 2b). ODI scores were available in five trials [16,19–22] where no significant difference was detected between the two groups (MD = 0.31, 95% CI = −0.66 to 1.27; P = 0.54) (Figure 2c).

Fusion rate and complications

The overall fusion rate was 91.8% (134/146) in the unilateral group and 96.0% (146/152) in the bilateral group (OR = 0.47, 95% CI = 0.18–1.27, P = 0.14, Figure 3a). No nonunion case was reported in the study of Dong [9]. The overall incidence of complications in the unilateral and bilateral groups was 5.48% (8/146) and 4.61% (7/152), respectively, and the difference was not significant (OR = 1.25, 95% CI = 0.44–3.59, P = 0.67, Figure 3b). No complications were observed in two studies [8,9].

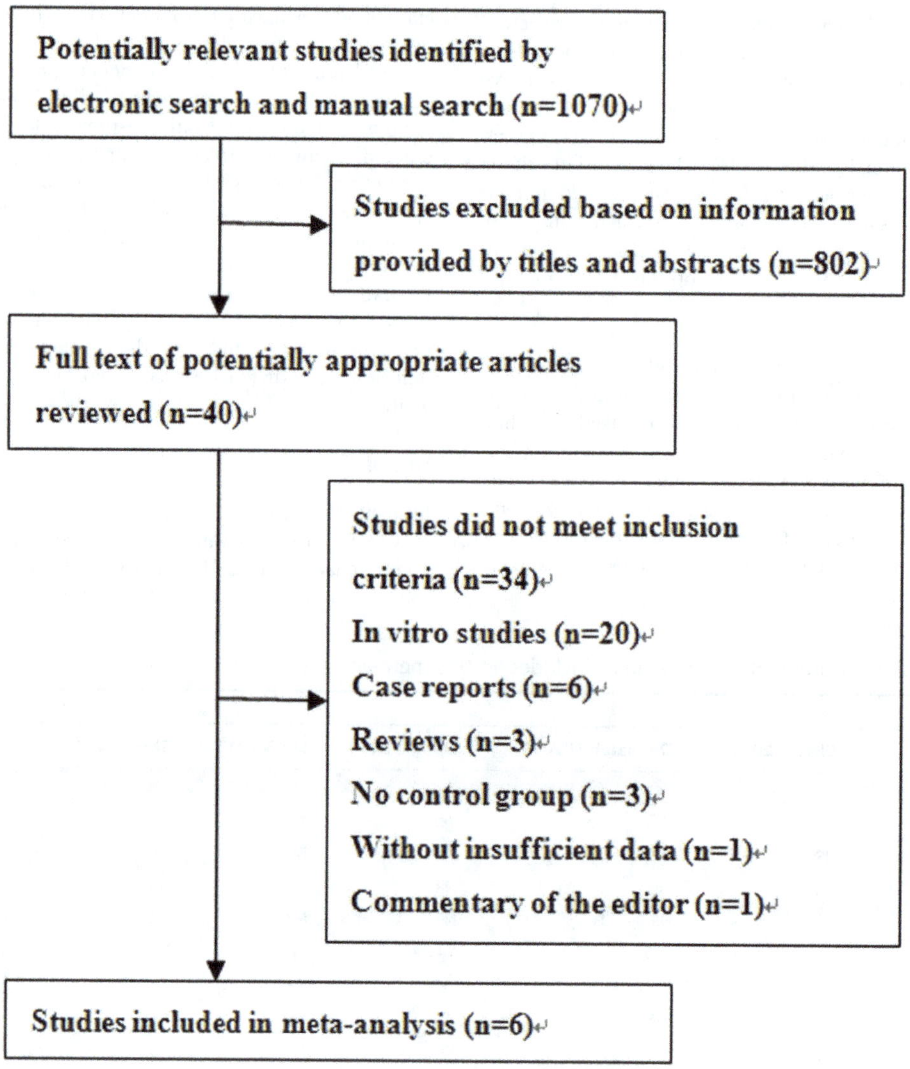

Figure 1. Flow diagram of study identification for this meta-analysis.

Table 2. Basic characteristics of the studies included in this meta-analysis.

Study	Time	Study design	Etiology	Case	Age	Follow-up	Fusion Technique
Choi Y	2013	RCT	disc herniation, spinal stenosis, degenerative spondylolisthesis, spondylolytic spondylolisthesis, and recurrent disc herniation	U:26	U: 53.39	U: 27.5 months	TLIF
				B:27	B: 56.22	B: 28.9 months	
Dahdaleh N	2013	RCT	single-level degenerative spondylosis or spondylolisthesis, Grade 1 or 2	U: 16	U: 62.2	U: 11.4 months	TLIF
				B: 20	B: 57.3	B: 12.4 months	
Dong J	2014	RCT	single-segment degenerative lumbar instability	U: 20	U: 54.0	U: 36 months	PLIF
				B: 19	B: 56.6	B: 36 months	
Lin B	2013	RCT	spinal canal stenosis,spondylolisthesis (grade I or II), and lumbar disk herniation	U: 43	U: 67	U: 26 months	TLIF
				B: 42	B: 65.5	B: 26 months	
Shen X	2013	RCT	Unilateral lumbar disc herniation, Foraminal stenosis	U: 31	U: 57.3	U: 26.6 months	TLIF
				B: 34	B: 58.9	B: 26.6 months	
Sonmez E	2013	CCT	single level recurrent disc herniation	U: 10	U: 47.3	U: 2 year	TLIF
				B: 10	B: 45.6	B: 2 year	

U unilateral fixation, B bilateral fixation.

Table 3. Methodological quality of the included studies assessed with the PEDro scale.

Study	Item PEDro score										Total score
	2	3	4	5	6	7	8	9	10	11	
Choi Y	+	−	+	−	−	+	+	+	+	+	7/10
Dahdaleh N	+	−	+	−	−	−	+	+	+	+	6/10
Dong J	+	−	+	−	−	−	+	+	+	+	6/10
Lin B	+	−	+	−	−	−	+	+	+	+	6/10
Shen X	+	−	+	−	−	−	+	+	+	+	6/10
Sonmez E	−	−	+	−	−	−	+	+	+	+	5/10

Operation time, blood loss and hospital stay

Operation time was assessed in four eligible studies and the results of the meta-analysis are presented in Figure 4a. Overall, unilateral PS fixation required a significantly less operative time as compared with bilateral PS fixation (MD = −30.17, 95% CI = −55.37 to −4.98; P = 0.02). Shown as a forest plot in Figure 4b are the results of meta-analysis of intra-operative blood loss; the amount of blood loss was significantly smaller in the unilateral group than in the bilateral group (MD = −99.06, 95% CI = −161.40 to −36.71; P = 0.002). Three studies reported the mean length of hospital stay where no significant difference was detected between the unilateral and bilateral groups (MD = 0.38, 95% CI = −0.83 to 1.58; P = 0.54).

Discussion

Bilateral PS fixation after lumbar interbody fusion is accepted as a standard procedure. Providing rigid fixation, bilateral PS fixation has a great biomechanical stability and clinical benefits. However, the rigidity of bilateral PS fixation can lead to device-related osteoporosis of the vertebrae [13] and makes the adjacent segment prone to load- and motion-induced degeneration [14]. To achieve optimal biomechanical conditions in the fused segment and minimize adverse effects in the adjacent levels caused by instrumentation, the use of less rigid systems of fixation has been advocated [15]. Some recent clinical and biomechanical studies on the suitability of unilateral PS fixation have demonstrated that a reliable fusion with fewer pedicle screws can be achieved [16,17]. Nevertheless, unilateral PS fixation may be detrimental to spine stability and the promotion for fusion as suggested by an *in vitro* study [18]. Therefore, the use of unilateral or bilateral PS fixation remains a matter of debate.

Numerous previous biomechanical and clinical studies attempted to comparatively evaluate unilateral and bilateral PS fixation approach and inconsistent results were obtained. Chen et al. [16] demonstrated that unilateral PS fixation was good enough to maintain the stability of the spine in a biomechanics study. Goel et al. [19] reported that the unilateral PS system was effective to reduce stress shielding of the vertebra and diminish peak stress arising in the adjacent levels above and below the fusion. Toyone and coauthors [20] recently reported that unilateral PS fixation was associated with a low incidence of adjacent-segment degeneration following posterior lumber interbody fusion. However, an increasing number of published studies have raised concerns over the clinical benefits of unilateral fixation. Yucesoy et al. [21] reported that unilateral PS fixation was inadequate to stabilize a 2-level unilateral lesion when compared with bilateral fixation. Aoki et al. [22] observed that unilateral fixation caused postoperative cage migration more frequently than bilateral fixation in patients who had scoliotic curvature with a Cobb angle >10°. In addition, Slucky et al. showed that unilateral PS fixation supplied only half of the improvement in stiffness compared bilateral PS fixation and caused significant off-axis rotational motions, which could hinder stability and the promotion for fusion after transforaminal lumbar interbody fusion (TLIF) [18].

However, unilateral PS fixation supplemented with translaminar facet screw fixation on the contralateral side offered stability comparable to that offered by bilateral PS fixation. Several other biomechanical and clinical studies also showed that supplementation of a contralateral facet screw might exert a similar effect as bilateral PS fixation on the stiffness or range of motion following TLIF [23–25]. Therefore supplementation of a contralateral facet

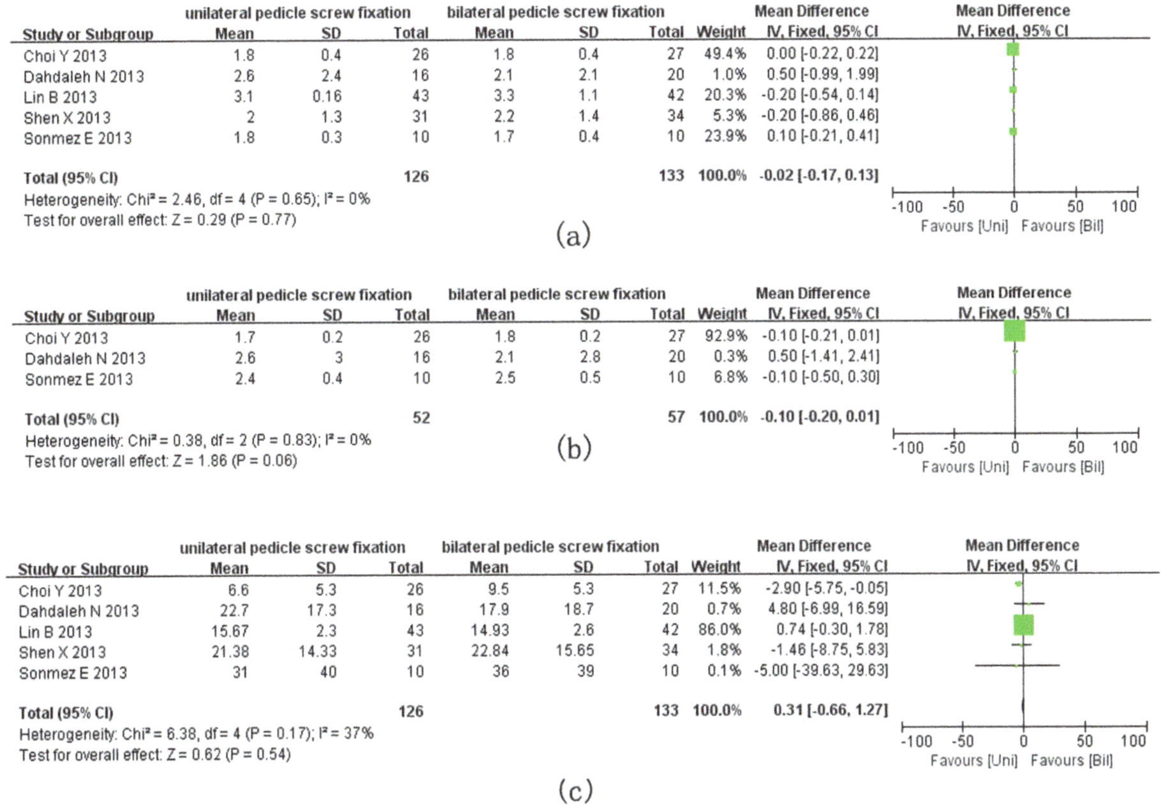

Figure 2. Forest plots for VAS for back pain (a), VAS for leg pain (b) and ODI (c) in patients undergoing unilateral and bilateral PS fixations respectively.

screw may possibly compensate the limitations of unilateral PS fixation in lumbar interbody fusion.

Spinal fusion can be achieved by both posterolateral and/or interbody fusion techniques [26]. However, conventional spinal fusion is related to significant muscle stripping and retraction that

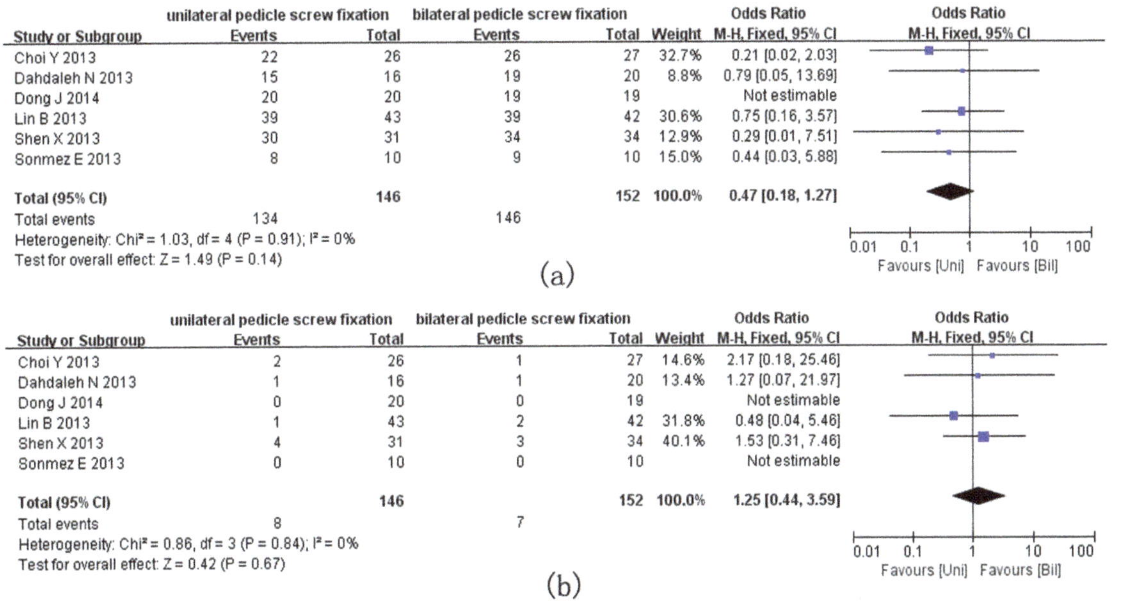

Figure 3. Forest plots for fusion rate (a) and incidence rate of complications (b) in patients undergoing unilateral and bilateral PS fixations respectively.

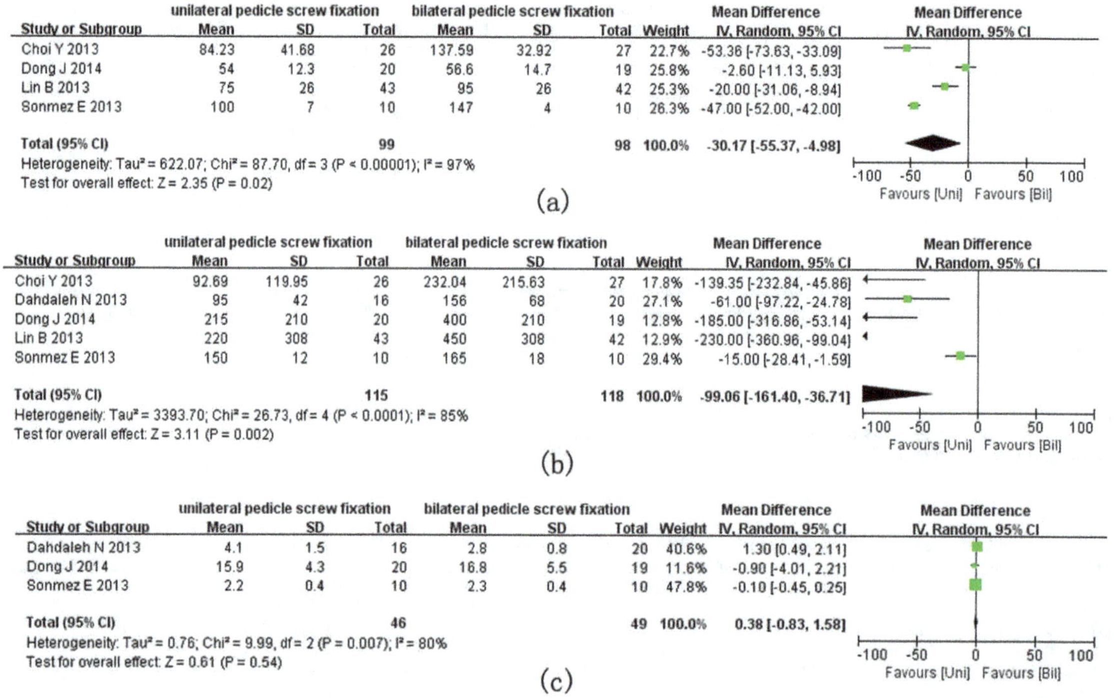

Figure 4. Forest plots for operation time (a), blood loss (b) and hospital stay (c) in patients undergoing unilateral and bilateral PS fixations respectively.

can adversely affect both short- and long-term patient outcomes [1]. In contrast, minimally invasive spinal fusion is performed by a muscle-dilating approach, which may significantly minimize or diminish the iatrogenic soft tissue injury, intra-operative blood loss, postoperative pain and the duration of hospital stays [27]. Accordingly, many surgeons prefer minimally invasive methods, such as TLIF with unilateral PS fixation [1,4,28], and believe that unilateral PS fixation is sufficient to accomplish spinal fusion. The objective of this meta-analysis was to systematically compare the efficiency and safety of unilateral and bilateral PS fixation procedures in MIS lumbar interbody fusion for one-level lumbar degenerative disease.

Our analysis suggested that there were no differences between unilateral PS fixation and bilateral PS fixation in VAS and ODI. This finding was in agreement with the results from some previous studies [9–11] where the patient outcomes were evaluated either using other assessment systems such as the Japanese Orthopaedic Association (JOA), 36-Item Short Form Healthy Survey version 2 (SF-36v2) and mProlo scores respectively or using radiographic parameters such as the whole lumbar lordosis, the segmental lordosis, fusion level disc space angle, lumbar scoliosis angle, and segmental scoliosis angle [11].

There were significantly less blood loss and significantly shorter operation time in the unilateral PS fixation group as compared with the bilateral PS fixation group in our meta-analysis. Unilateral PS fixation dissects soft tissue and insert pedicle screws only on one side and therefore it takes less time and decreases blood loss. Moreover, less soft tissue dissection may allow for early recovery [28]. However, the average length of hospital stay was similar in the two groups in our meta-analysis, which was inconsistent with the observation of a previous study where the hospital stay was shorter for unilateral fixation than for bilateral fixation due to early recovery and rehabilitation [7]. One of the reasons for the discrepancy might be the small number of studies included in our meta-analysis. Another reason might be the high heterogeneity among the included studies; in one study the hospital stay was longer in the unilateral group than in the bilateral group because of pulmonary edema in some patients.

Despite no statistical difference, the overall fusion rate was slightly lower in the unilateral group (91.8%) than in the bilateral group (96%). It was likely that less biomechanical stability in unilateral instrumentation might have negatively impacted the fusion. Because of this, supplementation of a contralateral facet screw has been proposed as a solution to compensate for the insufficient stability of unilateral PS fixation. The incidences of complications in unilateral and bilateral groups were 5.48% (8/146) and 4.61% (7/152), respectively. No single complication was identified in two studies. This finding was inconsistent with results from many previous studies where insufficient stability of unilateral PS fixation increased the incidence of cage migration [12,22].

Our study has a number of weaknesses. First of all, in some of the included studies, there were methodological limitations including failure to collect data prospectively, nonconsecutive enrollment of patients, inadequate baseline comparisons, and improper blinding or non-blinding. And these limitations somewhat reduced the level of evidence for this meta-analysis. Secondly, heterogeneity existed among the studies particularly when the continuous outcome measure variables were pooled. The heterogeneity might be attributable to differences among the included studies in the study design, study quality, patients' characteristics, and the diverse technical specifications. Thirdly, multiple assessment tools and fusion criteria were used in the included studies that might have confounded the combined results. Lastly, incomplete data recording was observed in some of the included studies. Pooling of such data might lead to bias.

In summary, through contrasting and combining results from 5 RCTs and 1 CCT on unilateral versus bilateral PS fixation in MIS lumbar fusion, this meta-analysis has shown that unilateral PS fixation may significantly reduce the intraoperative blood loss and shorten the operation time, somewhat improve the clinical outcome scores of ODI and VAS and fusion rate, and significantly decrease the incidence rate of complications while not affecting hospital stay as compared with bilateral PS fixation in patients with one-level lumbar degenerative disease. These findings suggest that unilateral PS fixation in MIS lumbar fusion is as effective and safe as but less time-consuming than bilateral PS fixation for one level lumbar degenerative disease. Nevertheless, this approach warrants further evaluations in high quality RCTs with large sample size and long-term follow-up before its wider clinical application.

Supporting Information

Checklist S1 PRISMA Checklist.

Author Contributions

Analyzed the data: CC YY. Contributed to the writing of the manuscript: ZL. Conceived and designed the meta-analysis: QF. Performed the study: ZL. Screened data for analysis: BQW PFL. Conducted data extraction: FZ JSL ZM.

References

1. Foley KT, Holly LT, Schwender JD (2003) Minimally invasive lumbar fusion. Spine (Phila Pa 1976) 28: S26−S35.
2. Sim HB, Murovic JA, Cho BY, Lim TJ, Park J (2010) Biomechanical comparison of single-level posterior versus transforaminal lumbar interbody fusions with bilateral pedicle screw fixation: segmental stability and the effects on adjacent motion segments: laboratory investigation. Journal of Neurosurgery: Spine 12: 700–708.
3. Kasai Y, Inaba T, Kato T, Matsumura Y, Akeda K, et al. (2010) Biomechanical study of the lumbar spine using a unilateral pedicle screw fixation system. Journal of Clinical Neuroscience 17: 364–367.
4. Deutsch H, Musacchio Jr MJ (2006) Minimally invasive transforaminal lumbar interbody fusion with unilateral pedicle screw fixation. Neurosurgical Focus 20: 1–5.
5. Ding W, Chen Y, Liu H, Wang J, Zheng Z (2014) Comparison of unilateral versus bilateral pedicle screw fixation in lumbar interbody fusion: a meta-analysis. European Spine Journal 23: 395–403.
6. Verhagen AP, de Vet HC, de Bie RA, Kessels AG, Boers M, et al. (1998) The Delphi list: a criteria list for quality assessment of randomized clinical trials for conducting systematic reviews developed by Delphi consensus. Journal of clinical epidemiology 51: 1235–1241.
7. Lin B, Xu Y, He Y, Zhang B, Lin Q, et al. (2013) Minimally Invasive Unilateral Pedicle Screw Fixation and Lumbar Interbody Fusion for the Treatment of Lumbar Degenerative Disease. Orthopedics 36: e1071−e1076.
8. Hastaların İTY, Sonuçları YT (2013) Unilateral Percutaneous Pedicle Screw Instrumentation with minimally Invasive TLIF for the Treatment of Recurrent Lumbar Disk Disease: 2 Years Follow-Up. Turkish neurosurgery 23: 372–378.
9. Dong J, Rong L, Feng F, Liu B, Xu Y, et al. (2014) Unilateral pedicle screw fixation through a tubular retractor via the Wiltse approach compared with conventional bilateral pedicle screw fixation for single-segment degenerative lumbar instability: a prospective randomized study: Clinical article. Journal of Neurosurgery: Spine 20: 53–59.
10. Dahdaleh NS, Nixon AT, Lawton CD, Wong AP, Smith ZA, et al. (2013) Outcome following unilateral versus bilateral instrumentation in patients undergoing minimally invasive transforaminal lumbar interbody fusion: a single-center randomized prospective study. Neurosurgical Focus 35: E13.
11. Xiaolong S, Lei W, Hailong Z, Xin G, Guangfei G, et al. (2013) Radiographic Analysis of One-level Minimally Invasive Transforaminal Lumbar Interbody Fusion (MI-TLIF) With Unilateral Pedicle Screw Fixation for Lumbar Degenerative Diseases. Journal of spinal disorders & techniques.
12. Choi UY, Park JY, Kim KH, Kuh SU, Chin DK, et al. (2013) Unilateral versus bilateral percutaneous pedicle screw fixation in minimally invasive transforaminal lumbar interbody fusion. Neurosurgical Focus 35: E11.
13. McAfee PC, Farey ID, Sutterlin CE, Gurr KR, Warden KE, et al. (1991) The effect of spinal implant rigidity on vertebral bone density. A canine model. Spine (Phila Pa 1976) 16: S190–197.
14. Ha KY, Schendel MJ, Lewis JL, Ogilvie JW (1993) Effect of immobilization and configuration on lumbar adjacent-segment biomechanics. J Spinal Disord 6: 99–105.
15. Korovessis P, Papazisis Z, Koureas G, Lambiris E (2004) Rigid, semirigid versus dynamic instrumentation for degenerative lumbar spinal stenosis: a correlative radiological and clinical analysis of short-term results. Spine (Phila Pa 1976) 29: 735–742.
16. Chen HH, Cheung HH, Wang WK, Li A, Li KC (2005) Biomechanical analysis of unilateral fixation with interbody cages. Spine (Phila Pa 1976) 30: E92–96.
17. Xue H, Tu Y, Cai M (2012) Comparison of unilateral versus bilateral instrumented transforaminal lumbar interbody fusion in degenerative lumbar diseases. Spine J 12: 209–215.
18. Slucky AV, Brodke DS, Bachus KN, Droge JA, Braun JT (2006) Less invasive posterior fixation method following transforaminal lumbar interbody fusion: a biomechanical analysis. Spine J 6: 78–85.
19. Goel VK, Lim TH, Gwon J, Chen JY, Winterbottom JM, et al. (1991) Effects of rigidity of an internal fixation device. A comprehensive biomechanical investigation. Spine (Phila Pa 1976) 16: S155–161.
20. Toyone T, Ozawa T, Shiboi R, Kamikawa K, Watanabe A, et al. Adjacent Segment Degeneration Occured 3-Times More 5-Years After Bilateral Instrumented Plif Than Unilateral Instrumented Plif: 27; 2010. LWW. 27.
21. Yücesoy K, Yüksel KZ, Baek S, Sonntag VK, Crawford NR (2008) Biomechanics of unilateral compared with bilateral lumbar pedicle screw fixation for stabilization of unilateral vertebral disease.
22. Aoki Y, Yamagata M, Nakajima F, Ikeda Y, Shimizu K, et al. (2010) Examining risk factors for posterior migration of fusion cages following transforaminal lumbar interbody fusion: a possible limitation of unilateral pedicle screw fixation. J Neurosurg Spine 13: 381–387.
23. Chen S-H, Lin S-C, Tsai W-C, Wang C-W, Chao S-H (2012) Biomechanical comparison of unilateral and bilateral pedicle screws fixation for transforaminal lumbar interbody fusion after decompressive surgery–a finite element analysis. BMC musculoskeletal disorders 13: 72.
24. Awad BI, Lubelski D, Shin JH, Carmody MA, Hoh DJ, et al. (2013) Bilateral Pedicle Screw Fixation versus Unilateral Pedicle and Contralateral Facet Screws for Minimally Invasive Transforaminal Lumbar Interbody Fusion: Clinical Outcomes and Cost Analysis. Global spine journal 3: 225–230.
25. Hsiang J, Yu K, He Y (2013) Minimally invasive one-level lumbar decompression and fusion surgery with posterior instrumentation using a combination of pedicle screw fixation and transpedicular facet screw construct. Surgical neurology international 4.
26. Chen Z, Zhao J, Liu A, Yuan J, Li Z (2009) Surgical treatment of recurrent lumbar disc herniation by transforaminal lumbar interbody fusion. International orthopaedics 33: 197–201.
27. Holly LT, Schwender JD, Rouben DP, Foley KT (2006) Minimally invasive transforaminal lumbar interbody fusion: indications, technique, and complications. Neurosurg Focus 20: 1–5.
28. Beringer WF, Mobasser J-P (2006) Unilateral pedicle screw instrumentation for minimally invasive transforaminal lumbar interbody fusion. Neurosurgical Focus 20: 1–5.

7

Development of TaqMan-Based Quantitative PCR for Sensitive and Selective Detection of Toxigenic *Clostridium difficile* in Human Stools

Hiroyuki Kubota[1,2]*, Takafumi Sakai[2], Agata Gawad[1], Hiroshi Makino[2], Takuya Akiyama[1,2], Eiji Ishikawa[2], Kenji Oishi[1,2]

1 Yakult Honsha European Research Center for Microbiology ESV, Gent-Zwijnaarde, Belgium, **2** Yakult Central Institute, Tokyo, Japan

Abstract

Background: *Clostridium difficile* is the main cause of nosocomial diarrhea, but is also found in asymptomatic subjects that are potentially involved in transmission of *C. difficile* infection. A sensitive and accurate detection method of *C. difficile*, especially toxigenic strains is indispensable for the epidemiological investigation.

Methods: TaqMan-based quantitative-PCR (qPCR) method for targeting 16S rRNA, *tcdB*, and *tcdA* genes of *C. difficile* was developed. The detection limit and accuracy of qPCR were evaluated by analyzing stool samples spiked with known amounts of *C. difficile*. A total of 235 stool specimens collected from 82 elderly nursing home residents were examined by qPCR, and the validity was evaluated by comparing the detection result with that by *C. difficile* selective culture (CDSC).

Results: The analysis of *C. difficile*-spiked stools confirmed that qPCR quantified whole *C. difficile* ($TcdA^+TcdB^+$, $TcdA^-TcdB^+$, and $TcdA^-TcdB^-$ types), TcdB-producing strains ($TcdA^+TcdB^+$ and $TcdA^-TcdB^+$ types), and TcdA-producing strains ($TcdA^+TcdB^+$ type), respectively, with a lower detection limit of 10^3 cells/g of stool. Of the 235 specimens examined, 12 specimens (5.1%) were *C. difficile*-positive by qPCR: $TcdA^+TcdB^+$ strain in six specimens and $TcdA^-TcdB^-$ strain in the other six. CDSC detected *C. difficile* in 9 of the 12 specimens, and toxigenic types of the isolates from the 9 specimens were consistent with those identified by qPCR, supporting the validity of our qPCR method. Moreover, the qPCR examination revealed that the carriage rate of whole *C. difficile* and that of toxigenic strains in the 82 subjects over a 6-month period ranged from 2.4 to 6.8% and 1.2 to 3.8%, respectively. An average qPCR count of *C. difficile* detected was $10^{4.5}$ cells/g of stool, suggesting that *C. difficile* constituted a very small fraction of intestinal microbiota.

Conclusion: Our qPCR method should be an effective tool for both clinical diagnosis and epidemiological investigation of *C. difficile*.

Editor: Michel R. Popoff, Institute Pasteur, France

Funding: This work was funded by Yakult Honsha European Research Center for Microbiology ESV (http://institute.yakult.co.jp/english/about/labo/). The funder provided support in the form of salaries for authors [HK, TS, AG, HM, TA, EI, KO], but did not have any additional role in the study design, data collection and analysis, decision to publish, or preparation of the manuscript. The specific roles of these authors are articulated in the 'author contributions' section.

Competing Interests: HK, AG, TA and KO are paid employees of Yakult Honsha European Research Center for Microbiology ESV. TS, HM, and EI were the paid employees at the time of this study.

* Email: hiroyuki.kubota@yher.be

Introduction

Clostridium difficile is the most common cause of healthcare-associated infectious diarrhea [1]. This bacterium can be categorized into three types on the basis of its production of two major toxins, TcdA and TcdB, namely i) TcdA-positive, TcdB-positive (A^+B^+) type; ii) TcdA-negative, TcdB-positive (A^-B^+) type; and iii) TcdA-negative, TcdB-negative (A^-B^-) type. Toxigenic strains, A^+B^+ and A^-B^+ types, are responsible for *C. difficile* infection (CDI). The elderly are particularly at increased risk of CDI possibly because of age-related changes in intestinal microbiota, weakened immune systems, and the presence of underlying diseases [2]. On the other hand, several surveys have reported that toxigenic *C. difficile* was detected in stools of asymptomatic elderly people [3–5]; such asymptomatic carriers may play a role in the transmission of CDI [5]. Selective detection of toxigenic *C. difficile* strains is therefore important, not only for clinical diagnosis but also for epidemiological investigations of *C. difficile* for infection control. Moreover, the quantification method of toxigenic *C. difficile* is useful in basic research such as studies to evaluate correlation of *C. difficile* count in the intestine and severity of the CDI symptom or to find an association between *C. difficile* colonization and the presence or absence of other intestinal bacteria.

C. difficile, including toxigenic strains in stool specimens, is traditionally detected by the culture method using selective medium. The *C. difficile* selective culture (CDSC) is a valuable method with advantages, such as high detection sensitivity and availability of isolates for characterization. However, the culture method is generally labor-intensive and time-consuming. In addition, since the culture method identifies predominant strains of *C. difficile* in stools, toxigenic strains that coexist with a larger population of non-toxigenic strains can be overlooked, which can fall into a false-negative result of toxigenic *C. difficile* detection. PCR-based methods have solved these shortcomings and have been widely used to detect toxigenic *C. difficile* in stools [6–9]. Several kinds of commercially available PCR kits are reported to be useful and reliable [10,11]. However, their quantitative application remains insufficient. A recent study indicated the possibility of quantification by showing that the threshold cycle (C_T) values of a commercial PCR targeting the *tcdB* gene were inversely correlated with *C. difficile* culture counts [12].

The purpose of this study was to develop a sensitive quantification method of toxigenic *C. difficile* and to evaluate its validity. We developed a new TaqMan real-time quantitative PCR (qPCR) method using sets of primers and a double-labeled fluorescent probe targeting the 16S rRNA, *tcdA*, and *tcdB* genes, and analyzed *C. difficile* in stools collected from elderly residents of nursing homes by means of qPCR.

Materials and Methods

Reference strains and culture conditions

All of the *C. difficile* strains (DSM 1296^T, ATCC 43255, ATCC 43596, ATCC 43598, ATCC 700057, CCUG 20309, CCUG 37780, CCUG 37785, NTCT 13307, NTCT 13366) and the other organisms belonging to the *Clostridium* genus that we used were cultured anaerobically in modified Gifu anaerobic medium broth (Nissui Pharmaceutical Co., Ltd., Tokyo, Japan) supplemented with 1% glucose (1% Glc-mGAM) at 37°C. Total bacterial cell counts of fresh cultures were determined by using the 4′, 6-diamidino-2-phenylindole (DAPI) staining method in accordance with the method of Jansen *et al.* [13]. On the basis of the DAPI counts, each fresh culture was diluted to obtain 1 mL of bacterial suspension containing 10^9 cells. Twenty microliters of suspension containing 2×10^7 cells was stored at −80°C until use for DNA extraction.

Development of primers and probes

The primers and probes listed in Table 1 were newly developed for this study. 16S rRNA gene-targeted primers (CD16SrRNA-F/R) and a probe (CD16SrRNA-P) for the detection of whole *C. difficile* (both toxigenic and non-toxigenic strains) were designed as follows. The sequences of *C. difficile* strains and other clostridial species were obtained from Ribosomal Database Project (http://rdp.cme.msu.edu/). Multiple alignments of these genes with the Clustal X program (http://www.clustal.org/clustal2/) were used to identify highly conserved regions as targets of the *C. difficile* specific primers and probe. For the detection of TcdA-producing strains (A^+B^+) and TcdB-producing strains (A^+B^+ and A^-B^+), respective primers-probe sets targeting *tcdA* (tcdA-F/R/P) and *tcdB* (tcdB-F/R/P) were developed by using a procedure similar to that with CD16SrRNA-F/R/P. The sequences of *tcdA* and *tcdB* of *C. difficile* and other Large Clostridial Toxin genes as references obtained from GenBank were used for multiple alignments and identification of target sites. The accession numbers of gene sequences used for the design of the primers and probes were listed in Table S1.

Stool specimens

Stool specimens were collected from 82 elderly residents from four nursing homes in France (11 males and 71 females; ages 66 to 94 years [average ± standard deviation, 84±6.2 years]). Stools were collected once every 3 months, three times in total (S_1, S_2, and S_3) from each subject. Since no subjects had abdominal symptoms at these samplings, no diarrheal stools or CDI-suspected stools were included. The subject ID was composed of five digits: the first two digits specified the site number (from 01 to 04) and the latter three digits specified the subject number (from 001).

Ethics statement

This study was conducted in compliance with the Declaration of Helsinki, good clinical practice (ICH topic E6; CPMP/ICH/135/95), and applicable regulatory requirements (French Public Health Code). The Independent Ethics Committee in Caen in France, COMITE DE PROTECTION DES PERSONNES NORD OUEST III, approved this study. Written informed consent forms were obtained from the subjects or their legal representatives.

Preparation of stool specimens for each analysis

Stool specimens within 24 h after defecation were collected and immediately examined for *C. difficile* toxins by enzyme immunoassay (EIA) at study sites. A portion of each stool was concurrently collected into an empty tube, and stored at −20°C until transportation. The stool samples were transported in a frozen state from the sites to our laboratory, and stored at −20°C until use for the following pretreatment for qPCR and CDSC.

After being thawed, each stool was weighed and suspended in 9 volumes of Dulbecco's PBS (−) (Nissui Pharmaceutical) to make a 10% (w/v) stool homogenate (100 mg stool/mL). One hundred microliters of stool homogenate was used immediately for CDSC. Two milliliters of the 10% stool homogenate was centrifuged at 16,000×*g* for 5 min, and the supernatant was discarded. The stool pellets (200 mg) were stored at −80°C until use for DNA extraction.

DNA extraction

DNA was extracted from pure cultured bacteria and stool pellets by using a FastDNA SPIN Kit for Feces (MP Biomedicals, Illkirch, France) in accordance with the manufacturer's instructions, with the exception that the first wash step with glass beads, sodium phosphate buffer, and PLS solution provided in the kit was skipped only in the extraction from pure culture bacteria. This is because the wash resulted in reduction in yield probably due to a difficulty of precipitation of bacterial cells with only glass beads in the buffer. DNA extracted from the pure cultured bacteria (2×10^7 cells) or 200 mg of stool pellets was finally dissolved in 100 µL of provided buffer.

qPCR

qPCR was performed in 384-well optical plates on an ABI PRISM 7900HT Sequence Detection System (Life Technologies, Foster City, CA). Ampdirect Plus (Shimadzu, Kyoto, Japan), a commercial PCR buffer, was used to neutralize inhibitory factors in stool DNA templates. Each reaction mixture of 20 µL was composed of 0.4 units of ExTaq DNA polymerase (TaKaRa Bio Inc., Shiga, Japan), 10 µL of 2×Ampdirect plus, 0.4 µL of Rox dye (Life Technologies), 0.2 µM of each specific primer, 0.2 µM of the fluorescent probe, and 5 µL of template DNA. The amplification program consisted of one cycle at 95°C for 30 s and then 50 cycles at 95°C for 5 s and 56°C for 50 s.

Selectivity of qPCR using new primers-probe sets

The selectivity of qPCR using the newly designed primers-probe sets was determined. DNA fractions extracted from pure cultures of each strain shown in Table 2 at doses corresponding to 10^5 cells per reaction were applied to qPCR with 16SrRNA-F/R/P, tcdA-

Table 1. Oligonucleotide sequences used in this study.

Target gene	Oligonucleotide	Sequence (5′-3′)	Position	Amplicon size (bp)
16s rRNA	CD16SrRNA-F	GCAAGTTGAGCGATTTACTTCGGT	59–82[a]	155
	CD16SrRNA-P	FAM-TGCCTCTCAAATATATTATCCCGTATTAG-TAMRA	156–184[a]	
	CD16SrRNA-R	GTACTGGCTCACCTTTGATATTYAAGAG	186–213[a]	
tcdA	tcdA-F	CAGTCGGATTGCAAGTAATTGACAAT	6051–6076[b]	102
	tcdA-P	FAM-TTGAGATGATAGCAGTGTCAGGATTG-TAMRA	6124–6152[b]	
	tcdA-R	AGTAGTATCTACTACCATTAACAGTCTGC	6091–6116[b]	
tcdB	tcdB-F	TACAAACAGGTGTATTTAGTACAGAAGATGGA	6079–6110[c]	240
	tcdB-P	FAM-TTTKCCAGTAAAATCAATTGCTTC-TAMRA	6159–6182[c]	
	tcdB-R	CACCTATTTGATTTAGMCCTTTAAAAGC	6291–6318[c]	

[a]GenBank accession number NR074454.
[b]GenBank accession number M30307.
[c]GenBank accession number X53138.

F/R/P, and tcdB-F/R/P. C_T values within ±3.3 of that obtained with the standard strain (*C. difficile* DSM 1296^T) were considered positive (+), whereas C_T values of more than 50 were considered negative (−) (Table 2). To evaluate the accuracy of quantitative detection among the target *C. difficile* strains, each analytical curve of the 10 *C. difficile* strains was generated by using the respective primers-probe sets (Table 3).

Comparison of analytical curve of *C. difficile*-spiked stool with that of *C. difficile* pure culture

A stool specimen lacking any amplification by qPCR using CD16SrRNA-F/R/P was selected, as this response suggested that the specimen lacked indigenous populations of *C. difficile*. The *C. difficile*-negative stool was diluted with Dulbecco's PBS (−) to make a 10% (w/v) stool homogenate (100 mg stool/mL). The number of cells in a pure culture of *C. difficile* DSM 1296^T in 1% Glc-mGAM broth was counted by using DAPI staining, and serial dilutions of the pure culture ranging from 10^4 to 10^9 cells/mL were prepared. Twenty microliters of the serial dilutions (containing *C. difficile* cells ranging from 2×10^2 to 2×10^7) were spiked into the 2 mL of the *C. difficile*-negative stool homogenates (containing 200 mg of stool) to obtain stool specimens with *C. difficile* at final concentrations ranging from 10^3 to 10^8 cells/g of stool. DNA extracted from the stool specimens was applied to qPCR, and the obtained C_T values were used to generate an analytical curve of the *C. difficile*-spiked stool. DNA extracted from 2×10^7 cells of pure cultured *C. difficile* and its serial dilutions were applied to qPCR to generate a standard analytical curve of the *C. difficile* pure culture. These two analytical curves were compared to evaluate the lower detection limit and detection accuracy of this qPCR method.

Determination of bacterial count by qPCR

Whole *C. difficile*, TcdA-producing strains, and TcdB-producing strains were enumerated by qPCR with 16SrRNA-F/R/P, tcdA-F/R/P, and tcdB-F/R/P, as follows. *C. difficile* DSM 1296^T A^+B^+ strain was selected as a standard strain for generating standard analytical curves for all three target *C. difficile* groups. Five microliters of 10-fold serial dilutions of DNA extracted from the pure culture of the *C. difficile* strain were applied to PCR to obtain a standard analytical curve ranging from 10^1 to 10^5 cells/5-μL reaction. Five microliters of the DNA solution extracted from 200 mg of stool and its 2- and 4-fold dilutions were applied to PCR as a template containing the corresponding DNA from 10, 5, or 2.5 mg of stool. The consequent C_T values of the stool specimens were applied to the standard analytical curve, and the corresponding bacterial counts (cells/g of stool) were calculated as qPCR counts.

Determination of toxigenic types of *C. difficile* predominating in individual stool specimens

By comparing the three qPCR counts targeting the 16S rRNA gene for whole *C. difficile* (A^+B^+, A^-B^+, and A^-B^- types), *tcdB* for TcdB-producing strains (A^+B^+ and A^-B^+ types), and *tcdA* for TcdA-producing strains (A^+B^+ type), the toxigenic types of *C. difficile* predominating in each stool specimen were determined as follows. When the differences among the three qPCR counts were within 0.3 $\log_{10}$ cells/g of stool (a 2-fold difference in real values), the toxigenic type of the dominant *C. difficile* strain was identified as A^+B^+. When the difference between the qPCR counts of the 16S rRNA gene and *tcdB* was within 0.3 $\log_{10}$ cells/g of stool and these counts were higher than that of *tcdA* by at least 0.3 $\log_{10}$ cells/g of stool, the toxigenic type was identified as A^-B^+. When the qPCR count of the 16S rRNA gene was higher than those of *tcdA* and *tcdB* by at least 0.3 $\log_{10}$ cells/g of stool, the toxigenic type was identified as A^-B^-.

Enzyme immunoassay (EIA)

C. difficile toxins in stools were detected with a commercial EIA kit, the Xpect *Clostridium Difficile* Toxin A/B Test (Remel Inc., Lenexa, KS), in accordance with the manufacturer's instructions.

C. difficile selective culture (CDSC)

In accordance with the method described by Wren [14], *C. difficile* was isolated by stool culture with cefoxitin cycloserine egg yolk (CCEY) agar. CCEY agar (BioConnections Ltd., Knypersley United Kingdom) supplemented with 40 mL of egg yolk emulsion (BioConnections), two vials of cefoxitin-cycloserin (BioConnections), and 10 mL of lysed horse blood per liter was prepared in-house and stored at 4°C for a maximum of 1 week before use. The 10% (w/v) stool homogenate was mixed with an equal volume of absolute ethanol and left at room temperature for 30 to 60 min. In an anaerobic glovebox (Coy Laboratory Products Inc., Grass Lake, MI), 100 μL of the alcohol-treated stool or its 10-fold dilution was inoculated onto the CCEY plates and cultured under anaerobic conditions at 37°C for 48 to 72 h. Suspected colonies of

Table 2. Specific detection of target *C. difficile* strains by qPCR with newly developed oligonucleotide sets.

Taxon	Strain	Toxin production type[a]	Reactions with following oligonucleotide sets[b]:		
			CD16SrRNA-F/R/P	tcdB-F/R/P	tcdA-F/R/P
Clostridium difficile	DSM 1296^T	A^+ B^+	+	+	+
	ATCC 43255	A^+ B^+	+	+	+
	ATCC 43596	A^+ B^+	+	+	+
	NTCT 13307	A^+ B^+	+	+	+
	NTCT 13366	A^+ B^+	+	+	+
	ATCC 43598	A^- B^+	+	+	−
	CCUG 20309	A^- B^+	+	+	−
	ATCC 700057	A^- B^-	+	−	−
	CCUG 37780	A^- B^-	+	−	−
	CCUG 37785	A^- B^-	+	−	−
Clostridium bifermentans	DSM 14991^T	na	−	−	−
Clostridium histolyticum	DSM 2158^T	na	−	−	−
Clostridium innocuum	DSM 1286^T	na	−	−	−
Clostridium novyi	DSM 14992^T	na	−	−	−
Clostridium perfringens	DSM 756^T	na	−	−	−
Clostridium ramosum	DSM 1402^T	na	−	−	−
Clostridium septicum	DSM 7534^T	na	−	−	−
Clostridium sordellii	DSM 2141^T	na	−	−	−
Clostridium sphenoides	DSM 632^T	na	−	−	−
Clostridium tertium	DSM 2485^T	na	−	−	−

[a]na, not applicable.
[b]The reactivity of qPCR for the target bacteria with each primers-probe set was investigated by using DNA extracts corresponding to 10^5 cells per reaction from each pure culture of the listed strains. Reactivity was judged by using the criteria described in the Materials and Methods. In addition, negative PCR results were obtained for the following bacterial strains, representing the major intestinal bacteria: *Blautia productus* JCM 1471^T, *Faecalibacterium prausnitzii* ATCC 27768^T, *Bacteroides vulgatus* ATCC 8482^T, *Bacteroides ovatus* JCM 5824^T, *Fusobacterium varium* ATCC 8501^T, *Collinsella aerofaciens* ATCC 25986^T, *Prevotella melaninogenica* ATCC 25845^T, *Veillonella parvula* GIFU 7884^T, *Bifidobacterium longum* ATCC 15707^T, *Bifidobacterium adolescentis* ATCC 15703^T, *Bifidobacterium catenulatum* ATCC 27539^T, *Lactobacillus gasseri* DSM 20243^T.

C. difficile were selected on the basis of their morphological characteristics and subjected to rapid identification by real-time PCR with the CD16SrRNA-F/R/P set. Obtained *C. difficile* isolates were examined by PCR for identification of toxigenic types and by cell cytotoxicity neutralization assay (CCNA) for the detection of TcdB.

Identification of toxigenic type of *C. difficile* isolates by PCR

Toxigenic types of *C. difficile* isolates were identified by comparing the size of PCR amplicons for the respective toxin genes, in accordance with the method described by Kato *et al.* [15]. An NK11/NK9 primer set for *tcdA* and an NK104/NK105 primer set for *tcdB* were used for amplification.

TcdB detection of *C. difficile* isolates by CCNA

The cytopathic effect of the isolates was examined with a *C. difficile* Toxin/Antitoxin Kit (Techlab, Blacksburg, VA). *C. difficile* isolates were subcultured in BHI broth anaerobically at 37°C for 5 days. The suspension was then centrifuged at 16,000×*g* for 5 min and the supernatant filtered with a 0.45-µm membrane filter. The filtrate was added to precultured Vero-B4 cells with or without *C. difficile* antitoxin. After incubation of the culture at 37°C for 24 or 48 h, the presence or absence of TcdB was determined by judging the cytopathic effects. The following criteria were employed: when at least 90% of the cells were rounded in the absence of antitoxin and the cytopathic effect was neutralized by the antitoxin, the culture was regarded as TcdB positive; when no cytopathic effect was observed in the cells both with and without antitoxin, the culture was regarded as TcdB negative.

Results

Selectivity of qPCR using primers-probe sets targeting the 16S rRNA, *tcdA*, and *tcdB* genes

For selective detection of whole *C. difficile* (A^+B^+, A^-B^+, and A^-B^- types), TcdB-producing strains (A^+B^+ and A^-B^+ types), and TcdA-producing strains (A^+B^+ type), respective primers-probe sets targeting 16S rRNA, *tcdB*, and *tcdA* genes were newly designed (Table 1). The selectivity of qPCR using the three designed primers-probe sets was assessed by using DNA extracted from each pure culture (Table 2). qPCR using each primers-probe set detected the respective target strains selectively, without any amplification of non-targeted strains. To evaluate the accuracy of quantitative detection among the target *C. difficile* strains, each analytical curve was compared (Table 3). The analytical curves of the 10 *C. difficile* strains (five A^+B^+ strains, two A^-B^+ strains, and three A^-B^- strains) with 16SrRNA-F/R/P had almost equal slopes. Similarly, for the seven TcdB-producing strains (five A^+B^+ and two A^-B^+ strains) with tcdB-F/R/P and the five TcdA-

Table 3. Comparison of qPCR analytical curves among *C. difficile* strains.

C. difficile strain	Toxin production type	CD16SrRNA-F/R/P		tcdB-F/R/P		tcdA-F/R/P	
		Analytical curve[a]	ΔC_T value at $x=0$[b]	Analytical curve[a]	ΔC_T value at $x=0$[b]	Analytical curve[a]	ΔC_T value at $x=0$[b]
DSM 1296[T]	$A^+ B^+$	$y=-3.46x+40.0$	–	$y=-3.63x+44.4$	–	$y=-3.43x+42.9$	–
ATCC 43255	$A^+ B^+$	$y=-3.48x+39.9$	−0.1	$y=-3.58x+43.9$	−0.5	$y=-3.54x+43.0$	0.1
ATCC 43596	$A^+ B^+$	$y=-3.44x+39.1$	−0.9	$y=-3.63x+43.4$	−1.0	$y=-3.58x+42.6$	−0.3
NTCT 13307	$A^+ B^+$	$y=-3.42x+40.4$	0.4	$y=-3.64x+44.5$	0.1	$y=-3.57x+43.6$	0.7
NTCT 13366	$A^+ B^+$	$y=-3.46x+41.1$	1.1	$y=-3.67x+45.2$	0.8	$y=-3.56x+44.4$	1.5
ATCC 43598	$A^- B^+$	$y=-3.47x+40.2$	0.2	$y=-3.58x+44.6$	0.2	Not amplified	Not applicable
CCUG 20309	$A^- B^+$	$y=-3.43x+41.2$	1.2	$y=-3.66x+45.0$	0.6	Not amplified	Not applicable
ATCC 700057	$A^- B^-$	$y=-3.52x+42.1$	2.1	Not amplified	Not applicable	Not amplified	Not applicable
CCUG 37780	$A^- B^-$	$y=-3.47x+40.3$	0.3	Not amplified	Not applicable	Not amplified	Not applicable
CCUG 37785	$A^- B^-$	$y=-3.44x+40.7$	0.7	Not amplified	Not applicable	Not amplified	Not applicable

[a]Each analytical curve of different *C. difficile* strains was generated with serial dilutions ranging from 10 to 10^5 cells per reaction. X-axis is bacterial cells applied to the reaction ($\log_{10}$ cells/reaction) and Y-axis is the C_T values obtained.
[b]Differences in C_T values compared with that of the type strain (DSM 1296[T]) are indicated.

producing strains (five A^+B^+ strains) with tcdA-F/R/P, the slopes of the analytical curves were equivalent. The differences in the intercepts of the analytical curves with 16SrRNA-F/R/P between the type strain and the others ranged from −0.9 to +2.1, suggesting that each target strain could be enumerated within approximately a 4-fold difference. The difference in the intercepts ranged from −1.0 to +0.8 in the case of analytical curves with tcdB-F/R/P and from −0.3 to +1.5 in the case of those with tcdA-F/R/P, thus providing further evidence of the accurate quantification of toxigenic strains. These results indicated that the newly developed TaqMan-based qPCR method was capable of detecting the target *C. difficile* strains selectively and with high accuracy.

Lower detection limit and detection accuracy of qPCR

The lower detection limit and detection accuracy of qPCR for *C. difficile* in stools were evaluated by analyzing stool samples spiked with *C. difficile* vegetative cells at a final concentration of 10^3 to 10^8 cells/g of stool. The analytical curve of the *C. difficile*-spiked stool was compared with the standard analytical curve of the *C. difficile* pure culture (Figure 1A–C). In the case of all the three primers-probe sets, the obtained analytical curves were nearly equivalent over the range of 10^3 to 10^8 cells, confirming that qPCR with the standard analytical curve of the pure culture allowed accurate detection of *C. difficile* in stools. These results also indicated that our qPCR method enabled quantitative detection of *C. difficile* in stools with a lower detection limit of 10^3 cells/g of stool.

Comparison of results of toxigenic *C. difficile* detection by qPCR and CDSC

To verify the validity of the new TaqMan-based qPCR method, we compared the results of *C. difficile* detection in stool specimens by qPCR with those by CDSC as a reference method. Stool specimens were collected from 82 elderly people in four different nursing homes once every 3 months for 6 months, i.e. a total of three times (S_1, S_2, and S_3 sampling). A total of 235 specimens were examined for *C. difficile* by qPCR and CDSC (Table 4). *C. difficile* was detected in 12 of the 235 specimens by qPCR, whereas this organism was isolated by CDSC from 9 specimens; there were thus three discrepancies between the methods. *C. difficile* toxins were not detected in any of the 235 specimens by EIA (data not shown).

Details of the test results from the 12 *C. difficile*-positive specimens from eight subjects are shown in Table 5. Whole *C. difficile* counts (16S rRNA target) ranged from 10^3 to 10^5 cells level/g of stool, with the exception of one specimen, #02010-S_3, which had a much higher count. The mean qPCR counts of whole *C. difficile*, TcdB-producing strains, and TcdA-producing strains were 4.5±1.3, 4.6±0.4, and 4.5±0.6 $\log_{10}$ cells/g of stool, respectively. On the basis of the qPCR counts for the three genes within each specimen, the toxigenic type of the predominating *C. difficile* was identified as A^+B^+ in six specimens (#02007-S_2, #03008-S_1, #03008-S_2, #03008-S_3, #03024-S_2, #04003-S_3) and as A^-B^- type in the other six specimens (#02010-S_3, #02011-S_3, #04011-S_2, #04026-S_1, #04026-S_2, #04026-S_3). The PCR analysis on CDSC revealed that the isolates from six specimens were of A^+B^+ type and those from the remaining three specimens were A^-B^- type. The A^+B^+ isolates from the six specimens were confirmed by cell cytotoxicity assay to be capable of producing TcdB, although the toxin was not detected in any of the stool specimens by EIA. The toxin-production profiles of these isolates, as determined by CDSC analysis, were consistent with those determined by qPCR. In terms of the results of toxigenic *C. difficile* detection, both qPCR and CDSC gave the same six positive specimens, indicating that qPCR was as efficient in detecting toxigenic *C. difficile* in stools as CDSC.

C. difficile carriage in the elderly in nursing homes

We obtained detection rates and qPCR counts of whole *C. difficile*, TcdB-producing strains, and TcdA-producing strains in elderly residents of different nursing homes at three samplings (S_1:82 specimens; S_2:79 specimens; and S_3:74 specimens) (See Table S2). Detection rates of whole *C. difficile* in S_1, S_2, and S_3 specimens from the four nursing homes were 2/82 (2.4%), 5/79 (6.3%), and 5/74 (6.8%), respectively. The detection rates of TcdA-producing strains were 1/82 (1.2%), 3/79 (3.8%), and 2/72 (2.7%), respectively, and those of TcdB-producing strains were exactly the same. On the basis of the qPCR counts, we determined the toxigenic types of the predominating *C. difficile* in each specimen; the rates of carriage of the respective types by the 82 subjects are shown in Figure 2. Whereas site 01 had no *C. difficile* carrier throughout the 6-month period, the other sites had some carriers of either the A^+B^+ strain or the A^-B^- strain, or both. The overall carriage rate of *C. difficile* in the 82 subjects fluctuated

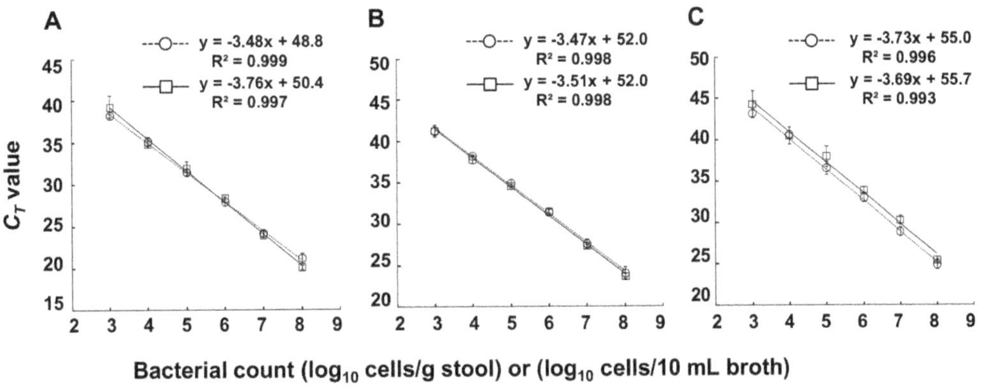

Figure 1. qPCR quantification of *C. difficile* DSM 1296^T (A^+B^+ strain) spiked into a human stool. Stool samples taken from a healthy adult and supplemented with serial dilutions of *C. difficile* DSM 1296^T (A^+B^+ strain) at final concentrations ranging from 10^3 to 10^8 cells/g of stool were examined by qPCR using CD16SrRNA-F/R/P (A), tcdA-F/R/P (B), or tcdB-F/R/P (C). Cell counts of the spiked *C. difficile* were determined by DAPI staining. The obtained analytical curve of the *C. difficile*-spiked stool (□) was compared with the standard analytical curve of the *C. difficile* pure culture (○).

Table 4. Comparison of detection results of *C. difficile* between qPCR and *C. difficile* selective culture (CDSC).

qPCR result[a]	No. of specimens with CDSC result[b]		Total
	C. difficile **positive**	*C. difficile* **negative**	
C. difficile **positive**	9	3	12
C. difficile **negative**	0	223	223
Total	9	226	235

[a]"*C. difficile* positive/negative" was defined by presence/absence of qPCR amplification with the 16S rRNA primers-probe set.
[b]"*C. difficile* positive/negative" was defined by presence/absence of *C. difficile* isolation by means of stool culture.

below 10% during the 6-month test period, except in one case (S_3 at site 02).

As a result of review of medical records, 19 (23%) of 82 subjects received at least one course of antibiotic treatment in the study period of 6 months. *C. difficile* was detected in only one of the 19 subjects (#02010). The number of subjects who had hospitalization during the study period was six (7.3%), only one of which, the same #02010, was *C. difficile*-positive. The subject underwent several antibiotic treatments and short-term hospitalizations between S_2 and S_3 sampling.

Discussion

We designed new oligonucleotide sets targeting the 16S rRNA, *tcdB*, and *tcdA* genes for the quantification of whole *C. difficile* (A^+B^+, A^-B^+, and A^-B^- types), TcdB-producing strains (A^+B^+ and A^-B^+ types), and TcdA-producing strains (A^+B^+ type), respectively. Most clinically isolated TcdA-negative, TcdB-positive strains (A^-B^+ type) possess *tcdA* that has a 1.8-kbp deletion in 8.0 kbp of the intact full length sequence [16–19], and therefore does not produce functional TcdA. We designed *tcdA*-specific primers and a probe against this deleted region, and confirmed that our PCR correctly identified intact *tcdA* genes and did not detect *tcdA* genes that were rendered non-functional due to the deletion (Table 2). Moreover, these newly developed primers-probe sets were designed against the highly conserved region of each gene and consequently included no mismatches with their target sequences. Indeed, qPCR was capable of detecting all the strains in the target group with almost equal reactivity (Table 3). Up to the present, many sets of primers and probes targeting toxin genes have been reported [6,20–22]. However, *in silico* comparison of those oligonucleotides with their target gene sequences currently available in the database revealed that most of them included at least a few mismatches against some of their targets (data not shown); this may result in inaccurate quantification due to strain-dependent differences in reactivity. It can be expected that our qPCR method overcame this potential defect.

The lower detection limit of *C. difficile* in stools remained to be solved. We previously reported that reverse transcription (RT)-qPCR targeting the rRNA molecule achieved sensitive detection of *C. difficile* with a lower detection limit of $10^{2.4}$ cells/g of stool [23]. However, this application was limited to *C. difficile* species because such a low detection limit was accomplished only by targeting rRNA molecules present in high copy numbers (10^3 to 10^4 molecules per single cell) [24,25]. Here, we developed a detection system for toxigenic strains that was based on qPCR targeting the toxin genes. To lower the limit of detection by qPCR, we subjected a highly concentrated stool DNA fraction to PCR in the presence of an agent that neutralized PCR amplification inhibitors. In general, extraction of DNA from larger amounts of stool and dissolution in smaller amounts of buffer can yield highly concentrated DNA, but the product will contain increased amounts of stool-derived PCR inhibitors. In our study, a stool DNA fraction that was prepared by using a commercial DNA extraction kit (FastDNA SPIN Kit for Feces) and contained DNA from as much as 10 mg of stool was subjected to qPCR without dilution because the commercial PCR buffer (Ampdirect Plus) neutralized the effect of the PCR inhibitors. This combination successfully lowered the detection limit to 10^3 cells/g of stool (Figure 1). We confirmed that an application of the extracted stool DNA solution to PCR without Ampdirect plus gave no amplification (data not shown). The qPCR counts of *C. difficile* in most subjects fell into a low range (e.g. 10^3 or 10^4 cells/g of stool; Table 5), indicating that the lower detection limit of 10^3 cells/g of stool is important in the in-depth investigation of *C. difficile* present in stools of asymptomatic subjects.

In our examinations, the consistent result of *C. difficile* detection was obtained in 232 out of 235 specimens between qPCR and CDSC (Table 4), supporting the validity of our TaqMan PCR as a sensitive method to detect *C. difficile* in stools. The other three specimens were qPCR positive but CDSC negative. One possible reason of this discrepancy is the difference of *C. difficile* forms targeted by the methods. *C. difficile* has typically two forms; one is the active and infectious form, vegetative cells, and the other is the inactive form, spores. In our CDSC examination, *C. difficile* spores were exclusively detected since alcohol treatment killed vegetative cells. In contrast, we confirmed that our qPCR method mainly detected vegetative cells because the DNA extraction efficiency from spores was approximately 1,000-times as low as that from vegetative cells (data not shown). The discrepant result between qPCR and CDSC in the three specimens may therefore reflect that *C. difficile* present in the stools was composed of the majority of vegetative cells and the minority of spores, and that a smaller amount of spores were undetectable by CDSC. In our study, CDSC was performed for the purpose of detecting only spores because it was thought to be difficult to meet all the requirements for the detection of vegetative cells by culture, such as collection of fresh stools with less exposure to aerobic environment, more rapid transportation of stool from study sites to our laboratory, and immediate examination. An application of a cultural procedure for the detection of vegetative cells as well as spores could have provided further information. In addition, modification of DNA extraction method to improve the extraction efficiency from spores would make it possible to compare detection results of the same target, both vegetative cells and spores, between qPCR and culture methods. Another possible reason of the discrepancy is an issue of living and dead cells. In general, while a culture method detects only living cells, conventional qPCR detects both living and dead cells, which could result in the higher detection rate of *C. difficile* by qPCR.

Table 5. Comparison of detection results of toxigenic *C. difficile* or toxins by qPCR, *C. difficile* selective culture (CDSC), and enzyme immunoassay (EIA).

Subject ID	Specimen	qPCR				CDSC			EIA
		Counts (log_{10} cells/g of stool)			Toxigenic type[a]	*C. difficile* isolation	Isolates test		
		16S rRNA	*tcdA*	*tcdB*			Toxigenic type[b, c]	Cell cytotoxicity[c]	
02007	S_2	4.4	4.5	4.7	$A^+ B^+$	Yes	$A^+ B^+$	Pos	Neg
02010	S_3	8.0	<3.0	<3.0	$A^- B^-$	Yes	$A^- B^-$	Neg	Neg
02011	S_3	3.3	<3.0	<3.0	$A^- B^-$	No	na	na	Neg
03008	S_1	5.1	5.1	5.1	$A^+ B^+$	Yes	$A^+ B^+$	Pos	Neg
	S_2	4.4	4.4	4.6	$A^+ B^+$	Yes	$A^+ B^+$	Pos	Neg
	S_3	4.5	4.6	4.7	$A^+ B^+$	Yes	$A^+ B^+$	Pos	Neg
03024	S_2	3.5	3.5	3.8	$A^+ B^+$	Yes	$A^+ B^+$	Pos	Neg
04003	S_3	5.0	5.0	4.9	$A^+ B^+$	Yes	$A^+ B^+$	Pos	Neg
04011	S_2	4.3	<3.0	<3.0	$A^- B^-$	No	na	na	Neg
04026	S_1	4.7	<3.0	<3.0	$A^- B^-$	Yes	$A^- B^-$	Neg	Neg
	S_2	3.5	<3.0	<3.0	$A^- B^-$	No	na	na	Neg
	S_3	3.0	<3.0	<3.0	$A^- B^-$	Yes	$A^- B^-$	Neg	Neg
Mean		4.5	4.5	4.6					
SD		1.3	0.6	0.4					

[a]Toxigenic types were identified on the basis of qPCR counts for the three genes, according to the criteria described in Materials and Methods.
[b]The toxigenic type of isolates was determined on the basis of PCR amplification of *tcdA* and *tcdB* by using the method of Kato *et al* [15].
[c]na, not applicable.

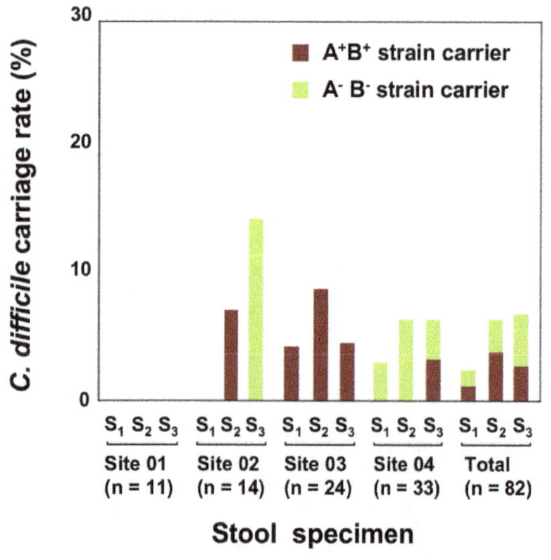

Figure 2. *C. difficile* carriage rates in four nursing home populations. On the basis of the qPCR counts for three genes (16S rRNA, *tcdA*, and *tcdB*), the toxigenic types (A^+B^+, A^-B^+, or A^-B^-) of *C. difficile* predominating in individual specimens were identified. The rates of carriage of each toxigenic type of *C. difficile* at three stool samplings (S1, S2, and S3) were calculated with respect to each nursing home (n = 11, 14, 24, and 33, respectively) and the total population (n = 82).

Recently, selective detection of living cells by PCR in combination with cell membrane-impermeable dyes, which modify DNA of dead cells and inhibit PCR amplification, has been reported [26,27]. We consider it necessary to apply such living cell-specific detection system to our qPCR method for the detection of authentic living bacterial cells in stools. Other reasons such as false-positive results of qPCR may also lead to discrepancy. Although the primers-probe set was carefully checked to specifically detect *C. difficile*, it remains a possibility of non-specific reaction with other unknown bacteria. Despite these differences in the methodological character of qPCR and CDSC, the highly comparable results of *C. difficile* detection were obtained (Table 4), suggesting the effectiveness of our qPCR targeting vegetative cells as the detection method of *C. difficile* in stools.

The *C. difficile* carriage rate in long-term care facilities (LTCFs) is considered higher than that in community-dwelling adults but lower than that in hospital inpatients [28]. In our previous study of 83 LTCFs residents in Japan [23], we revealed that the carriage rate of *C. difficile* was as high as 43%. Riggs *et al.* [5] reported a 51% carriage rate of toxigenic *C. difficile* in 68 inpatients of LTCFs in Ireland, as determined by using a culture method. However, in our present study of 82 nursing home residents in France, the carriage rates of *C. difficile* and toxigenic *C. difficile*, as determined by TaqMan-based qPCR over 6 months, ranged from 2.4% to 6.8% and 1.2% to 3.8%, respectively-much lower than those reported in the studies above. Nevertheless, the *C. difficile* carriage rates reported in other culture-based examinations are comparable to our current results [3,4,29,30]. For example, Walker *et al.* [30] reported that the carriage rates of whole *C. difficile* and toxigenic *C. difficile* in 225 LTCF residents in the United States were 7.1% and 4.0%, respectively. In a later study by Arvand *et al.* [29], these carriage rates in 240 elderly nursing home residents in Germany were 4.6% and 4.2%, respectively. LTCFs include various facilities, such as nursing homes, rehabilitation facilities, inpatient behavioral health facilities, and long-term chronic care hospitals. Because environmental contamination with *C. difficile* occurs commonly in hospitals [31,32], subjects in facilities close to hospital environments are likely to have more chances to acquire the organism. Certainly, the facilities in our study, which had relatively low *C. difficile* carriage rates, were nursing homes, whereas those in our previous study, which had higher carriage rates, were chronic care facilities. Thus, difference in the types of LTCFs may explain these variations in *C. difficile* carriage rates.

Exposure to antibiotics and frequent or prolonged hospitalization are the major risk factors for acquisition or colonization of *C. difficile* [31,33,34]. In our study, subject #02010, who had several antibiotic treatments and hospital stays between S_2 and S_3, acquired *C. difficile* at S_3, and the qPCR count was over 10^8 cells/g of stool– much higher than in the other subjects (Table 5). It is likely that overgrowth of *C. difficile* newly acquired from the hospital environment was observed by the TaqMan-based qPCR, although this was not a case of CDI because the strain was non-toxigenic. All eight of our *C. difficile*-positive subjects, including the four toxigenic *C. difficile* carriers, had no abdominal symptoms. The mean qPCR count of *C. difficile* in these asymptomatic carriers was 4.5 $\log_{10}$ cells/g of stool (Table 5). Naaber *et al.* [35] examined stools from patients with antibiotic-associated diarrhea by using *C. difficile* species-level qPCR. They reported increased numbers of *C. difficile*, ranging from 5.6 to 11.2 $\log_{10}$ cells/g of stool. They also revealed that the mean qPCR count in *C. difficile*-toxin-positive stools was higher than that in toxin-negative stools (9.3 vs. 6.3 $\log_{10}$ cells/g of stool). Riggs *et al.* [5] also reported that the mean *C. difficile* count in 18 patients with CDI was higher than that in 20 asymptomatic carriers (5.6 vs. 3.6 CFU/g of stool). Thus, the bacterial number in stools may be useful for predicting the status of *C. difficile* carriers (i.e. symptomatic or asymptomatic) and the severity of symptoms. Our TaqMan-based qPCR method would be appropriate for such assessments because it enables accurate monitoring of *C. difficile* counts with an appropriate lower detection limit. We believe that use of this method could provide valuable information for the control of CDI.

In conclusion, we developed a sensitive and selective detection system for *C. difficile* in human stools that uses TaqMan-based qPCR. Application of qPCR to the examination of stools from nursing home residents revealed in detail the prevalence of *C. difficile*, including toxigenic strains, indicating that this method can be an effective tool for both clinical diagnosis and epidemiological investigation.

Acknowledgments

We are grateful to Dr. Mr Xavier Deplanque and Dr. Véronique Vacher of Naturalpha SAS for coordinating the clinical stool collection study. We are also grateful to Dr. Isabelle Jeanmaire and Dr. Philippe Platel of the nursing homes in France for managing the clinical study as investigators. We thank Dr. Kazunori Matsuda of Yakult Honsha European Research Center for Microbiology ESV for his help in preparing this manuscript.

Author Contributions

Conceived and designed the experiments: HK TS HM EI KO. Performed the experiments: HK TS AG HM TA. Analyzed the data: HK HM KO. Contributed reagents/materials/analysis tools: HK TS AG HM TA KO. Wrote the paper: HK TS AG HM TA EI KO.

References

1. Rupnik M, Wilcox MH, Gerding DN (2009) *Clostridium difficile* infection: new developments in epidemiology and pathogenesis. Nat Rev Microbiol 7: 526–536.
2. Simor AE, Bradley SF, Strausbaugh LJ, Crossley K, Nicolle LE (2002) *Clostridium difficile* in long-term-care facilities for the elderly. Infect Control Hosp Epidemiol 23: 696–703.
3. Ryan J, Murphy C, Twomey C, Paul Ross R, Rea MC, et al. (2010) Asymptomatic carriage of *Clostridium difficile* in an Irish continuing care institution for the elderly: prevalence and characteristics. Ir J Med Sci 179: 245–250.
4. Rivera EV, Woods S (2003) Prevalence of asymptomatic *Clostridium difficile* colonization in a nursing home population: a cross-sectional study. J Gend Specif Med 6: 27–30.
5. Riggs MM, Sethi AK, Zabarsky TF, Eckstein EC, Jump RL, et al. (2007) Asymptomatic carriers are a potential source for transmission of epidemic and nonepidemic *Clostridium difficile* strains among long-term care facility residents. Clin Infect Dis 45: 992–998.
6. Belanger SD, Boissinot M, Clairoux N, Picard FJ, Bergeron MG (2003) Rapid detection of *Clostridium difficile* in feces by real-time PCR. J Clin Microbiol 41: 730–734.
7. Guilbault C, Labbe AC, Poirier L, Busque L, Beliveau C, et al. (2002) Development and evaluation of a PCR method for detection of the *Clostridium difficile* toxin B gene in stool specimens. J Clin Microbiol 40: 2288–2290.
8. Peterson LR, Manson RU, Paule SM, Hacek DM, Robicsek A, et al. (2007) Detection of toxigenic *Clostridium difficile* in stool samples by real-time polymerase chain reaction for the diagnosis of *C. difficile*-associated diarrhea. Clin Infect Dis 45: 1152–1160.
9. Sloan LM, Duresko BJ, Gustafson DR, Rosenblatt JE (2008) Comparison of real-time PCR for detection of the tcdC gene with four toxin immunoassays and culture in diagnosis of *Clostridium difficile* infection. J Clin Microbiol 46: 1996–2001.
10. Pancholi P, Kelly C, Raczkowski M, Balada-Llasat JM (2012) Detection of toxigenic *Clostridium difficile*: comparison of the cell culture neutralization, Xpert *C. difficile*, Xpert *C. difficile*/Epi, and Illumigene *C. difficile* assays. J Clin Microbiol 50: 1331–1335.
11. Huang H, Weintraub A, Fang H, Nord CE (2009) Comparison of a commercial multiplex real-time PCR to the cell cytotoxicity neutralization assay for diagnosis of *clostridium difficile* infections. J Clin Microbiol 47: 3729–3731.
12. Dionne LL, Raymond F, Corbeil J, Longtin J, Gervais P, et al. (2013) Correlation between *Clostridium difficile* Bacterial Load, Commercial Real-time PCR Cycle Thresholds, and Results of Diagnostic Tests Based on Enzyme Immunoassay and Cell-Culture Cytotoxicity Assay. J Clin Microbiol 51: 3624–3630.
13. Jansen GJ, Wildeboer-Veloo AC, Tonk RH, Franks AH, Welling GW (1999) Development and validation of an automated, microscopy-based method for enumeration of groups of intestinal bacteria. J Microbiol Methods 37: 215–221.
14. Wren M (2010) *Clostridium difficile* isolation and culture techniques. Methods Mol Biol 646: 39–52.
15. Kato H, Kato N, Watanabe K, Iwai N, Nakamura H, et al. (1998) Identification of toxin A-negative, toxin B-positive *Clostridium difficile* by PCR. J Clin Microbiol 36: 2178–2182.
16. Pituch H, Rupnik M, Obuch-Woszczatynski P, Grubesic A, Meisel-Mikolajczyk F, et al. (2005) Detection of binary-toxin genes (cdtA and cdtB) among *Clostridium difficile* strains isolated from patients with *C. difficile*-associated diarrhoea (CDAD) in Poland. J Med Microbiol 54: 143–147.
17. Sambol SP, Merrigan MM, Lyerly D, Gerding DN, Johnson S (2000) Toxin gene analysis of a variant strain of *Clostridium difficile* that causes human clinical disease. Infect Immun 68: 5480–5487.
18. Kato H, Kato N, Katow S, Maegawa T, Nakamura S, et al. (1999) Deletions in the repeating sequences of the toxin A gene of toxin A-negative, toxin B-positive *Clostridium difficile* strains. FEMS Microbiol Lett 175: 197–203.
19. Rupnik M (2008) Heterogeneity of large clostridial toxins: importance of *Clostridium difficile* toxinotypes. FEMS Microbiol Rev 32: 541–555.
20. Lemee L, Dhalluin A, Testelin S, Mattrat MA, Maillard K, et al. (2004) Multiplex PCR targeting tpi (triose phosphate isomerase), tcdA (Toxin A), and tcdB (Toxin B) genes for toxigenic culture of *Clostridium difficile*. J Clin Microbiol 42: 5710–5714.
21. Houser BA, Hattel AL, Jayarao BM (2010) Real-time multiplex polymerase chain reaction assay for rapid detection of *Clostridium difficile* toxin-encoding strains. Foodborne Pathog Dis 7: 719–726.
22. Alonso R, Munoz C, Gros S, Garcia de Viedma D, Pelaez T, et al. (1999) Rapid detection of toxigenic *Clostridium difficile* from stool samples by a nested PCR of toxin B gene. J Hosp Infect 41: 145–149.
23. Matsuda K, Tsuji H, Asahara T, Takahashi T, Kubota H, et al. (2012) Sensitive quantification of *Clostridium difficile* cells by reverse transcription-quantitative PCR targeting rRNA molecules. Appl Environ Microbiol 78: 5111–5118.
24. Matsuda K, Tsuji H, Asahara T, Kado Y, Nomoto K (2007) Sensitive quantitative detection of commensal bacteria by rRNA-targeted reverse transcription-PCR. Appl Environ Microbiol 73: 32–39.
25. Matsuda K, Tsuji H, Asahara T, Matsumoto K, Takada T, et al. (2009) Establishment of an analytical system for the human fecal microbiota, based on reverse transcription-quantitative PCR targeting of multicopy rRNA molecules. Appl Environ Microbiol 75: 1961–1969.
26. Rudi K, Moen B, Dromtorp SM, Holck AL (2005) Use of ethidium monoazide and PCR in combination for quantification of viable and dead cells in complex samples. Appl Environ Microbiol 71: 1018–1024.
27. Nocker A, Cheung CY, Camper AK (2006) Comparison of propidium monoazide with ethidium monoazide for differentiation of live vs. dead bacteria by selective removal of DNA from dead cells. J Microbiol Methods 67: 310–320.
28. Poutanen SM, Simor AE (2004) *Clostridium difficile*-associated diarrhea in adults. CMAJ 171: 51–58.
29. Arvand M, Moser V, Schwehn C, Bettge-Weller G, Hensgens MP, et al. (2012) High prevalence of *Clostridium difficile* colonization among nursing home residents in Hesse, Germany. PLoS One 7: e30183.
30. Walker KJ, Gilliland SS, Vance-Bryan K, Moody JA, Larsson AJ, et al. (1993) *Clostridium difficile* colonization in residents of long-term care facilities: prevalence and risk factors. J Am Geriatr Soc 41: 940–946.
31. Simor AE (2010) Diagnosis, management, and prevention of *Clostridium difficile* infection in long-term care facilities: a review. J Am Geriatr Soc 58: 1556–1564.
32. Gerding DN, Muto CA, Owens RC Jr (2008) Measures to control and prevent *Clostridium difficile* infection. Clin Infect Dis 46 Suppl 1: S43–49.
33. Makris AT, Gelone S (2007) *Clostridium difficile* in the long-term care setting. J Am Med Dir Assoc 8: 290–299.
34. Johnson S, Gerding DN (1998) *Clostridium difficile*-associated diarrhea. Clin Infect Dis 26: 1027–1034; quiz 1035–1026.
35. Naaber P, Stsepetova J, Smidt I, Ratsep M, Koljalg S, et al. (2011) Quantification of *Clostridium difficile* in antibiotic-associated-diarrhea patients. J Clin Microbiol 49: 3656–3658.

8

Mortality Predictors in Renal Transplant Recipients with Severe Sepsis and Septic Shock

Mônica Andrade de Carvalho[1]*, Flávio Geraldo Rezende Freitas[1,2], Hélio Tedesco Silva Junior[1], Antônio Toneti Bafi[1,2], Flávia Ribeiro Machado[2], José Osmar Medina Pestana[1]

1 Unidade de Transplante, Disciplina de Nefrologia, Universidade Federal de São Paulo, São Paulo, SP, Brazil, **2** Disciplina de Anestesiologia, Dor e Terapia Intensiva. Universidade Federal de São Paulo, São Paulo, SP, Brazil

Abstract

Introduction: The growing number of renal transplant recipients in a sustained immunosuppressive state is a factor that can contribute to increased incidence of sepsis. However, relatively little is known about sepsis in this population. The aim of this single-center study was to evaluate the factors associated with hospital mortality in renal transplant patients admitted to the intensive care unit (ICU) with severe sepsis and septic shock.

Methods: Patient demographics and transplant-related and ICU stay data were retrospectively collected. Multiple logistic regression was conducted to identify the independent risk factors associated with hospital mortality.

Results: A total of 190 patients were enrolled, 64.2% of whom received kidneys from deceased donors. The mean patient age was 51±13 years (males, 115 [60.5%]), and the median APACHE II was 20 (16–23). The majority of patients developed sepsis late after the renal transplantation (2.1 [0.6–2.3] years). The lung was the most common infection site (59.5%). Upon ICU admission, 16.4% of the patients had ≤1 systemic inflammatory response syndrome criteria. Among the patients, 61.5% presented with ≥2 organ failures at admission, and 27.9% experienced septic shock within the first 24 hours of ICU admission. The overall hospital mortality rate was 38.4%. In the multivariate analysis, the independent determinants of hospital mortality were male gender (OR = 5.9; 95% CI, 1.7–19.6; p = 0.004), delta SOFA 24 h (OR = 1.7; 95% CI, 1.2–2.3; p = 0.001), mechanical ventilation (OR = 30; 95% CI, 8.8–102.2; p<0.0001), hematologic dysfunction (OR = 6.8; 95% CI, 2.0–22.6; p = 0.002), admission from the ward (OR = 3.4; 95% CI, 1.2–9.7; p = 0.02) and acute kidney injury stage 3 (OR = 5.7; 95% CI,1.9–16.6; p = 0.002).

Conclusions: Hospital mortality in renal transplant patients with severe sepsis and septic shock was associated with male gender, admission from the wards, worse SOFA scores on the first day and the presence of hematologic dysfunction, mechanical ventilation or advanced graft dysfunction.

Editor: Antonio De Maio, University of California, San Diego, United States of America

Funding: The project was supported by funding from the Coordenação de Aperfeiçoamento de Pessoal de Nível Superior (CAPES) programme and Hospital do Rim. The funders had no role in study design, data collection and analysis, decision to publish, or preparation of the manuscript.

Competing Interests: The authors have declared that no competing interests exist.

* Email: mactulha@hotmail.com

Introduction

Sepsis is the leading cause of death in non-cardiac intensive care units, although there is some evidence of a decline in mortality rates, at least in developed countries [1–4]. The scenario in emerging and limited-resources countries seems to be different with higher reported rates [5,6], although low mortality rates has also been reported [7]. The incidence of sepsis is increasing over the past years and the growing number of patients living with solid organ transplants is a factor that contributes to this finding [2–4,8].

The most common solid organ transplant procedure worldwide is the renal transplantation. It is the treatment of choice for end-stage renal disease. Compared with chronic dialysis, renal transplantation is cost-effective, offers improved quality of life and confers a progressive survival benefit [9,10]. The overall survival rate of kidney grafts has improved consistently during the past decades [11]. Moreover, the number of adult candidates on the waiting lists with kidney failure continues to increase [12]. Therefore, more renal transplant recipients with functioning grafts will be exposed to pathogens while in a sustained immunosuppressive state.

Because of immunosuppression, infection frequently occurs after kidney transplantation and greatly impacts patient morbidity and mortality. This explains why infection is the second leading cause of death in renal transplant recipients, following cardiovascular diseases [13]. The importance of infection as cause of death is higher in underdeveloped countries [14,15]. Surprisingly,

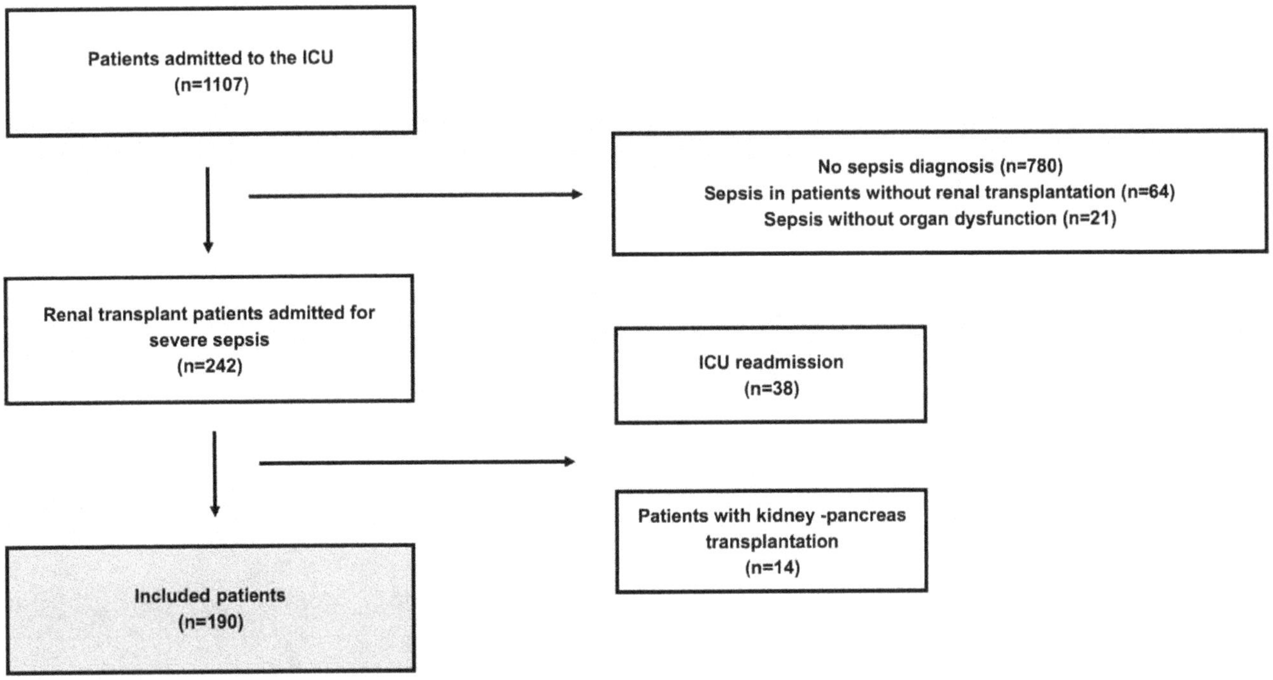

Figure 1. Study flowchart. ICU: intensive care unit.

relatively little is known about severe sepsis in this growing population. The aim of this study was to describe the characteristics of severe sepsis and septic shock in renal transplant patients who are admitted to the intensive care unit (ICU) and to evaluate the factors associated with hospital mortality.

Materials and Methods

This single center, retrospective, observational study was performed at a kidney transplant center in Brazil [16]. The institutional ethics committee approved the study and waived the informed consent requirement (Comitê de Ética em Pesquisa – Universidade Federal de São Paulo, reference number: 1736–10). All consecutive adult renal transplant recipients (older than 18 years) diagnosed with severe sepsis or septic shock who were admitted to our 12-bed ICU from June 1, 2010 to December 31, 2011 were included. We excluded pregnant patients, patients who underwent kidney-pancreas transplantation, and patients with "do not resuscitate" orders. All patients were included only in their first episode of sepsis.

Data were retrospectively collected through medical records by a single author (MAC). We recorded the following data: patient demographics, comorbid chronic illnesses, severe sepsis characteristics and the severity scores Sequential Organ Failure Assessment (SOFA) and Acute Physiology and Chronic Health Evaluation II (APACHE II). We also collected data on the initial treatment, life support and fluid balance as well as pre-transplant, peritransplant and post-transplant variables. We assessed adequacy of treatment according to the compliance to the 6-hours Surviving Sepsis Campaign bundle available during the study period [17], which are similar to the recent published 3-hour and 6-hour bundles of the 2012 revised guidelines [18]. All transplant patients in our hospital are under continuous surveillance. Thus, the hospital database has all information about outpatient's visits, hospital readmissions or death in other institutions. Thus, we collected not only the hospital mortality during the septic episode but also the one-year survival. The database was reviewed by two authors (FGRF and FRM). In cases of inconsistency, the sources documents were verified, and the data were corrected. Data were anonymized and de-identified prior to data analysis.

Severe sepsis was defined as a documented or presumed infection plus at least one organ failure secondary to infection. We did not use the systemic inflammatory response syndrome (SIRS) criteria, as depressed febrile response and diminished leukocytosis are frequently seen in solid-organ recipients [19]. Septic shock was defined as volume-refractory hypotension with the need for vasopressor. Organ dysfunction was diagnosed when one of the following factors was present: hypotension with systolic blood pressure <90 mmHg or mean arterial blood pressure <65 mmHg (cardiovascular); arterial oxygen partial pressure/oxygen inspiratory fraction (PaO_2/FiO_2) ratio ≤ 300 (respiratory); a bilirubin level $>$ twice the reference value (hepatic); a lactate level ≥ 1.5 times the reference value and a base deficit >5 (metabolic); an international normalized ratio (INR) >1.5 or a platelet count $<$ 100,000/mL (hematologic) and altered level of consciousness (neurologic). To define renal dysfunction, we used increased serum creatinine $>$ twice the baseline value. This cutoff was arbitrary chosen because of the lack of agreement on the definition of acute kidney injury (AKI) in this population. In parallel, we also used the definition recommended by Kidney Disease: Improving Global Outcomes (KDIGO) [20] to stage AKI during the ICU stay, without considering urine output.

The time to the sepsis diagnosis was defined as the number of hours elapsed between the onset of the first organ dysfunction and the recognition and management of sepsis by the healthcare provider, as described elsewhere [21]. The severe sepsis and septic shock treatment was analyzed based on compliance with the initial care bundle (within the first 6 hrs of presentation) [22].

Table 1. Patient characteristics and transplant variables.

	All Patients (n = 190)	Survivors (n = 117)	Non survivors (n = 73)	p value
Age (years)	51±13	50±13	52±13	0.300
Male gender	115 (60.5)	61 (52.1)	54 (73.9)	**0.002**
Body mass index (kg/m^2)	24±5	25±5	23±4	**0.003**
Comorbidities				
Hypertension	152 (80.0)	99 (84.6)	53 (72.6)	**0.040**
Diabetes mellitus	61 (32.1)	39 (33.3)	22 (30.1)	0.600
CAD	35 (18.4)	24 (20.5)	11 (15.0)	0.300
Stroke	8 (4.2)	6 (5.1)	2 (2.7)	0.700
CHF	5 (2.6)	3 (2.5)	2 (2.7)	1.000
Hepatitis C	13 (6.8)	7 (5.9)	6 (8.2)	0.500
Hepatitis B	6 (3.1)	3 (2.5)	3 (4.1)	0.600
COPD	6 (3.1)	1 (0.8)	5 (6.8)	**0.030**
ESRD etiology				0.220
Undetermined	67 (35.2)	41 (35.0)	26 (35.6)	
Glomerulonephritis	50 (26.3)	33 (28.2)	17 (23.2)	
Diabetes mellitus	36 (18.9)	18 (15.3)	18 (24.6)	
Hypertension	28 (14.7)	21 (17.9)	7 (9.5)	
Urologic disease	9 (4.7)	4 (3.4)	5 (6.8)	
Dialysis modality before transplant				0.480
Preemptive	8 (4.2)	7 (5.9)	1 (1.3)	
Hemodialysis	153 (80.5)	91 (77.7)	62 (84.9)	
Peritoneal	21 (11.0)	14 (11.9)	7 (9.5)	
Hemodialysis/peritoneal	8 (4.2)	5 (4.2)	3 (4.1)	
Time of dialysis (months)	34 (18–60)	32 (18–60)	36 (24–68)	0.170
Donor type				0.190
Deceased	122 (64.2)	71 (60.6)	51 (69.8)	
Living	68 (35.8)	46 (39.4)	22 (30.2)	
Donor gender [a]				0.330
Female	71 (42.0)	43 (40.6)	28 (44.5)	
Male	98 (58.0)	63 (59.4)	35 (55.5)	
Deceased donor [b]				
Cause of death [c]				0.930
Traumatic brain injury	33 (28.0)	21 (30.0)	12 (25.0)	
Subarachnoid hemorrhage	20 (16.9)	12 (17.1)	8 (16.6)	
Stroke	56 (47.5)	32 (45.7)	24 (50.0)	
Others	9 (7.6)	5 (7.2)	4 (8.4)	
Panel reactive antibodies [d]				0.660
0–50%	93 (84.5)	55 (83.3)	38 (86.3)	
>51%	17 (15.5)	11 (16.7)	6 (13.6)	
Final creatinine [e]				0.210
<1.5 mg/dL	31 (32.6)	21 (35.5)	10 (27.7)	
≥1.5 mg/dL	64 (67.4)	38 (64.5)	26 (72.3)	
Cold ischemia time (hours) [f]	23 (20–27)	23 (20–28)	22 (20–27)	0.630
Expanded criteria donor	31 (26.3)	13 (18.6)	18 (37.5)	**0.020**
Delayed graft function	82 (43.3)	44 (37.6)	38 (52.7)	**0.040**
Thymoglobulin use [g]	54 (28.5)	34 (29.0)	20 (27.7)	0.870
CMV disease treated	68 (35.9)	41 (35.0)	27 (37.5)	0.750
Current immunosuppression [h]				0.460
TAC+PRED+AZA	31 (16.3)	16 (13.6)	15 (20.5)	
TAC+PRED+MF	70 (36.8)	48 (41.0)	22 (30.1)	

Table 1. Cont.

	All Patients (n = 190)	Survivors (n = 117)	Non survivors (n = 73)	p value
CSA+PRED+AZA	17 (8.9)	12 (10.2)	5 (6.8)	
CSA+PRED+MF	7 (3.6)	4 (3.4)	3 (4.1)	
TAC/CSA+PRED+EVR/SRL	4 (2.1)	3 (2.5)	1 (1.7)	
SRL/EVR+PRED+MF	9 (4.7)	4 (3.4)	5 (6.8)	
Others	51 (26.8)	30 (25.6)	21 (28.7)	
Time between transplant and sepsis (years)	2.1 (0.6–7.2)	2.3 (0.6–7.8)	1.6 (0.6–7.0)	0.600
Acute rejection	55 (28.9)	34 (29.0)	21 (28.7)	0.960
Time rejection-sepsis (days) [i]	312 (130–776)	331(115–817)	282 (152–849)	0.900

CAD coronary artery disease, CHF: congestive heart failure, COPD: chronic obstructive pulmonary disease, ESRD: end-stage renal disease, CMV: *cytomegalovirus*, TAC: tacrolimus, PRED: prednisone, AZA: azathioprine, MF: mycophenolate, CSA: cyclosporine, EVR: everolimus, SRL sirolimus.
a) 21 missing data,
b) 122 deceased donors,
c) 4 missing data,
d) 12 missing data,
e) final creatinine refers to the donors' last serum creatinine level, 27 missing data,
f) 3 missing data,
g) patients who used thymoglobulin for treating rejection and/or induction in transplantation,
h) 1 missing data and i) time between the occurrence of rejection and sepsis (total of patients with rejection, 55 patients, 3 patients among the survivors and 6 among the non-survivors were excluded for missing data). The results are expressed as number (%) or median (IQR, 25%–75%) or mean ± standard deviation. Chi-squared test, Mann-Whitney U-test, and Student's t-test (univariate analysis).

Statistical methods

The categorical variables are described as percentages, and the continuous variables are described as measures of central tendency and dispersion, according to distribution, as assessed by the Kolmogorov-Smirnov test. We compare hospital survivors and non-survivor using the two-tailed t-test, Mann-Whitney U-test, chi-squared test, and Fisher's exact test, as appropriate. Multiple logistic regression was conducted to identify the independent risk factors associated with hospital mortality, including all variables with a p value <0.10 in the univariate analysis (using a stepwise forward regression model). The time until the sepsis diagnosis was categorized using the best cutoff value in the receiver operating characteristic (ROC) curve for mortality ($\geq$170 vs. $<$170 min). The number of organ dysfunctions ($\geq$2 vs. $<$2) and the KDIGO classification (stage 3 vs. stage $<$3) of acute kidney injury during ICU stay were also categorized. All variables were checked for confounding and collinearity. The model calibration was assessed using the Hosmer-Lemeshow test, which was considered to be appropriate if $p>0.10$. We did not include the variables with missing data $>$10%, as the lack of data would result in serious inconsistencies. The patients were followed for one year, and a mortality curve was generated using the Kaplan-Meier methodology. A p value <0.05 was considered to be significant. Data were analyzed using SPSS 19.0 for Windows (SPSS, Chicago, IL, USA).

Results

During the study period, 1107 patients were admitted to the ICU, 242 (21.9%) of whom were renal transplant patients who were admitted for severe sepsis. Of these patients, 190 were enrolled, as shown in Figure 1.

The patients' characteristics and transplant variables are summarized in Table 1. The leading causes of end-stage renal disease were glomerulonephritis (26.3%), diabetes mellitus (18.9%) and hypertension (14.7%), although most patients (35.2%) did not have an identifiable cause. The majority of kidneys transplanted were from deceased donors (64.2%). All patients had immunosuppression suspended at ICU admission and used hydrocortisone (50 mg every six hours). The majority of the patients developed sepsis late after the renal transplantation (2.1 years; range, 0.6–2.3 years). Fifty-five patients (28.9%) had histories of acute rejection that occurred at a median of 312 days (range, 130–776 days) before the ICU admission. The univariate analysis showed delayed graft function, and expanded criteria donor kidneys were associated with hospital mortality. No other clinical characteristic related to the transplant was significantly different between the survivors and non-survivors.

The lung was the most common site of infection (59.5%), followed by the urinary tract (16.8%) and abdomen (9.5%) (Table 2). We isolated the etiologic agents in the majority of the patients (57%). Most of these agents were bacteria (Gram-negative, 45.4%; Gram-positive: 20.4%). The other relevant agents were *Mycobacterium tuberculosis* (3.7%), Cytomegalovirus (3.7%) and fungi (24%), including *Pneumocystis jirovecii* (8.3%) (Table 3).

Upon ICU admission, 16.4% of the patients had $\leq$1 SIRS criterion (Figure 2). The most common SIRS criteria were tachypnea (74.7%) and tachycardia (67.9%). Two or more organ failures were present at admission in 61.5% of patients. Respiratory and hematological dysfunctions occurred more frequently in the non-survivors. Fifty-three patients (27.9%) experienced septic shock within the first 24 hours of ICU admission; however, 96 (50.5%) patients experienced septic shock during their ICU stays. The time for severe sepsis diagnosis was longer in the non-survivors. The patients who developed sepsis in the ward had worse outcomes than those patients in the emergency room (Table 2). The compliance rate with each component of the 6-hour bundle is shown in Table 2. The compliance rate for fluid administration (20 ml/kg crystalloid for hypotension or lactate $\geq$36 mg/dl) was higher among the survivors.

The clinical and biological variables at the ICU admission and during the ICU stay are shown in Table 3. In the univariate analysis, most of the variables were significantly different between the survivors and non-survivors. Note that more positive fluid

Table 2. Severe sepsis characteristics and treatment.

	All patients (n = 190)	Survivors (n = 117)	Non-survivors (n = 73)	p value
Site of infection				**0.006**
Respiratory	113 (59.5)	66 (56.4)	47 (64.3)	
Urinary	32 (16.8)	28 (23.9)	4 (5.4)	
Abdominal	18 (9.5	8 (6.8)	10 (13.7)	
Others	27 (14.2)	15 (12.8)	12 (16.4)	
SIRS criteria				
Tachypnea	142 (74.7)	84 (71.7)	58 (79.4)	0.230
Tachycardia	129 (67.9)	80 (68.3)	49 (67.1)	0.850
Leukocytosis	50 (26.3)	28 (23.9)	22 (30.1)	0.340
Leukopenia	31 (16.3)	16 (13.6)	15 (20.5)	0.210
Fever	46 (24.2)	32 (27.3)	14 (19.1)	0.200
Hypothermia	12 (6.3)	7 (5.9)	5 (6.8)	1.000
Organ failures				
Respiratory	84 (44.2)	43 (36.7)	41 (56.1)	**0.008**
Cardiovascular	78 (41.1)	49(41.8)	29 (39.7)	0.760
Renal	77 (40.5)	51 (43.5)	26 (35.6)	0.270
Hematologic	64 (33.9)	30 (25.6)	34 (46.6)	0.030
Neurologic	50 (26.3)	26 (22.2)	24 (32.8)	0.100
Metabolic	13 (7.9)	5 (4.8)	8 (12.9)	0.070
Hepatic	9 (4.7)	6 (5.1)	3 (4.1)	1.000
Admission				**<0.0001**
Emergency	110 (57.9)	83 (70.9)	27 (36.9)	
Ward	80 (42.1)	34 (29.0)	46 (63.0)	
Number of organs dysfunctions (≥2)	117 (61.5)	65 (55.5)	52 (71.2)	0.030
Glycemia (mg/dl)[a]	149 (121–194)	151 (121–195)	141 (119–193)	0.360
Time to sepsis diagnosis (hours)	2.5 (1.1–5.2)	2 (0.9–4.2)	3.5 (1.5–6.3)	**<0.001**
Time to antibiotics (minutes)	55 (30–120)	60 (30–120)	45 (20–80)	**<0.001**
Duration of ICU stay (days)	6 (3–13)	6 (3–11)	7 (3–16)	0.130
Duration of hospital stay (days)	20 (12–35)	21 (14–38)	15 (8–31)	0.010
Compliance to severe sepsis bundle				
Measure lactate	164 (86.3)	103 (88.0)	61 (83.5)	0.300
Broad-spectrum antibiotics	173 (91.0)	107 (91.5)	66 (90.4)	0.800
Blood cultures before antibiotics	151 (79.5)	93 (79.4)	58 (79.5)	0.990
Fluid resuscitation [b]	54 (62.3)	39 (75)	15 (44.1)	**0.004**
CVP >8 mm Hg [c]	6 (15.8)	2 (11.1)	4 (22.2)	0.370
ScvO2 >70% [c]	14 (36.8)	7 (38.9)	7 (38.9)	1.000
Initial care bundle	74 (39.0)	45 (38.5)	29 (39.7)	0.800

SIRS: systemic inflammatory response syndrome. ICU: intensive care unit. CVP: central venous pressure, $ScvO_2$: central venous oxygen saturation.
a) median glycemia during the first 24 h of sepsis,
b) indication to administer 20 ml/kg crystalloid for hypotension or lactate ≥36 mg/dl (n = 86),
c) indication to measure CVP or measure $ScvO_2$ (n = 38). The results are expressed as number (%) or median (IQR: 25%–75%). Chi-squared test and Mann-Whitney U-test (univariate analysis).

balance at 72 hours was also associated with hospital mortality; however this variable was not included in multiple logistic regression due to missing data.

The basal creatinine values (before severe sepsis) were 1.93±1.44 mg/dL. Four patients were under dialysis before ICU admission because of acute Kidney dysfunction. Seventy seven (40.5%) had renal dysfunction (increased serum creatinine > twice the baseline value). Staging AKI according KDIGO, 48 (25.3%) patients reaching Stage 1, 27 (14.2%) a Stage 2, and 94 (49.5%) a Stage 3. There was a strong association between acute kidney injury stage 3 and hospital mortality (Table 4). During ICU stay, 77 (40.5%) patients underwent dialysis (conventional hemodialysis or sustained low-efficiency dialysis). The need for dialysis was higher among non-survivors (75.3% vs. 18.8%, p< 0.001). The need for dialysis was not included in our multivariate analysis because of its collinearity with AKI stage 3.

The overall hospital mortality rate was 38.4% (32.1% in severe sepsis patients and 54.7% in patients with septic shock in the first

Table 3. Frequencies of infectious agents identified.

	Frequency, n (%)
Gram-negative	**49 (45.4)**
Escherichia coli	16 (15.0)
Klebsiella pneumonia	13 (12.0)
Pseudomonas aeruginosa	8 (7.4)
Acinetobacter baumanii	6 (5.5)
Enterobacter sp	3 (2.7)
Proteus mirabilis	2 (1.8)
Citrobacter sp	1 (0.9)
Gram-positive	**22 (20.4)**
Staphylococcus aureus	10 (9.2)
Enterococcus sp	7 (6.5)
Staphylococcus epidermidis	3 (2.7)
Streptococcus pneumoniae	1 (0.9)
Streptococcus viridans	1 (0.9)
Fungi	**26 (24.0)**
Candida albicans	10 (9.2)
Pneumocystis jiroveci	9 (8.3)
Cryptococcus	2 (1.8)
Histoplasma capsulatum	3 (2.7)
Cândida sp	2 (1.8)
Others	**11 (10.2)**
Mycobacterium turbeculosis	4 (3.7)
Cytomegalovirus	4 (3.7)
Listeria monocytogenes	1 (0.9)
Neisseria meningitidis	1 (0.9)
Salmonella sp	1 (0.9)

24 hrs of ICU admission). In the multivariate analysis, the independent determinants of hospital mortality were male gender, delta SOFA score 24 h, mechanical ventilation, hematological dysfunction, admission from ward and AKI stage 3 (Table 5). We could assess the one-year mortality data in all patients and the rate was 42.6% (37.2% for severe sepsis and 56.6% for septic shock). Figure 3 shows the Kaplan-Meier curves for one-year survival after ICU admission.

Discussion

In our study, we were able to show that the independent risk factors for hospital mortality in renal transplant recipients with severe sepsis and septic shock admitted to ICU did not include the transplant characteristics. There was a lower incidence of SIRS criteria than previously described in other sepsis studies, and there was a higher frequency of opportunistic pathogens causing severe sepsis. We also demonstrated a low increment in the mortality rate one-year after discharge.

The hospital mortality rate for ICU renal transplant recipients varies greatly in the literature, and no study has specifically evaluated septic patients [23–29]. Old Brazilian sepsis data from private and public ICU have shown higher mortality rates than in the present study [21,30]. More recent data still shows a higher mortality rate in Brazil [5] than that reported in some studies conducted in developed countries [2–4]. There are some possible explanations for this worst performance. In emerging countries, there are roughly enough resources but there is still limitation in access of care both in private and in public health systems. Sepsis awareness among lay people is restricted which contributes to a delay in searching for care. The gap between scientific evidence and bedside and staff's lack of knowledge, a frequent challenge even in the developed nations, is probably deeper in such settings. Our better findings might be partially explained by a shorter time to sepsis diagnosis [21], which was also associated with survival in our univariate analysis. In addition, the early management of these patients, as assessed by the compliance to Surviving Sepsis Campaign 6-hours bundle [17,18], was higher than those previously described [21,22]. The importance of high compliance with the resuscitation bundle to reduce mortality rate was demonstrated in Brazilian private hospitals [7]. In our study, there was a significant lower compliance to fluid administration in non-survivors. Interesting, non-survivors had higher fluid balance at 72 h. This finding suggests that fluids may be essential in the earliest phases of treatment, but late administration may be harmful.

Previous sepsis cohort studies have shown an increment in the mortality rate for sepsis patients (from 7% to 43%) 12 months after the initial assessment (hospital or 28-days mortality) [31]. In our study, no relevant increase in the 12-month mortality rate was observed compared to the in-hospital mortality rate (42.6% and 38.4%, respectively). This interesting and previously unreported

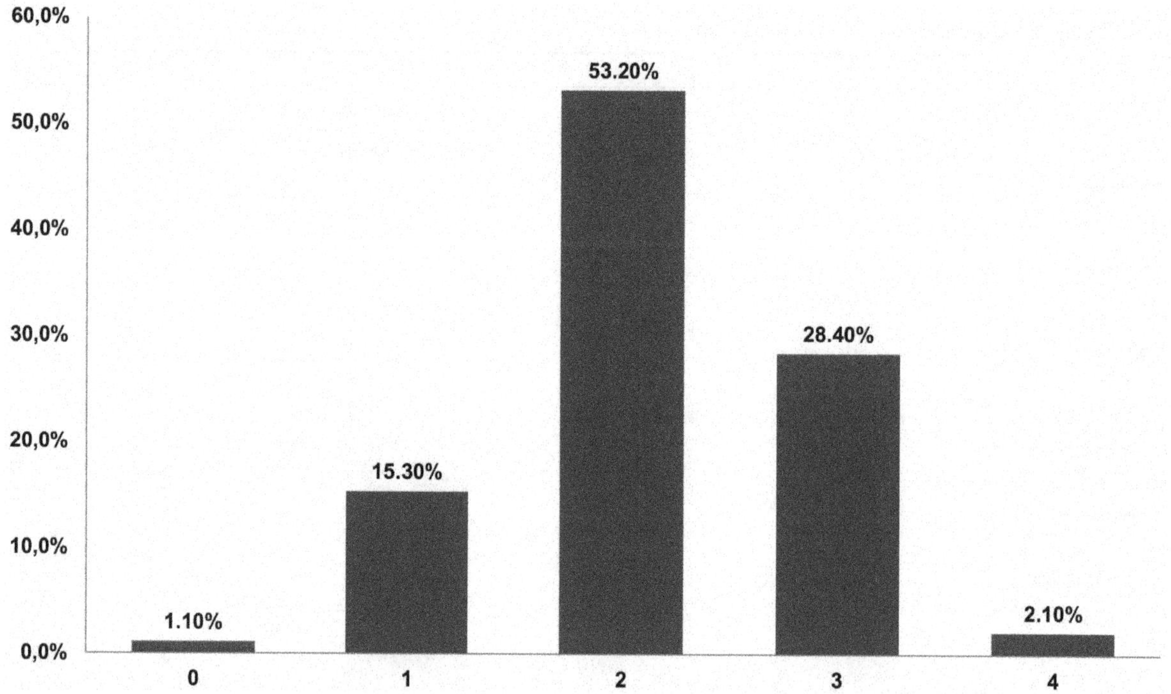

Figure 2. Frequency of systemic inflammatory response signs on intensive care unit admission.

finding might be explained, at least partially, by the fact that our patients were younger than those in other sepsis cohort studies [1,21]. Moreover, they were under continuous surveillance in a transplant center with adequate care during the entire follow-up period.

Considerable variations were present in our findings compared to other sepsis epidemiological studies. Our patients had fewer SIRS criteria. In a cohort, multicenter, observational study in European countries, Sprung *et al.* reported that approximately 90% of their septic patients had ≥3 SIRS criteria, while in our study only 30% of patients had ≥3 SIRS criteria [32]. Moreover, we found that 16.4% of the patients had ≤1 SIRS criteria. This profile of systemic inflammatory response has been previously suggested [19,33]. Sawyer *et al.* demonstrated that immunosuppressed solid organ transplant patients had significantly lower maximum temperatures and white blood cells counts compared to non-transplant patients [33]. These findings should be taken into account in sepsis studies involving transplant patients, as the need for meeting SIRS criteria to define sepsis could be flawed and may not adequately reflect the actual incidence of sepsis. In fact, the current SIRS criteria to define the presence of sepsis has been criticized even in immunocompetent patients [34].

In our study, the lung was the most common site of infection, which is in alignment with other sepsis cohort studies [22,35,36]. This finding was expected, as respiratory infection is the leading cause of ICU admission and acute respiratory failure in renal transplant recipients [23,26,29,37]. The second major source of sepsis was the urinary tract. Although this is the most common infectious complication after renal transplantation [38–40], urinary infection might not lead to severe sepsis as frequently as pneumonia even in these immunosuppressed patients. Interestingly, while the data may not be significant, urinary tract infection seems to be associated with lower mortality rates, as previously showed in immunocompetent patients [41]. We also found a higher frequency of microbiologically documented infection by opportunistic pathogens compared with non-transplant patients [1,8]. This finding was also expected, as infections caused by opportunistic pathogens in solid organ transplant recipient are frequent [42]. However, admissions for severe sepsis did not occur during periods of intensified immunosuppression (in the first months after transplantation or after treatment for acute rejection).

Our analysis showed that the classical factors usually associated with morbidity in this population, such as immunosuppressive regimens, previous rejection treatment and CMV disease, had no prognostic value. Although delayed graft function was associated with mortality, it did not remain in our final multivariate logistic regression model. The only other variable associated with mortality in the univariate analysis, expanded criteria donor, could not be included in the model as it was assessed only in the subgroup that received a deceased-donor kidney. This result aligns with other studies in critically ill renal transplant patients requiring ICU treatment [23,25,26,29].

Delta SOFA after 24 hours of ICU admission, the need of mechanical ventilation, the presence of hematologic dysfunction and admission from the ward and not from the emergency department were previously described as mortality risk factors in critically ill general septic patients [21,22,35,43–45]. The most controversial risk factor found in our study was male gender. Clinical sepsis studies evaluating gender-mortality relationships are inconsistent [46–49]. Recent studies have suggested that although the incidence of sepsis is greater in men, in-hospital mortality is significantly higher among women [48,49]. It is possible that gender influences outcomes differently in renal transplant patients. An example of these possible interactions is the reports that grafts from male donors show a trend towards better five-year survival compared to grafts from female donors [50]. Moreover, we did not have data about hormonal concentrations. The complexity of influencing factors did not allow us to evaluate the possible pathophysiological reasons for our finding.

Table 4. Severity scores at the ICU admission and the events during ICU stay.

	All patients (N = 190)	Survivors (N = 117)	Non survivors (N = 73)	p value
SOFA admission	5 (4–8)	5 (4–7)	6 (4–9)	**<0.0001**
SOFA at 24 h	5 (4–8)	4 (3–6)	7 (5–11)	**<0.0001**
SOFA at 72 h	5 (3–8)	4 (2–5)	8 (5–11)	**<0.0001**
Delta SOFA 24 h	0 (−1–1)	0 (−1–0)	1(0–3)	**<0.001**
Delta SOFA 72 h	−0.5 (−2–1)	−1 (−2–0)	2(−0.7–4)	**<0.001**
Lactate at admission (mg/dl)	10 (7–16)	10 (6–16)	10 (7–18)	**0.670**
Lactate at 6–12 h (mg/dl)	10 (7–16)	9 (6–13)	12 (8–25)	**0.001**
Lactate at 24 h (mg/dl)	8 (6–14)	8 (6–10)	13 (7–31)	**<0.0001**
Delta lactate 6–12 h (mg/dl)	1 (−3–4)	0 (−5–2)	4 (0–8)	**<0.001**
Delta lactate 24 h (mg/dl)	0 (−4–3)	−2 (−6–1)	3 (0–13)	**<0.001**
APACHE II score	20 (16–23)	18 (15–22)	21 (18–24)	**0.004**
Septic shock	53 (27.9)	24 (20.5)	29 (39.7)	**0.004**
Shock after 24 h	96 (50.5)	29 (24.7)	67 (91.7)	**0.004**
Mechanical ventilation	90 (47.4)	25 (21.3)	65 (89.0)	**<0.0001**
Hemodialysis	77 (40.5)	22 (18.8)	55 (75.3)	**<0.001**
AKI classification				**<0.0001**
Stage <3	96 (50.5)	80 (68.4)	16 (21.9)	
Stage 3	94 (49.5)	37 (31.6)	57 (78.1)	
Reinfection in ICU	34 (17.9)	18 (15.3)	16 (21.9)	0.200
Cumulative fluid balance				
First 6 h after severe sepsis[a]	500 (0–1500)	610 (0–1500)	250 (0–1500)	0.080
First 12 h after severe sepsis[b]	1500 (510–2640)	1500 (565–2569)	1175 (385–2736)	0.350
First 72 h after severe sepsis[c]	4634 (3192–6959)	4301 (3163–6208)	6099 (3657–8391)	**0.007**
First 6 h after septic shock[d]	1500 (774–2069)	1500 (790–2000)	1608 (750–2678)	0.710
First 12 h after septic shock[e]	2190 (1609–3231)	2000 (1394–3036)	2428 (1820–3330)	0.350
First 72 h after septic shock[f]	6928 (4598–8926)	5460 (2096–7117)	8750 (6928–13162)	**0.001**

SOFA: Sequential Organ Failure Assessment score, APACHE II: Acute Physiological and Chronic Health Evaluation II score, AKI: acute kidney injury (from KDIGO), ICU: intensive care unit.
a) n = 189,
b) n = 188,
c) n = 153,
d) n = 50,
e) n = 46,
f) n = 34. Results are expressed as number (%) or median (IQR: 25%–75%). Chi-squared test and Mann Whitney U-test (univariate analysis).

The degree of renal allograft dysfunction during ICU stay was also associated with hospital mortality. As there is no validated classification for AKI in renal transplant recipients, we used a KDIGO definition during the ICU stays [20]. Our results demonstrated that changes in graft function are important and associated with significant changes in outcomes. This result aligns with studies using RIFLE/AKIN definitions in which a worse RIFLE or AKIN class is associated with higher mortality and

Table 5. Multivariate logistic regression analysis in septic transplant patients with hospital mortality as dependent factor.

	OR (95% CI)	p value
Male gender	5.9 (1.7–19.6)	0.004
Delta SOFA 24 h (per point increase)	1.7 (1.2–2.3)	0.001
Mechanical ventilation	30.0 (8.8–102.2)	<0.0001
Hematological dysfunction	6.8 (2.0–22.6)	0.002
Sepsis admitted from ward	3.4 (1.2–9.7)	0.020
AKI stage 3	5.7 (1.9–16.6)	0.002

OR: odds ratio, CI: confidence interval, SOFA: Sequential Organ Failure Assessment, AKI stage 3: acute kidney injury stage 3.

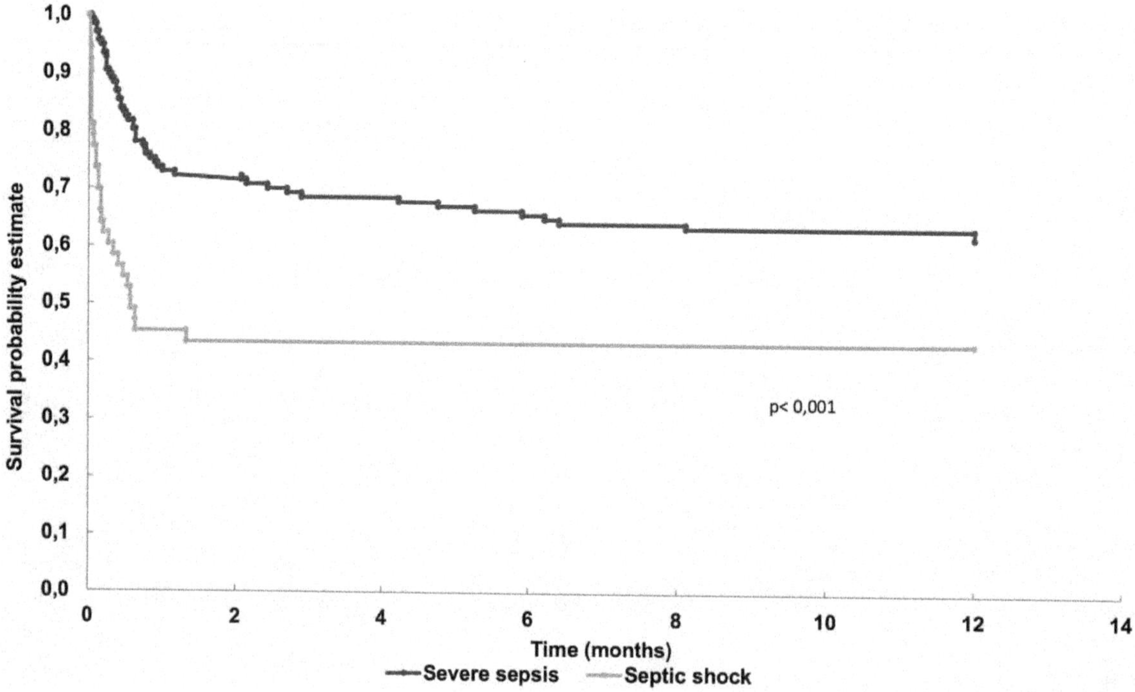

Figure 3. Kaplan-Meier curves (severe sepsis and septic shock) for one year survival after admission to the intensive care unit.

longer ICU or hospital stay [20]. This study is the first in renal transplant recipients to use a new approach of AKI classification to associate the degree of renal dysfunction with mortality. A previously reported by Nakamura *et al.*, higher acute kidney injury states correlate with lower graft survival rates. However, the authors did not present mortality as an outcome [51].

Our study had strengths and limitations. We included a homogeneous population of renal transplant recipients in a consecutive fashion. We assessed several transplant and sepsis characteristics, including treatment adequacy, which could interfere with patient outcomes. In addition, we used a new AKI classification approach. These contributions are relevant considering the paucity of data currently available in the literature. The study also has some limitations, the most important being the retrospective nature of our data collection. Second, our study has a single-center design, which limits the reproducibility of our findings. Third, we did not have a control group with septic non-transplanted patients and transplanted patients without sepsis. Fourth, we limited our analysis to ICU patients and did not include patients with severe sepsis in other hospital settings. The relevance of this limitation should have been minimized because in this institution, the vast majority of the septic patients are admitted to the ICU. Fifth, a better characterization of AKI is lacking. We do not have data regarding estimated glomerular filtration rate, time for dialysis onset or its duration, and long-term graft function. Moreover, we did not assess the role that acute rejection could have played in graft dysfunction. We also only consider creatinine and not diuresis in our AKI classification, which may have underestimated the number of patients with late stage diseases. However, controversy exists regarding the impact of this assessment in the score ability to predict prognosis [52]. Sixth, we have no data regarding adrenal insufficiency in our study. Besides the possibility of corticosteroid insufficiency related to critical illness or sepsis, previous chronic use of prednisone in nearly all patients could suppress the hypothalamic-pituitary-adrenal axis (HPA). This was the main reason for hydrocortisone administration. Another reason was the need for immunosuppressant drugs to prevent rejection, since all other immunosuppressant agents were discontinued at ICU admission.

Conclusion

Hospital mortality in renal transplant patients with severe sepsis and septic shock was associated with male gender, admission from the wards, worse SOFA scores on the first day and the presence of hematologic dysfunction, mechanical ventilation or advanced graft dysfunction. Transplant-related variables had no prognostic value.

Acknowledgments

We thank Creusa Maria Roveri Dal Bó for support with the statistical analyses.

Author Contributions

Conceived and designed the experiments: MAC FGRF JOMP. Performed the experiments: MAC FGRF ATB. Analyzed the data: MAC FGRF HTSJ FRM. Contributed reagents/materials/analysis tools: MAC FGRF HTSJ FRM. Wrote the paper: MAC FGRF HTSJ FRM.

References

1. Angus DC, Linde-Zwirble WT, Lidicker J, Clermont G, Carcillo J, et al. (2001) Epidemiology of severe sepsis in the United States: analysis of incidence, outcome, and associated costs of care. Crit Care Med 29: 1303–1310.
2. Kaukonen KM, Bailey M, Suzuki S, Pilcher D, Bellomo R (2014) Mortality related to severe sepsis and septic shock among critically ill patients in Australia and New Zealand, 2000–2012. Jama 311: 1308–1316.

3. Walkey AJ, Wiener RS, Lindenauer PK (2013) Utilization patterns and outcomes associated with central venous catheter in septic shock: a population-based study. Crit Care Med 41: 1450–1457.
4. Lagu T, Rothberg MB, Shieh MS, Pekow PS, Steingrub JS, et al. (2012) Hospitalizations, costs, and outcomes of severe sepsis in the United States 2003 to 2007. Crit Care Med 40: 754–761.
5. Latin American Sepsis Institute (2014) Surviving Sepsis Campaign. Available: http://www.ilas.org.br/upfiles/fckeditor/file/Relat%C3%B3rio%20Nacional%20fev%202014.pdf
6. Phua J, Koh Y, Du B, Tang YQ, Divatia JV, et al. (2011) Management of severe sepsis in patients admitted to Asian intensive care units: prospective cohort study. Bmj 342: d3245.
7. Noritomi DT, Ranzani OT, Monteiro MB, Ferreira EM, Santos SR, et al. (2014) Implementation of a multifaceted sepsis education program in an emerging country setting: clinical outcomes and cost-effectiveness in a long-term follow-up study. Intensive Care Med 40: 182–191.
8. Angus DC, Pereira CA, Silva E (2006) Epidemiology of severe sepsis around the world. Endocr Metab Immune Disord Drug Targets 6: 207–212.
9. Gallon LG, Leventhal JR, Kaufman DB (2002) Pretransplant evaluation of renal transplant candidates. Semin Nephrol 22: 515–525.
10. Davis CL (2004) Evaluation of the living kidney donor: current perspectives. Am J Kidney Dis 43: 508–530.
11. Sam R, Leehey DJ (2000) Improved graft survival after renal transplantation in the United States, 1988 to 1996. N Engl J Med 342: 1837–1838.
12. Knoll G (2008) Trends in kidney transplantation over the past decade. Drugs 68 Suppl 1: 3–10.
13. Adams PL (2006) Long-term patient survival: strategies to improve overall health. Am J Kidney Dis 47: S65–85.
14. Reis MA, Costa RS, Ferraz AS (1995) Causes of death in renal transplant recipients: a study of 102 autopsies from 1968 to 1991. J R Soc Med 1995, 88(1): 24–7.
15. Ingsathit A, Avihingsanon Y, Rattanasiri S, Premasathian N, Pongskul C, et al. (2010) Different etiologies of graft loss and death in Asian kidney transplant recipients: a report from Thai Transplant Registry. Transplant Proc 42: 4014–4016.
16. Medina-Pestana JO (2010) More than 1,000 kidney transplants in a single year by the "Hospital do Rim" Group in Sao Paulo - Brazil. Clin Transpl: 107–126.
17. Dellinger RP, Levy MM, Carlet JM, Bion J, Parker MM, et al. (2008) Surviving Sepsis Campaign: international guidelines for management of severe sepsis and septic shock: 2008. Intensive Care Med 34: 17–60.
18. Dellinger RP, Levy MM, Rhodes A, Annane D, Gerlach H, et al. (2013) Surviving sepsis campaign: international guidelines for management of severe sepsis and septic shock: 2012. Crit Care Med 41: 580–637.
19. Pelletier SJ, Crabtree TD, Gleason TG, Raymond DP, Oh CK, et al. (2000) Characteristics of infectious complications associated with mortality after solid organ transplantation. Clin Transplant 14: 401–408.
20. KDIGO AKI Work Group (2012) KDIGO clinical practice guideline for acute kidney injury. Kidney inter 2: 1–138.
21. Conde KA, Silva E, Silva CO, Ferreira E, Freitas FG, et al. (2013) Differences in sepsis treatment and outcomes between public and private hospitals in Brazil: a multicenter observational study. PLoS One 8: e64790.
22. Levy MM, Dellinger RP, Townsend SR, Linde-Zwirble WT, Marshall JC, et al. (2010) The Surviving Sepsis Campaign: results of an international guideline-based performance improvement program targeting severe sepsis. Crit Care Med 38: 367–374.
23. Klouche K, Amigues L, Massanet P, Garrigue V, Delmas S, et al. (2009) Outcome of renal transplant recipients admitted to an intensive care unit: a 10-year cohort study. Transplantation 87: 889–895.
24. Mouloudi E, Massa E, Georgiadou E, Iosifidis E, Katsika E, et al. (2012) Infections related to renal transplantation requiring intensive care admission: a 20-year study. Transplant Proc 44: 2721–2723.
25. Mouloudi E, Massa E, Georgiadou E, Iosifidis E, Kydona C, et al. (2012) Course and outcome of renal transplant recipients admitted to the intensive care unit: a 20-year study. Transplant Proc 44: 2718–2720.
26. Arulkumaran N, West S, Chan K, Templeton M, Taube D, et al. (2012) Long-term renal function and survival of renal transplant recipients admitted to the intensive care unit. Clin Transplant 26: E24–31.
27. Aldawood A (2007) The course and outcome of renal transplant recipients admitted to the intensive care unit at a tertiary hospital in Saudi Arabia. Saudi J Kidney Dis Transpl 18: 536–540.
28. Candan S, Pirat A, Varol G, Torgay A, Zeyneloglu P, et al. (2006) Respiratory problems in renal transplant recipients admitted to intensive care during long-term follow-up. Transplant Proc 38: 1354–1356.
29. Canet E, Osman D, Lambert J, Guitton C, Heng AE, et al. (2011) Acute respiratory failure in kidney transplant recipients: a multicenter study. Crit Care 15: R91.
30. Beale R, Reinhart K, Brunkhorst FM, Dobb G, Levy M, et al. (2009) Promoting Global Research Excellence in Severe Sepsis (PROGRESS): lessons from an international sepsis registry. Infection 37: 222–232.
31. Winters BD, Eberlein M, Leung J, Needham DM, Pronovost PJ, et al. (2010) Long-term mortality and quality of life in sepsis: a systematic review. Crit Care Med 38: 1276–1283.
32. Sprung CL, Sakr Y, Vincent JL, Le Gall JR, Reinhart K, et al. (2006) An evaluation of systemic inflammatory response syndrome signs in the Sepsis Occurrence In Acutely Ill Patients (SOAP) study. Intensive Care Med 32: 421–427.
33. Sawyer RG, Crabtree TD, Gleason TG, Antevil JL, Pruett TL (1999) Impact of solid organ transplantation and immunosuppression on fever, leukocytosis, and physiologic response during bacterial and fungal infections. Clin Transplant 13: 260–265.
34. Vincent JL, Opal SM, Marshall JC, Tracey KJ (2013) Sepsis definitions: time for change. Lancet 381: 774–775.
35. Vincent JL, Sakr Y, Sprung CL, Ranieri VM, Reinhart K, et al. (2006) Sepsis in European intensive care units: results of the SOAP study. Crit Care Med 34: 344–353.
36. Alberti C, Brun-Buisson C, Burchardi H, Martin C, Goodman S, et al. (2002) Epidemiology of sepsis and infection in ICU patients from an international multicentre cohort study. Intensive Care Med 28: 108–121.
37. Veroux M, Giuffrida G, Corona D, Gagliano M, Scriffignano V, et al. (2008) Infective complications in renal allograft recipients: epidemiology and outcome. Transplant Proc 40: 1873–1876.
38. Alangaden GJ, Thyagarajan R, Gruber SA, Morawski K, Garnick J, et al. (2006) Infectious complications after kidney transplantation: current epidemiology and associated risk factors. Clin Transplant 20: 401–409.
39. Pourmand G, Pourmand M, Salem S, Mehrsai A, Taheri Mahmoudi M, et al. (2006) Posttransplant infectious complications: a prospective study on 142 kidney allograft recipients. Urol J 3: 23–31.
40. Ak O, Yildirim M, Kucuk HF, Gencer S, Demir T (2013) Infections in renal transplant patients: risk factors and infectious agents. Transplant Proc 45: 944–948.
41. Knaus WA, Sun X, Nystrom O, Wagner DP (1992) Evaluation of definitions for sepsis. Chest 101: 1656–1662.
42. Fishman JA (2007) Infection in solid-organ transplant recipients. N Engl J Med 357: 2601–2614.
43. Ferreira FL, Bota DP, Bross A, Melot C, Vincent JL (2001) Serial evaluation of the SOFA score to predict outcome in critically ill patients. Jama 286: 1754–1758.
44. Moreno R, Vincent JL, Matos R, Mendonça A, Cantraine F, et al. (1999) The use of maximum SOFA score to quantify organ dysfunction/failure in intensive care. Results of a prospective, multicentre study. Working Group on Sepsis related Problems of the ESICM. Intensive Care Med 25: 686–696.
45. Dhainaut JF, Yan SB, Joyce DE, Pettila V, Basson B, et al. (2004) Treatment effects of drotrecogin alfa (activated) in patients with severe sepsis with or without overt disseminated intravascular coagulation. J Thromb Haemost 2: 1924–1933.
46. Dombrovskiy VY, Martin AA, Sunderram J, Paz HL (2007) Rapid increase in hospitalization and mortality rates for severe sepsis in the United States: a trend analysis from 1993 to 2003. Crit Care Med 35: 1244–1250.
47. Adrie C, Azoulay E, Francais A, Clec'h C, Darques L, et al. (2007) Influence of gender on the outcome of severe sepsis: a reappraisal. Chest 132: 1786–1793.
48. Sakr Y, Elia C, Mascia L, Barberis B, Cardellino S, et al. (2013) The influence of gender on the epidemiology of and outcome from severe sepsis. Crit Care 17: R50.
49. Pietropaoli AP, Glance LG, Oakes D, Fisher SG (2010) Gender differences in mortality in patients with severe sepsis or septic shock. Gend Med 7: 422–437.
50. Glyda Glyda M, Czapiewski W, Karczewski M, Pieta R, Oko A (2011) Influence of donor and recipient gender as well as selected factors on the five-year survival of kidney graft. Pol Przegl Chir 83: 188–195.
51. Nakamura M, Seki G, Iwadoh K, Nakajima I, Fuchinoue S, et al. (2012) Acute kidney injury as defined by the RIFLE criteria is a risk factor for kidney transplant graft failure. Clin Transplant 26: 520–528.
52. Lopes JA, Jorge S (2013) Comparison of RIFLE with and without urine output criteria for acute kidney injury in critically ill patients: a task still not concluded! Crit Care 17: 408.

9

Is the Readmission Rate a Valid Quality Indicator? A Review of the Evidence

Claudia Fischer[1]*, Hester F. Lingsma[1], Perla J. Marang-van de Mheen[2], Dionne S. Kringos[3], Niek S. Klazinga[3], Ewout W. Steyerberg[1]

1 Department of Public Health, Centre for Medical Decision Making, Erasmus MC, Rotterdam, the Netherlands, **2** Department of Medical Decision Making, Leiden University Medical Centre, Leiden, the Netherlands, **3** Department of Public Health, Amsterdam Medical Centre, Amsterdam, the Netherlands

Abstract

Introduction: Hospital readmission rates are increasingly used for both quality improvement and cost control. However, the validity of readmission rates as a measure of quality of hospital care is not evident. We aimed to give an overview of the different methodological aspects in the definition and measurement of readmission rates that need to be considered when interpreting readmission rates as a reflection of quality of care.

Methods: We conducted a systematic literature review, using the bibliographic databases Embase, Medline OvidSP, Web-of-Science, Cochrane central and PubMed for the period of January 2001 to May 2013.

Results: The search resulted in 102 included papers. We found that definition of the context in which readmissions are used as a quality indicator is crucial. This context includes the patient group and the specific aspects of care of which the quality is aimed to be assessed. Methodological flaws like unreliable data and insufficient case-mix correction may confound the comparison of readmission rates between hospitals. Another problem occurs when the basic distinction between planned and unplanned readmissions cannot be made. Finally, the multi-faceted nature of quality of care and the correlation between readmissions and other outcomes limit the indicator's validity.

Conclusions: Although readmission rates are a promising quality indicator, several methodological concerns identified in this study need to be addressed, especially when the indicator is intended for accountability or pay for performance. We recommend investing resources in accurate data registration, improved indicator description, and bundling outcome measures to provide a more complete picture of hospital care.

Editor: Wen-Chih Hank Wu, Providence VA Medical Center and Brown University, United States of America

Funding: This research has been funding by the Dutch Health Care Authority (NZa). The funders had no role in study design, data collection and analysis, decision to publish, or preparation of the manuscript.

Competing Interests: The authors have declared that no competing interests exist.

* Email: c.fischer@erasmusmc.nl

Background

Readmissions cause a high burden to healthcare systems and patients. In the US nearly 20% of Medicare patients are readmitted within 30 days after hospital discharge, associated with an estimated annual cost of $17billion [1]. Readmissions are thought to be related to quality of care, for instance due to postoperative complications. As readmissions vary widely across countries, regions and centers, at least part of them might be avoidable [2–6]. As a consequence, there is a high interest in the readmission rate as an indicator of quality of hospital care. Nevertheless, the actual way this indicator is used in different countries varies widely.

In the US, since 2009 all-cause hospital readmission rates for pneumonia, congestive heart failure, and acute myocardial infarction are publically reported by the Centers for Medicare and Medicaid Services (CMS) [7]. In 2010, the Patient Protection and Affordable Care Act (ACA) introduced the Hospital Readmissions Reduction Program (HRRP), for cost controlling. The program included financial penalties for hospitals having high readmission rates, which will be extended in the coming years [8]. In the UK, readmission rates for specific diseases have been published since 1998 by the National Centre for Health Outcomes Development (NCHOD) to improve quality [9]. It was found that the crude emergency readmission rate had increased from about 8% in 1998 to about 10% in 2006 [9]. In response, the NHS started a new regulation for reimbursement payments in 2011: hospitals receive no reimbursement for emergency readmissions within 30 days of discharge following an elective admission. All other emergency readmissions are reimbursed for only 25% [10]. Since the year 2006 also the Australian government monitors 28-day readmission rates to gain more insight in quality of care [11].

Readmissions are used for different aims, such as cost control or as balancing measure for length of hospital stay or other outcome measures. However, in recent years the focus has primarily been on using it as an easily available measure of the quality of hospital care. Despite its use by policymakers for both quality improvement and cost control, the validity of readmission rates as a measure of quality of hospital care is not evident [12].

However, in order to consider a quality indicator to evaluate care for external purposes it needs to fulfill certain criteria in regards to its reliability and validity. An indicator needs to show relevance, based on its impact on health, its importance for policy and its susceptibility to being influenced by the health care system. The assessment of an indicator needs to be feasible. The data needed to calculate an indicator need to be available, reliable and need to be seen in relation to the burden of reporting. Further, an indicator needs to show scientific soundness [13]. In the case of the readmission rate, this suggests, that readmissions are determined by quality of hospital care, measured by structures and processes. This implies that we are interested in avoidable readmissions.

We aim to give an overview of the different methodological aspects in the definition and measurement of readmission rates that need to be considered when interpreting readmission rates as a reflection of quality of hospital care for external purposes.

Methodology

A systematic computerized literature search was applied in the bibliographic databases Embase, Medline OvidSP, Web-of-Science, Cochrane central and PubMed for the period of 1st January 2001 to 27th May 2013.

With the search terms we aimed to cover quality indicators, quality measurement and readmission. This resulted in the following search strategy, which was adapted for the different bibliographic databases: ('clinical indicator'/de OR 'performance measurement system'/exp OR 'quality control procedures'/de OR 'quality control'/de OR 'medical audit'/de OR (((qualit* OR perform* OR safet* OR governance) NEAR/3 (indicat* OR measure* OR assessment* OR control* OR marker* OR metric*)) OR ((clinical OR medical) NEAR/3 (indicator* OR audit*))):ab,ti) AND ('hospital readmission'/de OR (readmiss* OR rehospital* OR ((re OR return) NEAR/3 (hospital* OR admiss*))):ab,ti).

Studies were included when they were written in English, focused on methodological aspects of readmission rates as a quality indicator for hospital care and full texts were available. We included only studies in major disease fields. Hence, studies focusing on rare diseases, just describing readmission rates over time or using readmissions as outcome measures of interventions were excluded.

Of the references identified in the literature search, titles and abstracts were screened and articles that did not meet the inclusion criteria were excluded. The full text of the remaining potentially eligible articles was reviewed to assess whether they should be included. In case of doubt, the article was discussed among the authors and if necessary, an independent researcher was consulted.

We discuss the methodological aspects that emerged from the literature review that are important for the validity of the readmission rates as an indicator of quality of care.

Results

Our search strategy resulted in 1609 unique references of which titles and abstracts were screened. Based on title and abstract 1189 studies were excluded. Of the remaining 420 articles another 318 were excluded based on full text review (Figure 1). We provide a detailed description of the included studies in the appendix S1, and below we discuss the most important findings.

The context in which readmission rates are used

Prior to using the readmission rate as a measure of quality of care, the context in which the indicator will be used needs to be clearly defined. The rationale for using readmission rates is one aspect of this context. The readmission rate can be used with the primary aim to improve quality of care or rather for reasons of cost control. Next, specification of the clinical processes of which quality of care is assessed is important. Currently, readmission rates are mostly intended to measure quality of care in hospitals. Which implies that the risk of being readmitted is determined by the quality of care delivered during the hospital stay. Yet, literature shows that the conditions after patients' discharge, like the presence of a social network after discharge [14] as well as patients' capacity for managing their own care, influence the likelihood of being readmitted [15,16]. As a result, hospitals pay attention to improving transitional care [17–24], for instance by patient education to prepare the patient for discharge and to coordinate outpatient follow up [23]. Although such a transition phase may help, the actual post-discharge phase is not really in a hospital's reach anymore. Another example are readmissions in chronic diseases, such as heart failure. These patients are readmitted often because of their comorbidities or because their condition becomes too severe to be treated by the general practitioner, irrespective from the quality of delivered care during their hospital stay [1]. Hence, the quality of care processes captured by readmission rates will often be broader than only in-hospital care [25].

In summary, using readmission rates as a quality measure requires a clear definition of the context, including the rationale of measuring readmissions, the related care processes and the patient groups.

Methodological aspects

Based on the literature we defined several methodological aspects that need to be considered when using the readmission rates as a quality indicator (table 1). These range from fundamental issues like the definition and the effect of competing outcomes, to more practical issues as the possibility to adjust for case-mix and the data reliability. These issues and their effects will be described in the next paragraphs. In the final paragraph we will focus on studies that have specifically tested the validity of readmission rates as a quality indicator.

Indicator definition

Type of readmission. The definition of readmissions determines the number of readmissions that will be counted (numerator). Planned procedures, such as staged operations, are readmissions that are not determined by quality of care and therefore should not be included in the numerator of the quality indicator [26,27]. However, this basic distinction is not always made [28]. Hence, capture quality of care related readmissions requires a more specific definition (such as disease specific or emergency readmissions) rather than all-cause readmissions. [29].

A frequently suggested alternative is to count unplanned readmission rates. However, not all unplanned readmissions are a result of poor quality of care as certain complications cannot be avoided. Research has shown that just about 25% of all readmissions are avoidable/preventable. Therefore, ideally, the addition on whether a readmission was avoidable/preventable. Although high variation in overall readmission rate can be observed, this is not the case for the rate of preventable readmissions [2,29]. Therefore, ideally it is defined, whether a readmission was avoidable/preventable (through proper care

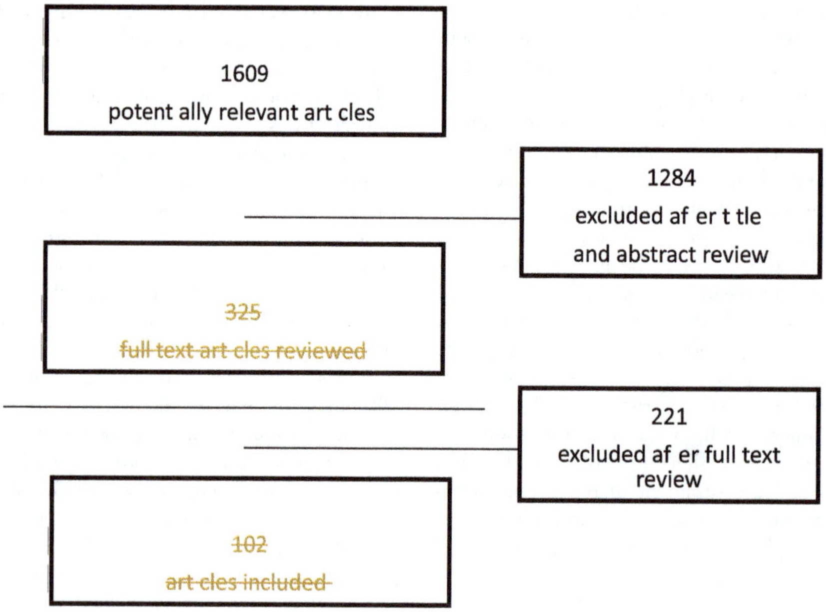

Figure 1. Flow chart of inclusion process.

delivery) [28,30] but the judgment on the preventability of a readmission remains subjective [2].

Time window. The time window after the index admission in which admissions are regarded as readmissions is not consistently defined in the literature. The indicator is generally calculated on basis of readmissions within one month (28 days UK, 31 days USA) regardless of the patient group and condition [28,31–33]. When choosing a time window, it needs to be considered that a too short time window might miss related readmissions while a large one increases the likelihood of included admissions unrelated to the index admission. For example, in cancer surgery a longer time frame would allow to provide a better overview of actual costs, but it would also include readmissions due to disease progression instead of poor quality of surgery [25]. Clearly, the type of disease the patient was originally treated for is largely influencing the optimal timeframe [32]. Therefore the timeframe for readmissions should be defined per disease.

The effect of competing outcomes

Association with (in-hospital) mortality. Mortality can be seen as a competing endpoint for readmissions: patients who die will not be readmitted [34,35]. Therefore patients who died during their hospital stay need to be excluded from the denominator of the readmission rate. Further, hospitals with high 30-day in-hospital mortality rates are not necessarily outliers on the readmission rate as well [36]. Research showed that the link between high readmission rates and mortality rates on hospital level is limited. A "modest" inverse relationship was merely found for heart failure patients, and no relation could be observed for pneumonia and acute myocardial infarction, suggesting that the two indicators measure different aspects of quality of care, which are not strongly related [37]. Therefore different outcome measures, such as the readmission rate and the mortality rate should be brought in relation with each other to gain insight in total hospital performance [36,37].

Association with length of in hospital stay. Length of stay is generally decreasing, partly because of efficiency gaining interventions, such as a "just-in-time bed availability system" to increase the bed turnover ratio [38,39]. Research suggests a link between length of stay and the risk of being readmitted [39–45]. For each day shorter in hospital, a 6% increase in likelihood of readmission was found [40]. Other studies fail to confirm this link [24,42,46–50], which might be due to inappropriate adjustment for disease severity [41,51].

Case mix adjustment

The likelihood that a patient is readmitted is not only affected by quality of care but also by characteristics of the patient. Between-hospital differences in readmission rates may be caused by differences in patient population and therefore readmission rates need to be adjusted for patient characteristics. Although many case-mix adjustment models for readmissions have been developed, there is little consensus on which patient characteristics affect the likelihood of a readmission [27,52]. Numerous studies, varying in their methodology, geographical characteristics, patient groups and considered variables, find different factors that increase the risk of re-admission. In general, two patient groups seem to be at a high risk of being readmitted: the sickest and poorest patients [2,20,51,53,54]. However, these factors are often not included as standard variables in case-mix adjustment models, as these models are often based on administrative data and therefore miss detailed clinical information.

In a review that evaluated 30 validated readmission risk prediction models, the authors concluded that most models had poor predictive ability. Almost all studies had c-statistics less than 0.70 [55], possibly due to missing demographic or clinical variables. In a more recent paper, the prediction model reached a higher predictive ability (c-statistic = 0.80) [41]. The authors concluded however that information on demographics, SES, prior utilization and diagnosis still had restricted predictive power [41]. Thus, current research provides limited guidance on which variables should be included in models to adjust for case-mix [41,55–57].

Table 1. Overview of methodological aspects challenging the validity of readmission rates for benchmarking.

	methodological aspect	problem	potential solution
Clinical setting	readmission rates are thought to reflect quality of hospital care (17–24)	care after discharge also influences readmission(14, 25)	clear definition of the indicator, the patient group and the clinical setting(hospital care, integrated care) aimed to measure increase insight in influence of post discharge phase/social factors on readmissions(14) relate readmission to other outcome measures such as mortality, emergency department and observation service use (14) evaluate home health care/nursing home information (15)
indicator definition			
Type of readmission	missing distinction between planned/ unplanned procedures (2, 26–29)	inclusion of readmissions unrelated to quality of care into the numerator (26) leads to overestimation of the rate of readmission (69)	specify definition of the indicator (27, 28, 31), define disease-specific/emergency readmissions instead of overall readmissions (2) include indication on preventability/avoidability of readmission in definition (2, 28–30)
time window	no consistent definition of the time window in which admission is considered as readmission(28) generally 28–31 day time frame used regardless of patient group/condition(31–33)	although 30 days seems generally sufficient (31, 33), for certain conditions it is a too short time window, while for others it increases the likelihood of including admissions unrelated to index admission(25, 32)	evaluate time frame based on condition under evaluation
effect of competing outcomes			
association with (in-hospital) mortality	a group of patients who receive poor quality of care are not readmitted, because they die or recover nevertheless (31, 34, 35)	not excluding patient who died from the denominator leads to a potential underestimation of rate of qoc related readmission	exclude patients who died during hospital stay from denominator link hospital data with death statistics, exclude patients from denominator who die outside hospital relate the readmissions with mortality rate in order to understand total hospital performance (36, 37)
association with length of in-hospital mortality	a decreased length of hospital stay increases readmissions (38, 39)	the exact mechanism with readmission is inconclusive (24, 39, 40, 42–50)	further research to understand the mechanism between length of stay and readmission
case mix adjustment using administrative data vs. clinical data	no consensus on which patient characteristics affect readmission likelihood(27, 52) two high risk groups defined: the sickest and the poorest (2, 51, 53, 54)	these factors are not standard variables in risk prediction models as often not available in administrative databases(36) current risk prediction models perform moderately (40)(39, 55–57)	apply proper case-mix adjustment for patient characteristics including socioeconomic status and disease severity(39, 51) further research on risk prediction models including linkage of primary care data and socioeconomic information
data reliability			
missing readmissions to other institutions	patients are readmitted to institutions other than index hospital (25, 35)	patients cannot always be followed between centers; only readmissions to same institutions are measured assessing "same hospital" readmissions, might be underestimation of the real number of readmissions(25)	further research on the proportion of patients readmitted to other hospitals than index hospital unique patient information to follow patients between centers
coding	coding practice influences the validity readmission rates(30, 58, 77–84) no conclusion on how to register readmissions potentially related to qoc in reliable way (2, 59–61)	missing distinction between planned/ unplanned procedures leads to overestimation of real readmission variation in coding leads to biased comparison between hospitals	increase investment in performance measurement systems(16) research on data reliability(28) standardized data registry (electronic data systems)(16, 62) engagement of the provider in measurement, analysis and interpretation of the indicator(16, 64)
completeness and accuracy of data source	reliable data collection systems are lacking(38) Readmissions are mainly calculated based on administrative data (16, 63) administrative data suffer from inaccuracy, like non-exact/incomplete registration of variables not relevant for financial concerns(39, 40, 64–69)	incomplete registration may lead to over/underestimation of real readmission inaccurate indication of readmissions related to qoc may lead to overestimation of readmissions (64, 65)	aim for minimum data set with complete registration registration of unique patient identifying information to enhance possibility for linking data(such as pharmacy data)(70) enhancing linkage opportunities increases possibility for better case-mix adjustment
validity of readmission rates as a quality measure	no gold standard on how to assess qoc in the literature huge variation in conclusions in regard to the validity of the readmission indicator (71–113)	potentially invalid conclusions on qoc	above described methodological conditions need to be taken into account when further investigating readmissions as a quality indicator additional data gathering for further investigation of outlier hospitals(93)

Data reliability

Missing readmissions to other institutions. Not all patients are readmitted to the same center where they had their index admission. This is mainly due to the centralization of complex operations in tertiary centers, such as in oncology [25]. When patients unexpectedly develop complications and are readmitted in their local center, they are not captured when only readmissions to the "same hospital" are counted [25]. Missing these patients leads to an underestimation of the true overall readmission rate.

Coding. The coding practice within a hospital has an essential impact on the validity of readmission rate as a quality indicator [58]. The way a "planned" procedure is defined is crucial for the comparability between hospitals. Ideally a planned readmission is coded in the registration system, for example, with an additional coding element "staged" at the index admission, which would indicate that a follow-up procedure is planned [59].

Urgent readmissions are sometimes considered as a potential proxy for the relatively subjective 'avoidable readmissions', as these are coded, for example an admission through the ER. Although low urgent readmission rates showed to be related to low avoidable readmission rates [60] it was shown that the "avoidability" of urgent readmissions also significantly varied by the time from discharge, with early readmissions being more likely to be avoidable [2,61].

Other causes for biased comparisons between hospitals are the different and unspecific definitions of the type of readmissions assessed, and variation in coding between hospitals. It is essential who is in charge of the coding process. For example administrative staff at the department or hospital level, the treating clinician, or specialized data coders. The variation in coding practice may affect both the readmission rates and the case-mix variables.

Completeness and accuracy of data source. Electronic health records and health information exchange networks result in more accurate and complete clinical data [62]. The major information source to calculate the readmission rate is administrative data. The advantage of administrative data is that this data is standard available and patient journeys can be followed (within hospitals) [63]. Nevertheless, one major limitation of administrative data is the data inaccuracy [64], which includes the non-exact or incomplete registration of variables that are not relevant for financial concerns [38,40,41]. Research showed that to a certain degree administrative data captures similar information compared to medical records, for example on all-cause readmissions [65–68]. However more specific information, like the identification of unplanned readmissions or index procedure related readmissions, showed to be more difficult to extract [66,69]. An accurate indication of whether a readmission is a part of treatment or due to a cancelled procedure and not a readmission related to a quality of care problem, would enhance the reliability of the data source [64,65].

The case-mix adjustment variables that have been investigated so far are most often present in administrative databases. However, clinical information such as disease severity is often lacking limiting case-mix adjustment possibilities. The addition of a unique patient identifier across different databases would enhance the possibility for linking data, such as pharmacy data [70] or clinical data. This would largely improve the possibilities for more precise definitions of readmissions and better case-mix adjustment.

Validity of readmission rates as a quality measure

No gold standard exists on how to assess quality of care. Usually different hospital structures and processes and their relation with patient outcomes are measured. The different definitions and proxies used in studies to quantify quality of hospital care influence whether an association between the readmission rate and 'quality' is found. For example, we found studies that relate readmissions to hospital volume, but neither can be regarded as a 'gold standard' of hospital quality.

Furthermore, the methodological aspects we discussed have a potential influence on the validity of the readmission rates as a quality indicator. These may contribute to the huge variation in conclusions with regard to the validity of readmission rates found in the literature. Different studies in different patient groups and conditions come to the conclusion that lower quality of hospital care is linked to a higher number of readmissions [71–94]. Especially safety-related events (such as postoperative complications) show a relation with readmissions [71,95]. Rosen and colleagues, who evaluated the correlation between patient safety indicators and readmissions, showed that patients who experienced a patient safety event had an increased risk of readmission [71]. Nevertheless, there are also studies that are inconclusive [96–101], show an inverse relationship [102,103] or no relationship at all between readmission rate and in-hospital quality of care [98,104–113]. Analysis of additionally collected data could help to gain insight into outlier hospitals in order to understand driving mechanisms behind high readmission rates [93].

Discussion

This review aimed to summarize the methodological aspects that need to be considered when using the readmission rate as a measure for quality of hospital care for external purposes. We found that the validity of readmission rates as a quality indicator is influenced by the clinical process that is assessed, the indicator definition, the extend of case-mix correction, the effect of competing outcomes and the data reliability. Ignoring or poorly handling these aspects may lead to a biased estimation of the overall readmission rate and a biased comparison of readmission rates between hospitals. As a result of variance in handling these methodological threats, studies on the validity of readmission rates as a quality indicator reach conflicting conclusions. We conclude that given the limitations of readmission rates, they need to be used with caution as a measure of in-hospital quality, even more when used as a tool for a pay for performance scheme.

Some of the discussed factors concerning the readmission rate could in principal be improved by investing resources in accurate data registry and refinements of indicator description. For instance, by using unique patient identifiers to follow patients across centers. That would help to avoid missing readmissions to other institutions. Another option would be to flag planned admissions, which are a part of the treatment plan or due to cancelled procedures, to measure just the quality of care related readmissions.

Other problems, such as the competing endpoint "mortality" are more complex. Patients who died in hospital need to be excluded from the patient group forming the denominator to calculate the readmission rate, as they are not at risk any more to be readmitted. These deaths are captured in the mortality rate. Therefore it is essential to combine outcome in order to provide a more complete picture of the quality of hospital care.

Nevertheless there are theoretical considerations whether a readmission is an indication of bad quality of care. First, a readmission is obviously a more positive outcome than dying. Secondly, if there is for example a chance of six percent that a complication occurs after discharge, it would mean that 100 patients need to be admitted longer, to avoid a complication in six patients [114]. It can be questioned whether by a longer length of hospital stay a complication really can be avoided or only detected at an earlier stage. It is also possible to inform the patient on the risk of developing a complication and decide together how to continue. Furthermore, it needs to be taken into account that readmissions are not always solely determined by quality of hospital care. For certain diseases, like heart failure, the patient's condition is the major driver behind repeated admissions. Patients with low socioeconomic status, elderly and patients with co-morbidities are at high risk of getting readmitted. Therefore case-mix adjustment is essential. Furthermore, the role of facilities outside the hospital and after the 30day time window, like community services, need to be involved in the conceptual framework of readmissions. When aiming to improve quality of care (in and outpatient) increased integration and cooperation between primary and secondary care is needed.

The literature study revealed inconclusive results for some methodological aspects, such as the relation with length of stay, or patient characteristics. The studies we assessed investigated different patient populations and often were based on hospital administrative data. A recent high quality study which was not included in our review investigated surgical readmissions of 479,471 patients from 3004 hospitals. The authors found that higher surgical volume was significantly related with lower composite readmission rates (upper volume quartile 12.7% vs. lower volume quartile 16.8% $P<0.0001$), and hospitals with the lowest surgical mortality rates had significantly lower readmission rates (lower mortality quartile 13.3% vs. upper mortality quartile 14.2% $P<0.0001$). But high adherence to surgical process measures was only marginally linked with lower readmission rates (highest quartile vs. lowest quartile, 13.1% vs. 13.6%; $P=0.02$), showing that it is still unclear whether low readmission rates are the result of good quality [115].

Furthermore, the risk of getting readmitted is also varying between patient groups and conditions. This supports the idea that outcome measures, like the readmission rate, are not a one size fits all measure. Even if quality of hospital care and the transition phase can potentially be improved, readmissions might be a more applicable measure for certain diseases than for others. For chronic diseases, where planned admissions are part of treatment strategies, readmissions are a less suitable performance measure. At least not until generally used data systems can identify planned admissions with high certainty. It requires clinical knowledge to determine whether (avoidable) readmissions may theoretically represent poor quality of care for specific diseases. Consequently more research is needed to build reliable algorithms to identify avoidable readmissions.

In sum, avoidable readmissions are of high relevance, as they are an adverse event to patients and family and are a high financial burden for healthcare systems. The assessment of the indicator shows difficulties, as the indicator definition is often not explicit enough to identify readmissions related to quality of care (avoidable readmissions). The data used to calculate the indicator is mainly administrative data, which generally includes incomplete and inaccurate data elements and lacks clinical information. Furthermore, in many countries readmissions to other institutions cannot be followed. Readmission rates are influenced also by other factors than quality of hospital care, which include length of stay, (in-hospital) mortality and patient characteristics. The magnitude of influence is partly not know as data is missing to investigate the association (e.g. no post discharge mortality, no clinical characteristics). Further, the scientific evidence of the indicator is limited, as existing research shows conflicting results with regard to the influence of quality of hospital care on the readmission rate (see Appendix S1). This, however, could be related to the prior mentioned methodological aspects that are variously.

Using outcome measures externally to measure and compare hospital performance has consequences. When financial consequences are linked to the outcome, unintended effects could occur. For example, hospitals may try to reduce their readmission to escape the penalty of exceeding the readmission rate by lowering admissions, moving readmissions after the 30-day window, or risk-avoidance in regards to high risk groups. These gaming efforts might reduce the focus on the actual intention: improving quality of hospital care.

A measure used for external purposes should be underpinned with solid evidence for its validity. However, the link between readmissions and the quality of hospital care seems not to be fully explained yet. Still, this does not imply that there is no room for improvement for hospitals in their readmission rate and the indicator could not be useful for internal use. Research should continue to gain insight in the driving mechanisms behind readmissions for the different conditions to improve our understanding how the readmission rate is a part of the quality of hospital care picture. In addition, the readmission rate needs to be brought into relation with other outcome indicators, and hence considered as part of a bundle, to understand all aspects of hospital performance [36].

The methodological aspects we identified need to be considered when using readmission rates as quality indicator. The use of readmission rates for external quality purposes, such as for pay for performance requires strict methodological criteria to avoid confounding. At its current state the rate of readmission does not fulfill the methodological requirements of a reliable and valid indicator. Therefore the indicator should not be used for external purposes. As this is nevertheless currently happening, readmission rates should be interpreted with great caution.

Author Contributions

Conceived and designed the experiments: CF NK DK HL. Performed the experiments: CF HL. Analyzed the data: CF HL. Contributed reagents/materials/analysis tools: CF HL PM ES DK NK. Wrote the paper: CF HL PM ES DK NK.

References

1. Jencks SF, Williams MV, Coleman EA (2009) Rehospitalizations among patients in the Medicare fee-for-service program. N Engl J Med. 360(14): 1418–28.
2. Van Walraven C, Bennett C, Jennings A, Austin PC, Forster AJ (2011) Proportion of hospital readmissions deemed avoidable: A systematic review. CMAJ. 183(7): E391–E402.
3. Krumholz HM, Merrill AR, Schone EM, Schreiner GC, Chen J, et al. (2009) Patterns of Hospital Performance in Acute Myocardial Infarction and Heart Failure 30-Day Mortality and Readmission. Circulation-Cardiovascular Quality and Outcomes. 2(5):407–13.
4. Jensen PH, Webster E, Witt J (2009) Hospital type and patient outcomes: an empirical examination using AMI readmission and mortality records. Health Econ. 18(12):1440–60.

5. Bernheim SM, Grady JN, Lin ZQ, Wang Y, Wang YF, et al. (2010) National Patterns of Risk-Standardized Mortality and Readmission for Acute Myocardial Infarction and Heart Failure Update on Publicly Reported Outcomes Measures Based on the 2010 Release. Circulation-Cardiovascular Quality and Outcomes. 3(5):459–67.
6. Schiotz M, Price M, Frolich A, Sogaard J, Kristensen JK, et al. (2011) Something is amiss in Denmark: a comparison of preventable hospitalisations and readmissions for chronic medical conditions in the Danish Healthcare system and Kaiser Permanente. BMC Health Serv Res. 11: 347.
7. Axon RN, Williams MV (2011) Hospital readmission as an accountability measure. JAMA. 2;305(5):504–5.
8. Desai AS, Stevenson LW (2012) Rehospitalization for heart failure: predict or prevent? Circulation. 24;126(4):501–6.
9. Department of Health. Emergency readmission rates (2008) London: Department of Health.
10. Department of Health. The operating framework. 2010. Available: https://www.gov.uk/government/uploads/system/uploads/attachment_data/file/151906/dh_122736.pdf.pdf. Accessed 2013 July 8.
11. Australian Government. Australian Institute of Health and Welfare. National Healthcare Agreement: PI 23-Unplanned hospital readmission rates, 2013 QS. Available: http://meteor.aihw.gov.au/content/index.phtml/itemId/507456. Accessed 2013 July 11.
12. Gu Q, Koenig L, Faerberg J, Steinberg CR, Vaz C, et al. (2014) The medicare hospital readmissions reduction program: potential unintended consequences for hospitals serving vulnerable populations. Health Serv Res. 49(3):818–37.
13. Mattke S, Kelley E, Scherer P, Hurst J, Lapetra MLG, et al. (2006) "Health Care Quality Indicators Project Initial Indicators Report", OECD Health Working Papers. Paris.
14. Kangovi S, Grande D (2011) Hospital readmissions - Not just a measure of quality. J Am Med Assoc. 306(16):1796–7.
15. Spector WD, Mutter R, Owens P, Limcangco R (2012) Thirty-day, all-cause readmissions for elderly patients who have an injury-related inpatient stay. Med Care. 50(10):863–9.
16. Forster AJ, van Walraven C (2012) The use of quality indicators to promote accountability in health care: the good, the bad, and the ugly. Open Med. 6(2):e75–9.
17. Shepperd S, Lannin NA, Clemson LM, McCluskey A, Cameron ID (2013) Discharge planning from hospital to home. Cochrane Database Syst Rev. 1: CD000313.
18. Lambrinou E, Kalogirou F, Lamnisos D, Sourtzi P (2012) Effectiveness of heart failure management programmes with nurse-led discharge planning in reducing re-admissions: A systematic review and meta-analysis. Int J Nurs Stud. 49(5):610–24.
19. Wong FKY, Ho MM, Yeung S, Tam SK, Chow SK (2011) Effects of a health-social partnership transitional program on hospital readmission: A randomized controlled trial. Soc Sci Med. 73(7):960–9.
20. Demir E, Chaussalet T, Adeyemi S, Toffa S (2012) Profiling hospitals based on emergency readmission: A multilevel transition modelling approach. Comput Methods Programs Biomed. 108(2):487–99.
21. Jha AK, Orav EJ, Epstein AM (2009) Public reporting of discharge planning and rates of readmissions. New Engl J Med. 361(27):2637–45.
22. Benbassat J, Taragin MI (2013) The effect of clinical interventions on hospital readmissions: a meta-review of published meta-analyses. Isr J Health Policy Res. 2(1):1.
23. Burke RE, Kripalani S, Vasilevskis EE, Schnipper JL (2013) Moving beyond readmission penalties: Creating an ideal process to improve transitional care. J Hosp Med. 8(2):102–9.
24. Chan FW, Wong FY, Yam CH, Cheung WL, Wong EL, et al. (2011) Risk factors of hospitalization and readmission of patients with COPD in Hong Kong population: analysis of hospital admission records. BMC Health Serv Res. 11: 186.
25. Rochefort MM, Tomlinson JS (2012) Unexpected Readmissions After Major Cancer Surgery. An Evaluation of Readmissions as a Quality-of-Care Indicator. Surg Oncol Clin North Am. 21(3):397–405.
26. McCormack R, Michels R, Ramos N, Hutzler L, Slover JD, et al. (2013) Thirty-day readmission rates as a measure of quality: causes of readmission after orthopedic surgeries and accuracy of administrative data. J Healthc Manag. 58(1):64–76; discussion -7.
27. Brooke BS, De Martino RR, Girotti M, Dimick JB, Goodney PP (2012) Developing strategies for predicting and preventing readmissions in vascular surgery. J Vasc Surg. 56(2):556–62.
28. Fischer C, Anema HA, Klazinga NS (2012) The validity of indicators for assessing quality of care: a review of the European literature on hospital readmission rate. Eur J Public Health. 22(4):484–91.
29. Van Walraven C, Jennings A, Forster AJ (2012) A meta-analysis of hospital 30-day avoidable readmission rates. J Eval Clin Pract. 18(6):1211–8.
30. Courtney EDJ, Ankrett S, McCollum PT (2003) 28-Day emergency surgical re-admission rates as a clinical indicator of performance. Ann R Coll Surg Engl. 85(2):75–8.
31. Rumball-Smith J, Hider P (2009) The validity of readmission rate as a marker of the quality of hospital care, and a recommendation for its definition. New Zealand Med J. 122(1289).
32. Demir E, Chaussalet TJ, Xie H, Millard PH (2008) Emergency readmission criterion: a technique for determining the emergency readmission time window. IEEE Trans Inf Technol Biomed. 12(5):644–9.
33. Maurer PP, Ballmer PE (2004) Hospital readmissions - are they predictable and avoidable? Swiss Medical Weekly. 134(41–42):606–11.
34. Gheorghiade M, Vaduganathan M, Fonarow GC, Bonow RO (2013) Rehospitalization for heart failure: Problems and perspectives. J Am Coll Cardiol. 61(4):391–403.
35. Grocott MPW (2010) Monitoring surgical outcomes: How and why? Curr Anaesth Crit Care. 21(3):129–36.
36. Almoudaris AM, Burns EM, Bottle A, Aylin P, Darzi A, et al. (2013) Single measures of performance do not reflect overall institutional quality in colorectal cancer surgery. Gut. 62(3):423–9.
37. Krumholz HM, Lin Z, Keenan PS, Chen J, Ross JS, et al. (2013) Relationship between hospital readmission and mortality rates for patients hospitalized with acute myocardial infarction, heart failure, or pneumonia. JAMA. 309(6):587–93.
38. Basu A, Howell R, Gopinath D (2010) Clinical performance indicators: Intolerance for variety? Int J Health Care Qual Assur. 23(4):436–49.
39. Heggestad T (2002) Do hospital length of stay and staffing ratio affect elderly patients' risk of readmission? - A nation-wide study of Norwegian hospitals. Health Services Research. 37(3):647–65.
40. Kaboli PJ, Go OT, Hockenberry J, Glasgow JM, Johnson SR, et al. (2012) Associations between reduced hospital length of stay and 30-day readmission rate and mortality: 14-year experience in 129 veterans affairs hospitals. Ann Intern Med. 157(12):837–45.
41. Shulan M, Gao K, Moore CD (2013) Predicting 30-day all-cause hospital readmissions. Health Care Manag Sci. 16(2):167–75.
42. Kramer AA, Higgins TL, Zimmerman JE (2013) The association between ICU readmission rate and patient outcomes. Crit Care Med. 41(1):24–33.
43. Ahmed J, Khan S, Lim M, Chandrasekaran TV, MacFie J (2012) Enhanced recovery after surgery protocols - compliance and variations in practice during routine colorectal surgery. Colorectal Disease. 14(9):1045–51.
44. Dobrzanska L, Newell R (2006) Readmissions: A primary care examination of reasons for readmission of older people and possible readmission risk factors. J Clin Nurs. 15(5):599–606.
45. Schneider EB, Hyder O, Brooke BS, Efron J, Cameron JL, et al. (2012) Patient readmission and mortality after colorectal surgery for colon cancer: Impact of length of stay relative to other clinical factors. J Am Coll Surg. 214(4):390–8.
46. Dunlay SM, Weston SA, Killian JM, Bell MR, Jaffe AS, et al. (2012) Thirty-day rehospitalizations after acute myocardial infarction: A cohort study. Ann Intern Med. 157(1):11–8.
47. Dallal RM, Trang A (2012) Analysis of perioperative outcomes, length of hospital stay, and readmission rate after gastric bypass. Surg Endosc Interv Tech. 26(3):754–8.
48. Lau ACW, Yam LYC, Poon E (2001) Hospital re-admission in patients with acute exacerbation of chronic obstructive pulmonary disease. Respiratory Medicine. 95(11):876–84.
49. Kiran RP, Delaney CP, Senagore AJ, Steel M, Garafalo T, et al. (2004) Outcomes and prediction of hospital readmission after intestinal surgery. J Am Coll Surg. 198(6):877–83.
50. Kociol RD, Liang L, Hernandez AF, Curtis LH, Heidenreich PA, et al. (2013) Are we targeting the right metric for heart failure? Comparison of hospital 30-day readmission rates and total episode of care inpatient days. Am Heart J.
51. Johnson T, Bardhan J, Odwazny R, Harting B, Skarupski K, et al. (2012) Hospital care may not affect the risk of readmission. Qual Manag Health Care. 21(2):68–73.
52. Van Walraven C, Wong J, Hawken S, Forster AJ (2012) Comparing methods to calculate hospital-specific rates of early death or urgent readmission. CMAJ. 184(15): E810–E7.
53. Khawaja FJ, Shah ND, Lennon RJ, Slusser JP, Alkatib AA, et al. (2012) Factors associated with 30-day readmission rates after percutaneous coronary intervention. Arch Intern Med. 172(2):112–7.
54. Goldfield NI, McCullough EC, Hughes JS, Tang AM, Eastman B, et al. (2008) Identifying potentially preventable readmissions. Health Care Financ Rev. 30(1):75–91.
55. Kansagara D, Englander H, Salanitro A, Kagen D, Theobald C, Kripalani S (2011) Readmission risk modeling: A systematic review. J Gen Intern Med. 26: S125.
56. Correll PK, Xuan W, Williamson M, Sundararajan V, Ringland C, et al. (2007) Reattendance at hospital for asthma in two Australian states, 2000–2003. Respirology. 12(2):220–6.
57. Giamouzis G, Kalogeropoulos A, Georgiopoulou V, Laskar S, Smith AL, et al. (2011) Hospitalization epidemic in patients with heart failure: Risk factors, risk prediction, knowledge gaps, and future directions. J Card Fail. 17(1):54–75.
58. Cram P, Ibrahim SA, Lu X, Wolf BR (2012) Impact of alternative coding schemes on incidence rates of key complications after total hip arthroplasty: a risk-adjusted analysis of a national data set. Geriatr orthop surg rehabil. 3(1):17–26.
59. Hannan EL, Zhong Y, Lahey SJ, Culliford AT, Gold JP, et al. (2011) 30-Day readmissions after coronary artery bypass graft surgery in New York State. JACC Cardiovasc Interventions. 4(5):569–76.

60. van Walraven C, Austin PC, Forster AJ (2012) Urgent readmission rates can be used to infer differences in avoidable readmission rates between hospitals. Journal of Clinical Epidemiology. 65(10):1124–30.
61. Bianco A, Mole A, Nobile CGA, Di Giuseppe G, Pileggi C, et al. (2012) Hospital Readmission Prevalence and Analysis of Those Potentially Avoidable in Southern Italy. Plos One. 7(11).
62. Ben-Assuli O, Shabtai I, Leshno M (2013) The impact of EHR and HIE on reducing avoidable admissions: controlling main differential diagnoses. BMC Med Inf Decis Mak. 13:49.
63. Holt PJE, Poloniecki JD, Hofman D, Hinchliffe RJ, Loftus IM, et al. (2010) Re-interventions, Readmissions and Discharge Destination: Modern Metrics for the Assessment of the Quality of Care. Eur J Vasc Endovasc Surg. 39(1):49–54.
64. Amin BY, Schairer W, Tu TH, Ames CP, Berven S, et al. (2012) Improving benchmarking in spine surgery: Suggested modifications of the UHC algorithm for calculating readmission rates following spine surgery. Neurosurgery. 71(2): E575–E6.
65. Lindenauer PK, Normand SLT, Drye EE, Lin Z, Goodrich K, et al. (2011) Development, validation, and results of a measure of 30-day readmission following hospitalization for pneumonia. J Hosp Med. 6(3):142–50.
66. Sellers MM, Merkow RP, Halverson A, Hinami K, Kelz RR, et al. (2013) Validation of New Readmission Data in the American College of Surgeons National Surgical Quality Improvement Program. Journal of the American College of Surgeons. 216(3):420–7.
67. Krumholz HM, Wang Y, Mattera JA, Wang YF, Han LF, et al. (2006) An administrative claims model suitable for profiling hospital performance based on 30-day mortality rates among patients with heart failure. Circulation. 113(13):1693–701.
68. Wallmann R, Llorca J, Gomez-Acebo I, Ortega AC, Roldan FR, et al. (2013) Prediction of 30-day cardiac-related-emergency-readmissions using simple administrative hospital data. Int J Cardiol. 164(2):193–200.
69. Adeyemo D, Radley S (2007) Unplanned general surgical re-admissions - How many, which patients and why? Ann R Coll Surg Engl. 89(4):363–7.
70. Parker JP, McCombs JS, Graddy EA (2003) Can pharmacy data improve prediction of hospital outcomes? Comparisons with a diagnosis-based comorbidity measure. Med Care. 41(3):407–19.
71. Rosen AK, Loveland S, Shin M, Shwartz M, Hanchate A, et al. (2013) Examining the Impact of the AHRQ Patient Safety Indicators (PSIs) on the Veterans Health Administration: The Case of Readmissions. Med Care. 51(1):37–44.
72. Mokhtar SA, El. Mahalli AA, Al-Mulla S, Al-Hussaini R (2012) Study of the relation between quality of inpatient care and early readmission for diabetic patients at a hospital in the eastern province of Saudi Arabia. East Mediterr Health J. 18(5):474–9.
73. Kergoat MJ, Latour J, Lebel P, Leclerc BS, Leduc N, et al. (2012) Quality-of-care processes in geriatric assessment units: principles, practice, and outcomes. J Am Med Dir Assoc. 13(5):459–63.
74. Auerbach AD, Hilton JF, Maselli J, Pekow PS, Rothberg MB (2009) Shop for quality or volume? Volume, quality, and outcomes of coronary artery bypass surgery. Ann Intern Med. 150(10): 696-704+W-123.
75. Stukel TA, Alter DA, Schull MJ, Ko DT, Li P (2010) Association between hospital cardiac management and outcomes for acute myocardial infarction patients. Med Care. 48(2):157–65.
76. Chen JY, Ma Q, Chen H, Yermilov I (2012) New bundled world: quality of care and readmission in diabetes patients. J Diabetes Sci Technol. 6(3):563–71.
77. Weber RS, Lewis CM, Eastman SD, Hanna EY, Akiwumi O, et al. (2010) Quality and performance indicators in an Academic Department of Head and Neck Surgery. Arch Otolaryngol Head Neck Surg. 136(12):1212–8.
78. Kent TS, Sachs TE, Callery MP, Vollmer Jr CM (2011) Readmission after major pancreatic resection: A necessary evil? J Am Coll Surg. 213(4):515–23.
79. Barbieri CE, Lee B, Cookson MS, Bingham J, Clark PE, et al. (2007) Association of procedure volume with radical cystectomy outcomes in a nationwide database. Journal of Urology. 178(4):1418–21.
80. Chung ES, Guo L, Casey DE Jr, Bartone C, Menon S, et al. (2008) Relationship of a quality measure composite to clinical outcomes for patients with heart failure. Am J Med Qual. 23(3):168–75.
81. Judge A, Chard J, Learmonth I, Dieppe P (2006) The effects of surgical volumes and training centre status on outcomes following total joint replacement: analysis of the Hospital Episode Statistics for England. J Public Health (Oxf). 28(2):116–24.
82. Boulding W, Glickman SW, Manary MP, Schulman KA, Staelin R (2011) Relationship between patient satisfaction with inpatient care and hospital readmission within 30 days. Am J Managed Care. 17(1):41–8.
83. Youn YJ, Yoo BS, Lee JW, Kim JY, Han SW, et al. (2012) Treatment performance measures affect clinical outcomes in patients with acute systolic heart failure: Report from the Korean Heart Failure Registry. Circ J. 76(5):1151–8.
84. VanSuch M, Naessens JM, Stroebel RJ, Huddleston JM, Williams AR (2006) Effect of discharge instructions on readmission of hospitalised patients with heart failure: Do all of the Joint Commission on Accreditation of Healthcare Organizations heart failure core measures reflect better care? Qual Saf Health Care. 15(6):414–7.
85. Showalter JW, Rafferty CM, Swallow NA, DaSilva KO, Chuang CH (2011) Effect of Standardized Electronic Discharge Instructions on Post-Discharge Hospital Utilization. Journal of General Internal Medicine. 26(7):718–23.
86. Polanczyk CA, Newton C, Dec GW, Di Salvo TG (2001) Quality of care and hospital readmission in congestive heart failure: An explicit review process. J Card Fail. 4:289–98.
87. Luthi JC, Lund MJ, Sampietro-Colom L, Kleinbaum DG, Ballard DJ, et al. (2003) Readmissions and the quality of care in patients hospitalized with heart failure. International Journal for Quality in Health Care. 15(5):413–21.
88. Joynt KE, Orav EJ, Jha AK (2011) The association between hospital volume and processes, outcomes, and costs of care for congestive heart failure. Ann Intern Med. 154(2):94–102.
89. Horwitz LI, Wang YF, Desai MM, Curry LA, Bradley EH, et al. (2012) Correlations among risk-standardized mortality rates and among risk-standardized readmission rates within hospitals. Journal of Hospital Medicine. . 7(9):690–6.
90. Hernandez AF, Hammill BG, Peterson ED, Yancy CW, Schulman KA, et al. (2010) Relationships between emerging measures of heart failure processes of care and clinical outcomes. Am Heart J. 159(3):406–13.
91. Bottle A, Aylin P (2009) Application of AHRQ patient safety indicators to English hospital data. Qual Saf Health Care. 18(4):303–8.
92. Halfon P, Eggli Y, van Melle G, Chevalier J, Wasserfallen JB, et al. (2002) Measuring potentially avoidable hospital readmissions. Journal of Clinical Epidemiology. 55(6):573–87.
93. Halfon P, Eggli Y, Pretre-Rohrbach I, Meylan D, Marazzi A, et al. (2006) Validation of the potentially avoidable hospital readmission rate as a routine indicator of the quality of hospital care. Med Care. 44(11):972–81.
94. Maeda JLK (2010) Evidence-Based Heart Failure Performance Measures and Clinical Outcomes: A Systematic Review. Journal of Cardiac Failure. 16(5):411–8.
95. Encinosa WE, Hellinger FJ (2008) The impact of medical errors on ninety-day costs and outcomes: An examination of surgical patients. Health Serv Res. 43(6):2067–85.
96. Shahian DM, Meyer GS, Mort E, Atamian S, Liu X, et al. (2012) Association of National Hospital Quality Measure adherence with long-term mortality and readmissions. BMJ Qual Saf. 21(4):325–36.
97. Fonarow GC, Abraham WT, Albert NM, Stough WG, Gheorghiade M, et al. (2007) Association between performance measures and clinical outcomes for patients hospitalized with heart failure. J Am Med Assoc. 297(1):61–70.
98. Stefan MS, Pekow PS, Nsa W, Priya A, Miller LE, et al. (2012) Hospital Performance Measures and 30-day Readmission Rates. J Gen Intern Med. 1–9.
99. Nathwani D, Williams F, Winter J, Winter J, Ogston S, et al. (2002) Use of indicators to evaluate the quality of community-acquired pneumonia management. Clin Infect Dis. 34(3):318–23.
100. Morse RB, Hall M, Fieldston ES, McGwire G, Anspacher M, et al. (2011) Hospital-level compliance with asthma care quality measures at children's hospitals and subsequent asthma-related outcomes. J Am Med Assoc. 306(13):1454–60.
101. Schopfer DW, Whooley MA, Stamos TD (2012) Hospital compliance with performance measures and 30-day outcomes in patients with heart failure. Am Heart J. 164(1):80–6.
102. Mansi IA, Shi R, Khan M, Huang J, Carden D (2010) Effect of compliance with quality performance measures for heart failure on clinical outcomes in high-risk patients. J Natl Med Assoc. 102(10):898–905.
103. Marcin JP, Romano PS (2004) Impact of between-hospital volume and within-hospital volume on mortality and readmission rates for trauma patients in California. Crit Care Med. 32(7):1477–83.
104. Patterson ME, Hernandez AF, Hammill BG, Fonarow GC, Peterson ED, et al. (2010) Process of care performance measures and long-term outcomes in patients hospitalized with heart failure. Med Care. 48(3):210–6.
105. Roccaforte R, Demers C, Baldassarre F, Teo K, Yusuf S (2005) Effectiveness of comprehensive disease management programmes in improving clinical outcomes in heart failure patients. A meta-analysis. Eur J Heart Fail. 7(7):1133–44.
106. Gawlas I, Sethi M, Winner M, Epelboym I, Lee JL, et al. (2012) Readmission After Pancreatic Resection is not an Appropriate Measure of Quality. Ann Surg Oncol. 1–7.
107. Jimenez-Puente A, Garcia-Alegria J, Gomez-Aracena J, Hidalgo-Rojas L, Lorenzo-Nogueiras L, et al. (2004) Readmission rate as an indicator of hospital performance: The case of Spain. Int J Technol Assess Health Care. 20(3):385–91.
108. Ricciardi MJ, Selzer F, Marroquin OC, Holper EM, Venkitachalam L, et al. (2012) Incidence and predictors of 30-day hospital readmission rate following percutaneous coronary intervention (from the national heart, lung, and blood institute dynamic registry). Am J Cardiol. 110(10):1389–96.
109. Auerbach AD, Maselli J, Carter J, Pekow PS, Lindenauer PK (2010) The relationship between case volume, care quality, and outcomes of complex cancer surgery. J Am Coll Surg. 211(5):601–8.
110. Rumball-Smith J, Blakely T, Sarfati D, Hider P (2013) The mismeasurement of quality by readmission rate: How blunt is too blunt an instrument?: A quantitative bias analysis. Med Care. 51(5):418–24.
111. Luthi JC, Burnand B, McClellan WM, Pitts SR, Flanders WD (2004) Is readmission to hospital an indicator of poor process of care for patients with heart failure? Qual Saf Health Care. 13(1):46–51.

112. Mayer EK, Bottle A, Aylin P, Darzi AW, Athanasiou T, et al. (2011) The volume-outcome relationship for radical cystectomy in England: An analysis of outcomes other than mortality. BJU Int. 108(8 B):E258–E65.
113. McConnell KJ, Lindrooth RC, Wholey DR, Maddox TM, Bloom N (2013)Management practices and the quality of care in cardiac units. JAMA Intern Med. 173(8):684–92.
114. Marang-van de Mheen PJ, Dijs-Elsinga J, Otten W, Versluijs M, Smeets HJ, et al. (2010) The importance of experienced adverse outcomes on patients' future choice of a hospital for surgery. Qual Saf Health Care. 19(6):e16.
115. Tsai TC, Joynt KE, Orav EJ, Gawande AA, Jha AK (2013) Variation in surgical-readmission rates and quality of hospital care. N Engl J Med. 369(12):1134–42.

Effects of Polypharmacy on Adverse Drug Reactions among Geriatric Outpatients at a Tertiary Care Hospital in Karachi: A Prospective Cohort Study

Bilal Ahmed[1]☯, Kashmira Nanji[2]☯, Rakshinda Mujeeb[1], Muhammad Junaid Patel[1]*

1 Department of Medicine, Aga Khan University, Karachi, Pakistan, **2** Department of Family Medicine, Aga Khan University, Karachi, Pakistan

Abstract

Background: Adverse drug reactions (ADRs) present a challenging and expensive public health problem. Polypharmacy is defined according to the WHO criteria as the, "concurrent use of five or more different prescription medication". Elderly are more prone to adverse reactions due to comorbid conditions, longer lists of medications and sensitivity to drug effects. The aim of the study is to estimate the incidence and strength of association of ADRs due to polypharmacy among the geriatric cohort attending outpatient clinics at a tertiary care center.

Methods: A hospital based prospective cohort study was conducted at ambulatory care clinics of Aga Khan University Hospital April 2012 to March 2013. One thousand geriatrics patients (age ≥65 years) visiting ambulatory clinics were identified. They were divided on the basis of exposure (polypharmacy vs. no polypharmacy). We followed them from the time of their enrollment (day zero) to six weeks, checking up on them once a week. Incidence was calculated and Cox Proportional Hazard Model estimates were used.

Results: The final analysis was performed on 1000 elderly patients. The occurrence of polypharmacy was 70% and the incidence of ADRs was 10.5% among the study cohort. The majority (30%) of patients were unable to read or write. The use of herbal medicine was reported by 3.2% of the patients and homeopathic by 3%. Our Cox adjusted model shows that polypharmacy was 2.3 times more associated with ADRs, con-current complementary and alternative medicine (CAM) was 7.4 times and those who cannot read and write were 1.5 times more associated with ADRs.

Conclusion: The incidence of ADRs due to poly pharmacy is alarmingly high. The factors associated with ADRs are modifiable. Policies are needed to design and strengthen the prescription pattern.

Editor: Robin Dore, David Geffen School of Medicine, United States of America

Funding: This work was supported by the University Research Council, Aga Khan University URC ID 102013MED. The funders had no role in study design, data collection and analysis, decision to publish, or preparation of the manuscript.

Competing Interests: The authors have declared that no competing interests exist.

* Email: junaiddrpatel@gmail.com

☯ These authors contributed equally to this work.

Background

Epidemiologic transition over the years has increased the percentage of elderly (aged greater than 65 years). The elderly people now constitute more than 60% of the world population, which in turn increases their hospital visits leading to multiple medications' use [1]. Approximately there are 841 million elderly (60 years and older) people in the world. By 2050, nearly 8 in 10 of the world's older population will be living in the less developed areas [2]. This increase in life expectancy has brought about increased numbers of certain chronic illnesses, which involves hospital admissions, multiple medications and its associated ADR's [3]. Inappropriate use of medicines is one of the challenges of the public health domain and may lead to serious (ADRs) [4]that account for 3% to 23% of hospital admissions, prolong hospital stays, and increase in morbidity and mortality [5].

According to WHO, polypharmacy is defined as the concurrent use of five or more different prescription medications. Previous studies have provided evidence that the probability of ADRs among geriatric patients is estimated at 6% when two drugs are taken, increases to 50% when five drugs are taken, and becomes 100% when eight or more drugs are taken simultaneously [6]. Polypharmacy has also been documented as a major risk factor for ADRs in the developed countries [7]. Ageing has a strong impact on the pharmacokinetics and pharmacodynamics, comorbidity, and patterns of medication that may contribute to an increased risk of adverse events. A study from Malaysia found higher incidence of polypharmacy among geriatric inpatients (62.8%) on admission and it was associated with the high prevalence of cardiovascular diseases and diabetes mellitus [8].

Few epidemiological studies investigating the role of polypharmacy among the geriatrics have been almost exclusively conducted in the developed countries [9,10]. However, there is a scarcity of evidence from Asian countries including Pakistan, and prospective studies investigating the association between polypharmacy and ADRs are almost lacking [11,12]. Hence, determining the true incidence along with strength of association of ADRs due to polypharmacy among geriatrics would help in designing guidelines and policies for this vulnerable population. We hypothesize that the risk of ADRs among the exposed (polypharmacy) was greater than that of the un-exposed group. The overall aims of the study were to estimate the incidence of ADRs and its association with polypharmacy among the geriatric cohort attending outpatient clinics at a tertiary care center in Karachi, Pakistan.

Methods

Study Design and Population

A prospective cohort study was conducted during April 2012 to March 2013 at Aga Khan University Hospital (AKUH) Karachi, Pakistan, a 563 bedded, Join Commission International (JCI) accredited tertiary care center providing state of the art health care facilities. The study recruited a cohort of 1000 geriatrics patients having age ≥65 years, using consecutive sampling technique, either male or female at their index visit to any sub-specialty ambulatory care clinics (Family Medicine, Medicine, Surgery, Obstetrics and Gynecology) and was followed for six weeks to collect relevant factual data for the incidence of ADRs due to polypharmacy. **Figure 1** shows the flow of participant in the study. Subjects who were transferred to inpatient departments directly from clinic or those who required hospital admission or known to be mentally disabled or were suffering from advanced neurological diseases like dementia or acute confusion were not recruited. Written informed consent was obtained from each participant at the time of recruitment, those who were not able to read or write, detailed explanation was provided about the study protocol by the data collector and thumb impression was obtained in presence of a family member.

Ethics Statement. Ethical approval for this study was obtained from the ethical review committee of Aga Khan University (AKU FWA 00001177).

Ascertainment of Polypharmacy

Trained interviewers screened and enrolled participants on the basis of standard definition of Polypharmacy which is defined by WHO as the, "concurrent use of five or more different prescription medications [13]." Multiple sources like computerized medical records, patient's medical files and pharmacy prescriptions were used for data extraction to avoid any miss outs. The unexposed group was defined as patients receiving less than five drugs at their index visit. Telephonic interviews were conducted once weekly till the sixth week by an interviewer to follow the participants if they had developed any ADRs. At the index visit, interviewer collected complete information related to dug history. Subjects' progress notes were also reviewed to determine any information related to the addition of new drugs, newly developed ADR's, and critical laboratory values *(see Appendix S1)*.

Ascertainment of Adverse Drug Reaction

We obtained information on ADRs defined as "the presence of undesired outcomes due to receiving medicines" from multiple sources [14]. Two physicians and one pharmacist independently reviewed each reported ADR to determine the likelihood that the event was connected to a medication. A thorough literature search was performed before labeling any case as an ADR [15]. Besides this, the standard ADR Reporting Form by the drug and poison information center at the Department of Pharmacy Services, AKU, was also used to record all the essential information regarding the adverse effects: suspected drugs, suspected reaction, date of onset, date when the adverse effects ceased and severity of the ADR experienced (fatal, non-fatal). Subjects with ADRs were formally referred to their primary investigators.

Drug characteristics by Anatomical Therapeutic Chemical

Drugs involved in the ADRs were coded into various drug classes according to Anatomical Therapeutic Chemical (ATC) classification based on WHO-ATC Index 2005 [16]. In the ATC classification system, the drugs are divided into different groups according to the organ or system on which they act and their chemical, pharmacological and therapeutic properties.

Covariables

Covariables were collected from administrative questionnaires at baseline. Covariables included age (65–70, 71–80 and >80 years), sex, educational status (Can't Read or Write, ≤5, 6–14, and >14 years of education), occupational status (unemployed/retired, employed), polypharmacy (no, yes), medication data with dose, frequency and duration, frequency of dose missing (no, yes) and non-prescription drugs (herbal, homeopathic, over the counter).

Statistical Methods

The sample size was calculated by taking into account the objectives of the study. We used Epi Info Version 6 to calculate the sample size. The calculations were based on the assumption that polypharmacy among the Pakistani geriatrics is 50% (as we do not have any information regarding these in our community). By taking into account all of these figures together with 99% confidence interval, and exposed to non-exposed ratio of 1:1 with 90% power and risk ratio of 1.3, the sample size came out to be n = 750. After adjusting 30% for non -responders the final required sample size was approximately 1000 geriatric participants.

In the analysis of cohort of 1000 geriatrics, we evaluated polypharmacy at baseline and cumulative incidence of ADRs, in relation to other baseline characteristics. The incidence of ADRs was calculated and Pearson chi-square tests were used to evaluate differences between categories. The Proportional hazard assumption was checked for all independent variables. A multivariable Cox regression analysis was used to study the independent association of variables with the presence of ADRs. The Relative Risk (RR) with 95% Confidence Intervals (CIs) was estimated. In the Cox model we adjusted for age, gender, employment status, use of nonprescription medications at baseline as potential confounding factors.

Statistical Package for Social Sciences (SPSS) Version 19 was used for analysis.

Results

We followed 1000 elderly patients for six weeks after enrollment, and identified 107 (10.7%) ADRs in the full cohort. The overall occurrence of ADRs due to polypharmacy was 70%. Males were reported to have greater incidence of ADRs (59%). We found slightly higher risks of ADRs among population of illiterate persons when compared to people with higher level of education. The hazard ratios for different levels of education status ranged from 0.8–1.7. Likewise, use of non-prescription medicines,

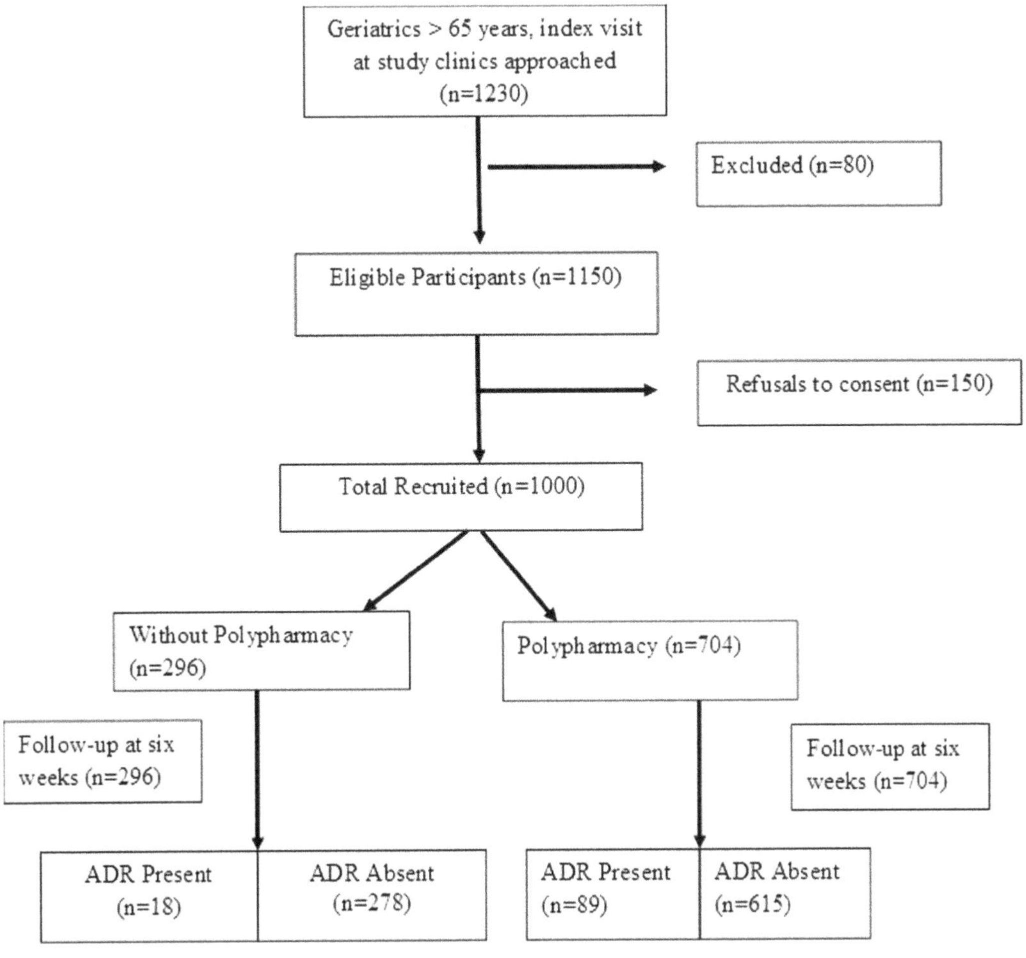

Figure 1. Flow of Study Participants.

including herbal and homeopathic medicines, carries much higher risk of ADRs. All other characteristics were comparable between ADRs positive and ADRs negative groups as shown in *table 1*. Later, we compared subjects according to exposure status however; none of the characteristics were statistically different between the two groups as shown in table 2.

After adjusting for age, gender and occupational status, an adjusted multivariable model indicated that polypharmacy, low level of education and use of concurrent homeopathic medicines were significantly associated with ADRs among geriatrics. Risk of ADRs among elderly patients with polypharmacy was 2.3 (95% CI: 1.4–3.9) higher than those who took lesser number of medicines. Low level of education (i.e. those who were unable to read or write and those with less education than primary schooling) was more likely to be associated with ADRs. However, as the level of education increases the association with ADRs turns out to be protective (RR = 0.7, 95% CI: 0.5–0.9). Risk of ADRs among geriatrics who took concurrent homeopathic medicines was higher compared to those who did not (RR = 7.4, 95% CI 3.2–8.8), as shown in *table 3*.

In table 4, we calculated the incidence of ADRs according to the exposure to various drug classes. The highest incidence was found for antitussives and anti-dopaminergic drugs in our study group.

Discussion

In this prospective cohort study the incidence of ADRs with polypharmacy was found to be 10.5%, moreover, we also found high rates of polypharmacy in geriatric outpatients which is consistent with previous researches. In the current study, 68.2% of the elderly patients were taking more than five medications a day. This is slightly higher than the rates previously reported for geriatric population. We observed a statistically significant association between low levels of education and the concurrent use of non-prescription medicines both before and after adjusting for potential confounders. With the hope of directing intervention efforts; many associations have been proposed for ADRs among the geriatric population (aged 65 years or older) since they are mostly prescribed with multiple medications which make them vulnerable to ADRs.

Investigators suggest that longer stay in hospital is one of the probable cause for the occurrence of ADRs in geriatrics and it is defined as an undesirable condition caused by the use of multiple medications [17].

The incidence of 10.6% ADRs found in this study is low as compared to other general or outpatient studies conducted in different countries [8,9,18]. This could be due to the difference in the methodological aspects of the study particularly the study population and the self-reporting of ADRs in the follow-ups which was conducted through telephonic calls in the current study. This

Table 1. Descriptive and Univariate Cox Analysis Along With 95% Confidence Intervals of Eligible Geriatrics Attending Tertiary Care Center.

Variable	ADR Negative	ADR Positive	*Unadjusted RR	95% CI
	n=893	n=107		
Age				
65–70	448 (50.2)	59 (55.1)	Reference	
71–80	359 (40.2)	42 (39.3)	1.8	0.77–4.13
Above 80	86 (9.6)	6 (5.6)	1.6	0.68–3.77
Gender				
Male	422 (47.3)	63 (58.9)	Reference	
Female	471 (52.7)	44 (41.1)	1.5	1.03–2.2
Level of Education				
More than 14 years	43 (4.8)	5 (4.7)	Reference	
Can't Read Or Write	269 (30.1)	36 (33.6)	1.7	1.3–2.8
Less than 5 years	119 (13.3)	25 (23.4)	1.6	1.3–4.3
6–14 years	462 (51.7)	41 (38.3)	0.8	0.2–0.9
Occupation				
Employed	421 (47.1)	45 (42.1)	Reference	
Unemployed	472 (52.9)	62 (57.9)	1.2	0.8–1.7
Use of Concurrent Homeopathic Medicine				
No	877 (98.2)	94 (87.9)	Reference	
Yes	16 (1.8)	13 (12.1)	4.6	2.5–8.2
Use of Concurrent Herbal Medicine				
No	873 (97.8)	95 (88.8)	Reference	
Yes	20 (2.2)	12 (11.2)	3.8	2.1–6.9
Poly-Pharmacy				
No	278 (31.1)	18 (16.8)	Reference	
Yes	615 (38.9)	89 (83.2)	2.1	1.2–3.4

**Relative risk obtained from Cox regression analysis.*

probably implies an underestimation of actual occurrence of adverse effects. Another reason for the lower frequency of ADRs observed in our study is probably due to the method of extracting information on the use of complementary and alternative medicines (herbal 3.2% and homeopathic 2.9%) which is missing in most of the studies recording ADRs along with poly-pharmacy. Interestingly, among these patients who were taking CAM, the occurrence of ADRs were similar i.e. 12%. Most studies conclude that most of the ADRs in outpatients turn out to be harmless; however this study opposes this fact where 13% patients (n = 14 out of 107) had to make a hospital visit as a result of ADRs [19].

The use of CAM i.e. herbal and homeopathic has become increasingly popular in both developed and the developing countries [20,21]. In this study, 14% of the elderly patients were using homeopathic and 13% were using herbal medications. This is lower than the rates reported in other studies where the use of CAM is as high as 66% [21]. One of the strong motivational factors to use CAM is their perceived remedial benefits, and safety profile. However, we can only speculate about the role and benefits of CAM in certain diseases as the role of CAM in chronic diseases is still controversial. In the current study those elderly who were taking concurrent homeopathic medication were 7 times more at risk of developing ADRs. The probable reason for this high risk of developing ADRs can be due to the fact that many commonly used CAM products have the potential to interfere with the intended action of concomitant prescription medications, which could lead to serious drug interactions and in turn increase the risk of ADRs. Nevertheless, it is important to educate the patients about the risks and benefits of CAM. Studies are required to determine the impacts of CAM, particularly its impact when used in conjunction with prescribed medicines.

It is evident that some drugs such as anticholinergic and antipsychotics can impair the physical and cognitive function in the elderly patients [22]. In the current study antipsychotics had an ADR incidence of 333 per 1000 population and anti-hypertensive had incidence of 128/1000. This implies that the more drugs with these effects that the elderly patients are exposed to (number and dose), the poorer will be their quality of life and they will be more prone to ADRs, as evident from the results of the current study that those elderly patients who were positive of polypharmacy had 2.3 times more risk of developing ADRs [23].

There are several strengths of our study; a cohort study design was carefully chosen which is ideal in predicting the causal association of exposure with the outcome so inferences can be drawn regarding causality of association between polypharmacy and other factors with the ADRs. We collected data from OPD prescriptions to avoid any miss outs. In addition, we estimated the incidence of ADRs due to polypharmacy, defined as the use of >5 scheduled medications in the line of WHO guidelines. The criteria of more than five medications used included only systemic and

Table 2. Characteristics of Eligible Participants Attending Tertiary Care Center, According To Exposure Status.

Variable	Polypharmacy (n) %	
	Yes	No
Age		
65–70	345 (49)	162 (54.7)
71–80	286 (40.6)	115 (38.9)
Above 80	73 (10.4)	19 (6.4)
Level of Education		
More than 14 years	35 (5)	13 (4.4)
Can't Read or Write	221 (31.4)	84 (28.4)
Less than 5 years	103 (14.6)	41 (13.9)
6–14 years	345 (49)	158 (53.4)
Gender		
Male	365 (51.8)	150 (50.7)
Female	339 (48.2)	146 (49.3)
Use of Concurrent Herbal Medicine		
No	686 (97.4)	282 (95.3)
Yes	18 (2.6)	14 (4.7)
Use of Concurrent Homeopathic Medicine		
No	691(98.2)	280 (94.6)
Yes	13 (1.8)	16 (5.4)

routinely administered medications. Moreover, there was no loss in following-up in our cohort. However, our study has certain limitations that need to be considered while interpreting the results. This was a hospital based study hence generalizability to public sector settings remain questionable. We followed our subjects for a duration of six weeks only, thus adverse effects arising after this time may not be captured and this might have underestimated our results.

To the best of our knowledge, this is the first Asian study to record the incidence of ADRs in geriatric outpatients with polypharmacy; our study confirms the notion that elderly patients are more likely to experience these adverse reactions as the result of age-related increase in the frequency of drug use, sensitivity to drug effects, and prevalence of predisposing conditions that can increase the frequency and severity of ADRs.

With the current state of health system utilization and health-seeking behavior in Pakistan, it is highly desirable to reduce the divergence by exploring more opportunities for integration of patient safety. As a way forward this study and its findings may encourage the physicians to implement judicious prescribing.

Appropriate educational, managerial or regulatory strategies are needed for evidence based prescribing. It is also important that medications for the elderly patients be reviewed periodically for indication, therapeutic aims, dose, efficacy and probable side effects. Moreover, the benefit and risks of treatment (drugs)

Table 3. Adjusted Multivariable Analysis Showing Relative Risk of Adverse Drugs Reactions Along With 95% CI.

Variables	Relative Risk	95% CI
Polypharmacy		
No	*Reference*	
Yes	2.3	1.4–3.9
Level of Education		
More than 14 years	*Reference*	
Can't Read Or Write	1.5	1.2–2.8
Less than 5 years	1.3	1.1–2.9
6–14 years	0.7	0.5–0.9
Use of Concurrent Homeopathic Medicine		
No	*Reference*	
Yes	7.4	3.2–8.8

Table 4. Incidence of Adverse Drug Reactions According To Drug Exposure.

Drugs Classification	ADR negative	ADR Positive	Incidence per 1000 population
Antitussives	1	2	666
Anti-dopaminergic	1	1	500
Antipsychotics	4	2	333
Anti-hypertensive	68	10	128
Antibiotics	98	14	125
Supplements	74	10	119
Cardiovascular	491	57	104
Anti-diabetics	73	6	75
Anti-lipidemic	13	1	71
NSAIDs	18	1	52
Anti-peptic ulcer	42	2	45
Statins	2	0	0
Anticoagulants	2	0	0

including the impact on functions and quality of life should be discussed with patients and their caregivers.

In conclusion, in this reasonably large hospital based prospective cohort study of geriatrics, the incidence of ADRs due to polypharmacy is high. Several factors including low level of education and use of non-prescription medications remain responsible for the high burden. While additional research with more sophisticated design is needed to confirm our findings, our data suggests that a comprehensive strategy for evidence based prescribing must be implemented.

Research in Context

Stimulated by JK. Nguyen's findings [9], we performed a hospital based prospective cohort study where we surveyed the geriatric population (>65 years) attending the outpatient clinics of Aga Khan University Hospital Karachi throughout the year 2012. The data was collected from different consulting clinics of Anesthesia, Family Medicine, Internal Medicine and Obstetrics. The sampled geriatric population was recruited from clinics and followed to collect relevant factual data for the incidence of adverse drug reactions due to polypharmacy. We used the operational definition for polypharmacy as the concurrent use of five or more different prescription medications.

We initiated the data collection by gathering demographic information where 30% of the total patients were not able to read or write and 53% of the patients were unemployed. The mean age was found to be 70 years (range 65–70). Later on, during the follow up phase, the patients were asked about self-medication and its frequency, 53% patients were self-medicating via OTC drugs. On asking whether a pharmacist provided them any valuable information regarding side/adverse effects of the dispensed drug, 35% patients reported a negative response. The overall occurrence of polypharmacy was 68% while the incidence of ADRs along with polypharmacy was found to be 10.5%. About 3.2% of the participants relied on herbal medicines and 3% on homeopathic medicines.

Our study supports the findings of JK. Nguyen and colleagues. Our Cox adjusted model shows that polypharmacy was 2.3 times more associated with ADRs. Con-current homeopathic use was 7.4 times and those who were unable to read and write were 1.5 times more at risk of developing ADRs.

Author Contributions

Conceived and designed the experiments: BA KN. Performed the experiments: BA KN RM. Analyzed the data: BA KN. Contributed to the writing of the manuscript: BA KN RM MJP.

References

1. Nobili A, Licata G, Salerno F, Pasina L, Tettamanti M, et al. (2011) Polypharmacy, length of hospital stay, and in-hospital mortality among elderly patients in internal medicine wards. The REPOSI study. European journal of clinical pharmacology 67: 507–519.
2. (2013) United Nations, Department of Economic and Social Affairs, Population Division (2013) World Population Ageing.
3. Trumic E, Pranjic N, Begic L, Fahir B (2012) Prevalence of Polypharmacy and Drug Interaction Among Hospitalized Patients: Opportunities and Responsabilities in Pharmaceutical Care. Materia socio-medica 24: 68.
4. Steinman MA, Seth Landefeld C, Rosenthal GE, Berthenthal D, Sen S, et al. (2006) Polypharmacy and prescribing quality in older people. Journal of the American Geriatrics Society 54: 1516–1523.
5. Hajjar ER, Hanlon JT, Artz MB, Lindblad CI, Pieper CF, et al. (2003) Adverse drug reaction risk factors in older outpatients. The American journal of geriatric pharmacotherapy 1: 82–89.
6. Chumney EC, Robinson LC (2006) The effects of pharmacist interventions on patients with polypharmacy. Pharmacy Practice 4: 103–109.
7. Hohl CMl, Dankoff J, Colacone A, Afilalo M (2001) Polypharmacy, adverse drug-related events, and potential adverse drug interactions in elderly patients presenting to an emergency department. Annals of emergency medicine 38: 666–671.
8. Najjar MF, Aziz NA, Hassan Y, Ghazali R, AlRazzaq A, et al. (2010) Predictors of polypharmacy and adverse drug reactions among geriatric in patients at Malaysian hospital. HealthMed 4.

9. Nguyen JK, Fouts MM, Kotabe SE, Lo E (2006) Polypharmacy as a risk factor for adverse drug reactions in geriatric nursing home residents. The American journal of geriatric pharmacotherapy 4: 36–41.
10. Haider SI, Johnell K, Thorslund M, Fastbom J (2007) Trends in polypharmacy and potential drug-drug interactions across educational groups in elderly patients in Sweden for the period 1992–2002. International journal of clinical pharmacology and therapeutics 45: 643–653.
11. Sabzwari SR, Qidwai W, Bhanji S (2013) Polypharmacy in elderly: A cautious trail to tread. JPMA The Journal of the Pakistan Medical Association 63: 624–627.
12. Lam DPY, Mak CF, Chan S, Yao RWY, Leung SSY, et al. (2010) Polypharmacy and inappropriate prescribing in elderly Hong Kong Chinese patients. Journal of the American Geriatrics Society 58: 203–205.
13. Viktil KK, Blix HS, Moger TA, Reikvam A (2007) Polypharmacy as commonly defined is an indicator of limited value in the assessment of drugâ€related problems. British journal of clinical pharmacology 63: 187–195.
14. Edwards IR, Aronson JK (2000) Adverse drug reactions: definitions, diagnosis, and management. The Lancet 356: 1255–1259.
15. Gandhi TK, Weingart SN, Borus J, Seger AC, Peterson J, et al. (2003) Adverse drug events in ambulatory care. New England Journal of Medicine 348: 1556–1564.
16. World Health O (2009) Collaborating centre for drug statistics methodology. Guidelines for ATC classification and DDD assignment 3.
17. Classen DC, Pestotnik SL, Evans RS, Lloyd JF, Burke JP (1997) Adverse drug events in hospitalized patientsExcess length of stay, extra costs, and attributable mortality. Jama 277: 301–306.
18. Budnitz DS, Shehab N, Kegler SR, Richards CL (2007) Medication use leading to emergency department visits for adverse drug events in older adults. Annals of Internal Medicine 147: 755–765.
19. Thomsen LA, Winterstein AG, SAndergaard B, HaugbÅlle LS, Melander A (2007) Systematic review of the incidence and characteristics of preventable adverse drug events in ambulatory care. Annals of Pharmacotherapy 41: 1411–1426.
20. Ernst E (2000) The role of complementary and alternative medicine. BMJ: British Medical Journal 321: 1133.
21. Herman PM, Craig BM, Caspi O (2005) Is complementary and alternative medicine (CAM) cost-effective? A systematic review. BMC Complementary and Alternative Medicine 5: 11.
22. Hilmer SN (2008) The dilemma of polypharmacy. Australian Prescriber 31: 2.
23. Field TS, Gurwitz JH, Harrold LR, Rothschild J, DeBellis KR, et al. (2004) Risk factors for adverse drug events among older adults in the ambulatory setting. Journal of the American Geriatrics Society 52: 1349–1354.

11

Neonatal Adaptation in Infants Prenatally Exposed to Antidepressants- Clinical Monitoring Using Neonatal Abstinence Score

Lisa Forsberg[1,2]*, Lars Navér[1,2], Lars L. Gustafsson[3], Katarina Wide[1,2]

1 Department of Pediatrics, Karolinska University Hospital, Stockholm, Sweden, **2** Department of Clinical Science, Intervention and Technology (CLINTEC), Karolinska Institutet, Stockholm, Sweden, **3** Department of Laboratory Medicine, Division of Clinical Pharmacology, Karolinska Institutet, Stockholm, Sweden

Abstract

Background: Intrauterine exposure to antidepressants may lead to neonatal symptoms from the central nervous system, respiratory system and gastrointestinal system. Finnegan score (Neonatal Abstinence Score, NAS) has routinely been used to assess infants exposed to antidepressants in utero.

Aim: The purpose was to study neonatal maladaptation syndrome in infants exposed to selective serotonin reuptake inhibitors (SSRI) or serotonin-norepinephrine reuptake inhibitors (SNRI) in utero.

Method: Retrospective cohort study of women using antidepressants during pregnancy and their infants. Patients were identified from the electronic health record system at Karolinska University Hospital Huddinge containing pre-, peri- and postnatal information. Information was collected on maternal and infant health, social factors and pregnancy. NAS sheets were scrutinized.

Results: 220 women with reported 3rd trimester exposure to SSRIs or SNRIs and who gave birth between January 2007 and June 2009 were included. Seventy seven women (35%) used citalopram, 76 used (35%) sertraline, 34 (15%) fluoxetine and 33 (15%) other SSRI/SNRI. Twenty-nine infants (13%) were admitted to the neonatal ward, 19 were born prematurely. NAS was analyzed in 205 patients. Severe abstinence was defined as eight points or higher on at least two occasions (on a scale with maximum 40 points), mild abstinence as 4 points or higher on at least two occasions. Seven infants expressed signs of severe abstinence and 46 (22%) had mild abstinence symptoms. Hypoglycemia (plasma glucose <2.6 mmol/L) was found in 42 infants (19%).

Conclusion: Severe abstinence in infants prenatally exposed to antidepressants was found to be rare (3%) in this study population, a slightly lower prevalence than reported in previous studies. Neonatal hypoglycemia in infants prenatally exposed to antidepressant may however be more common than previously described.

Editor: Gabriele Fischer, Medical University of Vienna, Austria

Funding: Funding provided by Swedish Research Council, grant number 2011-3440 www.vr.se to LLG, Swedish Research Council, grant number 2012-3466, www.vr.se to KW, The Mayflower Foundation, www.majblomman.se to KW LF and The Samariten Foundation, www.stiftelsensamariten.se to LF KW. The funders had no role in study design, data collection and analysis, decision to publish, or preparation of the manuscript.

Competing Interests: The authors have declared that no competing interests exist.

* Email: lisa.forsberg.1@ki.se

Background

Psychiatric conditions are common during and after pregnancy. A large US study showed a prevalence of 13% for both mood and for anxiety disorders in pregnant or postpartum women [1]. Antidepressants are commonly used to treat major depressive disorders as well as other psychiatric conditions such as anxiety and obsessive compulsive disorders. Selective serotonin reuptake inhibitors (SSRIs) are the most prescribed group of antidepressants, also in pregnant women [2]. Serotonin norepinephrine reuptake inhibitors (SNRIs) are also used during pregnancy with similar effects on prenatally exposed children as SSRIs [3]. A population based register study showed that 3% of all pregnant women in Sweden used antidepressants, mainly SSRIs, three months prior to conception, whereas the numbers decreased during pregnancy, down to 1% in the third trimester [2]. In Denmark, there has been an increase in antidepressant use in pregnancy. In 1997, 0.2% of all pregnant women had at some point during pregnancy been using antidepressants, in 2010 this figure had increased to 3.2% [4].

Use of paroxetine during early pregnancy has been linked to an increased risk of heart malformations, OR 1.66 (95% CI 1.09 to

2.53) and hypospadias, OR 2.45 (95% CI 1.12 to 4.64) [5]. A Canadian study found a significantly increased risk of heart malformations only in infants exposed to paroxetine daily doses higher than 25 mg [6]. A neonatal maladaptation syndrome in infants exposed to SSRIs during late pregnancy is well known. It includes symptoms such as jitteriness, feeding problems, respiratory distress, hypoglycemia [5,7,8]. The relative risk of persistent pulmonary hypertension, a potentially life threatening condition, is increased in infants prenatally exposed to SSRI, from 1.2 per 1000 live births in unexposed infants to 3 per 1000 live births in SSRI exposed neonates [9]. Maternal illness (depression, anxiety) may also contribute to milder neonatal symptoms usually resolving within a week [10]. The mode of action for neonatal maladaptation after SSRI/SNRI exposure is largely unknown. 'Abstinence' due to the discontinued distribution of the pharmacological substance at delivery as well as serotonergic overstimulation has been suggested [8].

Finnegan score, or Neonatal Abstinence Score sheet (NAS) was originally developed to diagnose abstinence in infants prenatally exposed to opioids [11], but has also been used to assess neonatal symptoms in SSRI exposed infants [12].

As stated above, antidepressants during pregnancy is a common clinical problem, of growing significance. Conducting clinical research in the field of perinatal pharmacological exposure is complicated due to many ethical considerations and an abundance of potential confounders. This study was initiated to shed light on the occurrence of neonatal abstinence/maladaptation after SSRI/SNRI exposure *in utero* and its prevalence, timing, severity and clinical features of this known but inadequately described condition.

Methods

The study design was a retrospective cohort study. The study patients were identified in the integrated electronic health record used in the delivery and prenatal care units as well as for outpatient maternal visits (Obstetrix^R 2.12.01.100, Siemens AG, Munich, Germany). Patients with diagnostic codes for psychiatric illness during pregnancy and exposure to fetus of pharmacological substances were selected as the study population.

Women fulfilling these criteria and who had been giving birth at the Karolinska University Hospital Huddinge between 1 January, 2007 and 30 June, 2009 were included. Patients with reported substance abuse (alcohol or drugs) or use of certain kinds of neurotropic medication (antiepileptic drugs, lithium, opioids) were excluded. Information about substance abuse was reported in the patient records but not systematically confirmed through urine toxicology or breathalyser. Patients where substantial parts of the prenatal care records could not be retrieved were also excluded.

Information regarding social situation, prenatal medication (antidepressants and other pharmacological substances), health status and pregnancy related complications were retrieved from the prenatal part of the electronic health record (Obstetrix^R). The information on use of antidepressants, bensodiazepines and other pharmacological substances was based on self-report or stated by the prescribing physician in the patient records. Obstetrix^R was also used to extract clinical information about the delivery, infant health including health problems in the maternal ward and admission to the neonatal ward. During the study period, all infants where the mother had reported antidepressant use during late pregnancy were routinely observed at the maternal ward for at least 72 hours and modified Finnegan score used regularly to detect signs of abstinence. The assessments were extracted from the electronic health record system and analyzed.

A modified Finnegan score or Neonatal Abstinence Score (NAS) in Swedish was used in this study [13]. A version re-translated into English from Swedish is showed in Fig. 1. The assessment includes four categories: central nervous system (CNS), respiratory, gastrointestinal and 'other symptoms'. The maximum score for each scoring occasion is 40 points, of which 21 are related to CNS items. Neonatal abstinence was in this study classified as either mild (score 4 and above on at least two occasions) or severe (score 8 and above on at least two occasions). A similar classification has been used previously [12].

Population data regarding rates of neonatal admission, rates of smoking in early pregnancy, caesarian section and maternal age with regard to the Stockholm county area and Karolinska University Hospital Huddinge were obtained from the Swedish Neonatal Quality Register (SNQ) and from the statistical unit at National Swedish Board of Health and Welfare. These data were obtained as processed data [14].

Statistical analyses were performed with Statistica^R 64, version 12 (StatSoft Scandinavia AB, Uppsala, Sweden). In the comparison between groups, chi square Pearson's test, ANOVA (Analysis of Variance) or Kruskal Wallis was used. Ordinal regression was used in the comparison of different levels of abstinence. Logistic regression or linear regression was used in the multiple regression models.

The study was a retrospective evaluation, based on patient records and conducted several years after the delivery of the infants. Neither written nor verbal informed consent was obtained. Data from patient records were extracted by one researcher and only relevant parts of the records were entered. The data was recorded in a data file with the confidentiality that is applied to patient records. Every individual was given a code number to strengthen the protection of confidentiality. No individual is possible to identify from the report. The study design was approved by the Regional Ethical Review Board in Stockholm (no. 2010/686-31).

Results

During the study period of 2.5 years between January 1, 2007 and June 30, 2009, 365 patients with diagnostic code for pharmacological exposure to fetus and psychiatric illness during pregnancy delivered at Karolinska University Hospital Huddinge. Use of SSRI/SNRI was confirmed in 277 patients. Thirty-four were excluded due to confirmed (or strongly suspected) substance abuse, opioid use or use of other psychotropic medication such as lithium or antipsychotics. Twenty patients could not be included due to missing data. One pair of twins was excluded. Two hundred and twenty patients remained; 54 gave birth in 2007, 103 in 2008 and 63 during the first six months of 2009. During 2007, 2008 and 2009 a total of 13755 infants were born at Karolinska University Hospital Huddinge [14].

Table 1 describes the women in the cohort with regard to social factors, health status and reported medication during pregnancy (antidepressants and other); divided by reported third trimester antidepressant use. The most common exposures were citalopram, sertraline and fluoxetine (Table 1). The remaining patients, in all 33 (15%), were exposed to escitalopram (13 patients), venlafaxine (11 patients), paroxetine (8 patients) and duloxetine (one patient). Depression and anxiety disorders were the most common reasons for antidepressant use.

Cigarette smoking in early pregnancy in the cohort was 13% (for all 2.5 years) as compared to 5.4% in 2007, 4.9% in 2008 and 4.7% in 2009 for women in early pregnancy in the whole Stockholm area. BMI was higher in the cohort, 24.4 kg/m^2,

	Time ⟶									
CNS		Score								
Cry	Highpitched, possible to soothe Highpitched, not possible to soothe	2 3								
Sleep	Sleeps < 3 h after feed Sleeps < 2 h after feed Sleeps < 1 h after feed	1 2 3								
Moro-reflex	Over active Very over active	2 3								
Tremor	Moderate tremors disturbed Severe tremors disturbed Moderate tremors undisturbed Severe tremors undisturbed	1 2 3 4								
	Scratch marks	1								
Tone	Increased muscle tone	2								
Seizures	Myoclonic jerks Generalised seizures	3 5								
Respiratory										
Yawning	Frequent yawning >3-4/interval	1								
Nose	Congested nose	1								
Sneezing	>3-4 times/interval Nasal flaring	1 2								
Tachypnea (>60/min)	No retractions With retractions	1 2								
Gastrointestinal										
Sucking behaviour	Excessive sucking	1								
Feeding	Poor feeding	2								
Vomiting	Regurgitation Projectile vomiting	2 3								
Stool	Loose Watery	2 3								
Other symptoms										
	Sweating	1								
Fever	37.2-38.2°C >38.2°C	1 2								
Colour	Mottling	1								
TOTAL SCORE										

Figure 1. Neonatal Abstinance Score. Modified from Finnegan to Swedish, (Sarman 2000) here re-translated.

compared to all women who gave birth in the Stockholm area 2007 (23.9), 2008 (23.9) and 2009 (23.8).

A total of 48% of the women had 'other illnesses' documented in the prenatal care records. Most of these illnesses were mild and manageable, such as musculoskeletal problems, asthma, migraine, thyroid diseases or gastrointestinal reflux disease. Some were potentially serious such as obesity or chronic hepatitis. Eleven patients had more severe conditions such as diabetes mellitus, inflammatory bowel disease, serious or potentially serious pulmonary, rheumatic or neurological diseases.

Birth weight and head circumference did not differ between the four different exposure groups (Table 2). Linear regression adjusting for maternal age, maternal smoking in early pregnancy, gestational age and infant sex showed no statistical significance regarding birth weight ($p = 0.75$). A model adjusting for only maternal smoking did not reach statistical significance. For head circumference the corresponding result was $p = 0.56$. A model adjusting for maternal smoking only did not show any statistically significant differences between the four antidepressant exposure groups. Prematurity (gestational age of 36 weeks and 6 days or less) was seen in 13% of the infants exposed to citalopram (Table 2). In

Table 1. Characteristics of study population, women with antidepressant treatment and delivery at Karolinska University Hospital Huddinge Jan 2007 to June 2009.

	All antidepressants	Citalopram	Sertraline	Fluoxetine	Other antidepressants**
	n = 220	n = 77 (35%)	n = 76 (35%)	n = 34 (15%)	n = 33 (15%)
Age of mother at delivery mean (years)	31.2	31.2	32.1	29.4	31.0
Maternal psychiatric diagnosis# (n)					
Depression	168	59	58	29	22
Anxiety disorder	80	29	27	8	16
Other psychiatric diagnoses##	34	7	12	10	5
Tobacco in early pregnancy* (n [%])					
No smoking	189 (86%)	69 (90%)	62 (82%)	29 (85%)	29 (88%)
<10 cigarettes per day	25 (11%)	7 (9%)	11 (14%)	4 (12%)	3 (9%)
>10 cigarettes per day	4 (2%)	1 (1%)	2 (3%)	1 (3%)	
Snuff	2 (1%)		1 (1%)		1 (3%)
Employment status* (n [%])					
Full time employed	87 (40%)	32 (42%)	33 (43%)	9 (26%)	13 (39%)
Part time employed	54 (25%)	19 (25%)	18 (24%)	5 (15%)	12 (36%)
Unemployed	72 (33%)	23 (30%)	23 (30%)	18 (53%)	8 (24%)
Missing data	7 (3%)	3 (4%)	2 (3%)	2 (6%)	
Body mass index* mean (kg/m^2)	24.4	24.0	24.7	24.9	24.1
Other illnesses* (n [%])	106 (48%)	33 (43%)	42 (55%)	12 (35%)	19 (58%)
Antidepressant dose in third trimester** median (range) (mg)	NA	20 (5–80)	50 (5–200)	30 (10–80)	NA
Use of benzodiazepine during pregnancy (n [%])	14 (6%)	4 (5%)	5 (7%)	3 (9%)	2 (6%)
Use of other medications during pregnancy (n [%])	136 (62%)	43 (56%)	44 (58%)	27 (79%)	22 (67%)
Mode of delivery (n [%])					
Vaginal delivery	155 (70%)	57 (74%)	48 (63%)	25 (74%)	25 (76%)
Cesarean section (planned)	24 (11%)	7 (9%)	11 (14%)	2 (6%)	4 (12%)
Cesarian section (acute)	20 (9%)	5 (6%)	9 (12%)	4 (12%)	2 (6%)
Vacuum extraction	21 (10%)	8 (10%)	8 (11%)	3 (9%)	2 (6%)

#one patient can have more than one diagnosis.
##other psychiatric diagnoses, all antidepressants (n): Phobia (4), Post-traumatic stress disorder (4), Eating disorder (9), Personality disorder (6), Obsessive compulsive disorder (7), Bipolar disorder type II (1), Attention deficit hyperactivity disorder (3).
*stated by mother at interview with midwife in prenatal care center, gestational week 10–14.
**other antidepressants (n = 33): escitalopram (13 patients), venlafaxine (11), paroxetine (8) and duloxetine (1).
***Highest dose in maternal care records during third trimester.
NA = not applicable.

a logistic regression model adjusting for maternal age, maternal tobacco use in early pregnancy and infant sex there were no statistically significant differences regarding prematurity between citalopram exposed infants (13%) and infants exposed to sertraline (7%, p = 0.85), fluoxetine (9%, p = 0.67) or other antidepressants (3%, p = 0.30).

Hypoglycemia in the neonate was defined as a blood glucose level <2.6 mmol/L. Hypoglycemia was diagnosed in 42 (19%) of all study infants. A logistic regression model (adjusting for 5 min Apgar, gestational age, tobacco use in early pregnancy and infant sex) showed significantly more infants with at least one hypoglycemic episode in the fluoxetine group, 12 (35%), compared to 8 (10%) in the citalopram group, p = 0.01. There were no significant differences between citalopram exposed infants and infants exposed to sertraline (p = 0.74) or other antidepressants (p = 0.70). A model adjusting for only 5 min Apgar and gestational age did not add further information.

The blood glucose values of all hypoglycemic infants (n = 42) ranged from 1.0 to 2.5 mmol/L (mean 2.0 mmol/L). In hypoglycemic infants exposed to citalopram (n = 8) the mean blood glucose was 2.0 (range 1.4 to 2.3). These numbers for hypoglycemic infants exposed to sertraline, fluoxetine and other antidepressants were 1.9 (range 1.0 to 2.5), 1.9 (range 1.0 to 2.5) and 2.1 (range 1.1 to 2.5) respectively. There were no significant differences between the groups, p = 0.6 (Kruskal Wallis).

Respiratory disorders included 'respiratory distress syndrome of newborn', 'transient tachypnea of newborn', 'other respiratory distress of newborn', pneumothorax, persistent fetal circulation and 'condition originating in the perinatal period', the latter an apneoic event. There were 14 cases (6.3%) of respiratory disorders and 4 of them were in prematurely born infants. No significant correlation was seen between occurrence of respiratory disorders and type of antidepressant exposure in third trimester, in logistic regression adjusting for 5 min Apgar score and gestational age (in weeks), p = 1.0.

Table 2. Neonatal characteristics of infants exposed to antidepressants in utero, born 1 Jan 2007 to 30 June 2009 at Karolinska University Hospital.

	All antidepressants	Citalopram	Sertraline	Fluoxetine	Other antidepressants**
	n = 220	n = 77	n = 76	n = 34	n = 33
Sex (male:female) (n[%])	106:114 [48:52]	38:39 [49:51]	36:40 [47:53]	16:18 [47:53]	16:17 [48:52]
Gestational age (weeks)					
mean [95% CI]	38.5 [38.3 to 38.7]	38.2 [37.8 to 38.5]	38.8 [38.4 to 39.1]	38.6 [38.1 to 39.1]	38.5 [38.0 to 39.1]
range	31–42	31–41	32–41	35–42	34–42
Prematurity (n [%]) *	19 [9]	10 [13]	5 [7]	3 [9]	1 [3]
Birth weight (gram)					
mean [95% CI]	3386 [3314 to 3458]	3302 [3177 to 3425]	3476 [3352 to 3600]	3385 [3217 to 3553]	3377 [3167 to 3588]
range	1790–5015	1790–4315	1905–5015	2110–4670	2305–4615
Head circumference (cm)					
n	217	75	75	34	33
mean [95% CI]	34.3 [34.1 to 34.5]	34.0 [33.6 to 34.4]	34.4 [34.1 to 34.8]	34.3 [33.7 to 34.8]	34.5 [33.9 to 35.1]
range	28–38	28–37.5	31–38	30–37	31–37.5
Hypoglycemia (n [%])	42 [19]†	8 [11]	15 [20]	12 [35]	7 [21]
Respiratory diagnosis (n [%])	14 [6]	5 [6]	5 [7]	2 [6]	2 [6]
Jaundice (n [%])	10 [5]	5 [6]	3 [4]	1 [3]	1 [3]
Neonatal care (n [%])	29 [13]	10 [13]	9 [12]	6 [18]	4 [12]

*gestational age <37+0.
**other antidepressants (n = 33): escitalopram (13 patients), venlafaxine (11), paroxetine (8) and duloxetine (1).
†p 0.02, statistical test (logistic regression, adjusting for gestational age, maternal tobacco use, infant sex and 5 min Apgar).

There were five children with Apgar score <7 at five minutes of age.

Jaundice was diagnosed in 10 children (4 born prematurely). There were no significant differences between groups for antidepressant exposure, in a logistic regression model adjusting for 5 min Apgar and gestational age, p = 1.0.

One hundred and fifty-eight infants (71%), received the diagnostic code Z001A 'healthy infant born in hospital'.

Twenty-nine (13%) of the infants exposed to antidepressants were admitted to the neonatal ward. During 2007, 2008 and 2009, 13755 infants were born at Karolinska University Hospital Huddinge [14] and 1418 (10.3%) of them admitted to the neonatal ward (data from Swedish Neonatal Quality Register). A univariate analysis showed no statistical difference between exposed and unexposed infants (born at Karolinska University Huddinge) regarding probability for neonatal admission (p = 0.16). Multivariate analysis (logistic regression adjusting for 5 min Apgar and gestational age) did not reveal any differences in admittance rates between the four exposure groups (p = 0.67).

No specific treatment for neonatal maladaptation syndrome was performed. The patients were treated with supportive care. Respiratory disorders were treated with CPAP (continuous positive airway pressure) if needed (8 cases) and hypoglycemia with intensified oral feeding, in some instances with i.v glucose, depending on the severity of the condition.

A total of 205 infants (93%) were scored with Neonatal Abstinence Score sheet (table 3). The mean time at 'peak score' i e highest recorded score in patients who had a score of four or higher at any time, was for infants exposed to citalopram 31.6 hours (range 2–90; SD 21.4), for sertraline exposure 37.4 (1–84; 21.7), fluoxetine exposure 37.1 (4–74; 21.3) and other antidepressants exposure 22.1 hours (3–64; 17.6). There were no statistically significant differences between the groups (Kruskal Wallis, p = 0.07).

CNS symptoms contributed with on average 67% of the points in the group with severe abstinence (two or more scores of eight or higher) and 58% in the group with mild abstinence (two or more scores of four or higher). Infants exposed to citalopram had mild abstinence in 18 cases (25%), severe abstinence in two cases. Comparing citalopram to sertraline exposure in ordinal regression, adjusting for 5 min Apgar and infant sex, infants exposed to sertraline had an odds ratio of 1.08 (95% confidence interval, 0.64 to 1.82). Odds ratio for fluoxetine compared to citalopram was 0.86 (95% CI, 0.45 to 1.63) and for other antidepressants compared to citalopram 1.3 (95% CI, 0.61 to 2.61). There were no significant differences in the occurrence of mild or severe abstinence between the different types of antidepressant exposure, adjusting for 5 min Apgar and infant sex, p = 0.85.

There were no significant differences in mean maternal SSRI dose in third trimester (analysis made for citalopram [p = 0.20], sertraline [p = 0.83] and fluoxetine [p = 0.18]) between infants with or without abstinence (Mann Whitney U test).

Twenty-nine infants in the study were admitted to the neonatal ward. Twenty four percent of them were not scored with NAS compared to 4% of the infants who remained in the maternity ward (p = 0.0007).

Discussion

This study shows that a majority of all infants born to mothers with SSRI or SNRI treatment during pregnancy are healthy in the neonatal period. Only 3% developed a severe abstinence syndrome and 22% signs of mild abstinence, the symptoms mainly arising from the central nervous system. Our results are in accordance with other studies with similar or slightly higher

Table 3. Analyses of Neonatal Abstinence Score in infants exposed to antidepressants in utero, born at Karolinska University Hospital Huddinge 1 Jan 2007 to 30 June 2009.

	All antidepressants	citalopram	sertraline	fluoxetine	Other antidepressants[≠]	p
Scoring performed (n[%])	205 [93%]	71 [92%]	71 [93%]	33 [97%]	30 [91%]	0.5[†]
Number of scoring occasions						
(mean [SD] [range])	8.4 [3.0] [2–27]	8.5 [2.7] [3–18]	8.4 [2.9] [2–20]	8.4 [4.4] [2–27]	8.3 [2.2] [5–13]	0.66[††]
Neonatal abstinence (n[%])						
No abstinence	152 [74%]	51 [72%]	53 [75%]	24 [73%]	24 [80%]	
*Mild abstinence**	46 [22%]	18 [25%]	16 [23%]	7 [21%]	5 [17%]	
*Severe abstinence***	7 [3%]	2 [3%]	2 [3%]	2 [6%]	1 [3%]	0.85***

*two or more scorings of 4–7.
**two or more scorings of 8 or above.
***Multiple ordinal regression, adjusted for infant sex and 5 min Apgar.
†Chi square test.
††Kruskal Wallis.
≠other antidepressants (n = 33): escitalopram (13 patients), venlafaxine (11), paroxetine (8) and duloxetine (1).

prevalence of the neonatal abstinence/maladaptation syndrome in infants with intrauterine SSRI/SNRI exposure. A study that used Finnegan score and similar definitions of severe and mild neonatal maladaptation syndrome found mild or severe neonatal maladaptation syndrome in 18/60 (30%) infants exposed to SSRI, compared to 0/60 control infants [12]. A slightly different definition of severe maladaptation (NAS score >12 or 3 scores >8) reported a prevalence of 4% in infants exposed to SSRI and 9% in infants exposed to venlafaxine [15]. Oberlander et al described symptoms of transient poor neonatal adaptation in 30% of a group of infants exposed to SSRI with or without the addition of clonazepam [16]. The reasons behind the differences in prevalence may be found in the different definitions of neonatal maladaptation syndrome as well as differences in study population (maternal age, socioeconomic status, health care, concomitant pharmacological treatment, use of tobacco and alcohol).

Hypoglycemia was common, 19% of all infants had blood glucose of 2.6 mmol/L or lower. Most of them were treated with intensified oral feeding. Other studies have found an association between prenatal antidepressant exposure and hypoglycemia [7]. The etiology behind this may be increased demands of energy in babies with abstinence. The prevalence reported in other studies have been lower, 1.4% in a register based cohort study [17] or 3/60 exposed infants in an Israeli cohort [12]. These large differences between studies may be explained by different definitions of hypoglycemia (the ICD-10 diagnosis of neonatal hypoglycemia, P70.4, requires blood glucose 2.2 mmol/L or lower) as well as differences in study protocols or in clinical practice. Hypoglycemia is also fairly common in all infants. In a clinical study of healthy term and preterm infants, 12% of the term and 14% of the preterm infants had a blood glucose of below 2.6 mmol/L during the first week of life [18]. In observational studies such as this one, the high rates of hypoglycemia may also be due to the fact that jitteriness and tremor can be perceived as symptoms of hypoglycemia leading to the measurement of blood glucose, increasing the chance of diagnosing a low blood glucose value. Hypoglycemia in infants is however a potentially serious condition [19,20] and needs to be further investigated, preferably in a randomized controlled study. Until then, screening of blood glucose in neonates prenatally exposed to antidepressants should be considered.

The mothers in this study had a more unfavorable health status than the average pregnant Stockholm County population with regard to higher proportion of smokers and higher BMI. This may also affect neonatal outcome. The catchment area of Karolinska University Hospital Huddinge includes many socioeconomically constrained areas, often associated with higher BMI and a higher proportion of smokers. Any comparison between this catchment area and the rest of Stockholm County must be done with caution. Studies on infants to mothers with opioid use during pregnancy have shown increased risk of neonatal abstinence as well as other negative neonatal outcomes in opioid exposed infants where there was a concomitant heavy cigarette consumption [21]. Smoking cessation and control of weight gain during pregnancy may be an important method in this patient group to improve infant (and maternal) health.

Several other studies report a high incidence of respiratory symptoms in infants exposed to SSRIs [5,22]. However, some experts argue that the increased risk of neonatal complications that have been attributed to SSRI exposure may be due to confounding factors [23]. Fourteen neonates in this study had a respiratory diagnosis but the study design did not allow a comparison to an unexposed population.

Different antidepressants have different pharmacokinetic properties. This may, in theory, influence the timing of symptoms of abstinence or serotonergic overstimulation in exposed neonates. Time to peak value (NAS) was therefore analyzed but failed to show any significant differences between the groups. Individual factors such as metabolic and transporter capacity of SSRI/SNRI in mother and child as well as placenta may be of greater influence on the occurrence of maladaptation and timing of symptoms [15,24–26]. Time to peak value ranged between 2 and 90 hours suggesting that infants exposed to antidepressants may have a relatively late onset of peak abstinence symptoms. With today's extremely short duration of hospital stay for newborns, the symptoms may even occur after discharge from hospital. Karolinska University Hospital Huddinge, as well as several other hospitals, has abandoned the policy of advising parents of infants prenatally exposed to antidepressants to stay at least 72 hours. In uneventful deliveries, the mother and infant usually leave the maternity ward within 48 hours.

Seven percent of the infants in the study were not subject to abstinence scoring. This may be due to the fact that the midwife nurse was not aware of the guidelines, that the infant was perceived to be healthy or that the scoring sheet was not properly stored. Also, NAS is often used as a screening tool and may therefore be considered unnecessary in sick infants in the neonatal ward who are subjected to more sophisticated surveillance methods. This may explain why scoring was not performed in a larger proportion of the infants admitted to the neonatal ward compared to the maternity care units.

The causal relationship between SSRI or SNRI exposure and high scoring values in the NAS is of course not established in each infant included in this study. Other illnesses or prenatal risk factors, unrelated to pharmacological exposure or maternal illness, may contribute. This study could not investigate an increased risk of neonatal symptoms in infants prenatally exposed to antidepressants compared to unexposed ones.

It can be argued that we recruited a too small study population. There may have been differences between the exposure groups had they been larger. The retrospective design of the study and the changed policy of the hospital (Neonatal Abstinence Score and increased surveillance of all infants prenatally exposed to SSRIs were abandoned in July 2009) made it impossible to perform this study on a larger cohort. The retrospective design is of course an important limitation to this study. A prospective design would have allowed us to for example confirm antidepressant use and exposure in mother and infant.

Monitoring neonates with prenatal exposure to drugs and abuse substances is a delicate task. There is a risk that health care professionals are being too interventional, introducing unnecessary concern regarding the infant's health. There is also a risk, with antidepressants becoming increasingly common in the pregnant population- and considered 'safe'- that knowledge about potentially serious complications is lost. A modified Neonatal Abstinence Score could be useful in detecting abstinence/maladaptation in this group. The CNS and respiratory categories are probably more useful than the gastrointestinal category. Most important is however knowledge among care givers regarding the possible symptoms that can arise after prenatal exposure to antidepressants.

Conclusions

Severe abstinence in a cohort of infants exposed to SSRI/SNRI in late pregnancy was rare since it occurred in only 3% of the cases. Neonatal hypoglycemia was observed in 19% of the infants which is higher than previously reported. Admission to the neonatal ward was seen in 13% of the infants and did not differ significantly from the admittance rate in other infants born in the same hospital during the studied period.

Author Contributions

Conceived and designed the experiments: LF LN LLG KW. Performed the experiments: LF LN KW. Analyzed the data: LF LN LLG KW. Contributed reagents/materials/analysis tools: LF KW LN. Wrote the paper: LF LN LLG KW.

References

1. Vesga-Lopez O, Blanco C, Keyes K, Olfson M, Grant BF, et al. (2008) Psychiatric disorders in pregnant and postpartum women in the United States. Arch Gen Psychiatry 65: 805–815.
2. Stephansson O, Granath F, Svensson T, Haglund B, Ekbom A, et al. (2011) Drug use during pregnancy in Sweden - assessed by the Prescribed Drug Register and the Medical Birth Register. Clin Epidemiol 3: 43–50.
3. Lennestal R, Kallen B (2007) Delivery outcome in relation to maternal use of some recently introduced antidepressants. J Clin Psychopharmacol 27: 607–613.
4. Jimenez-Solem E, Andersen JT, Petersen M, Broedbaek K, Andersen NL, et al. (2013) Prevalence of antidepressant use during pregnancy in Denmark, a nationwide cohort study. PLoS One 8: e63034.
5. Reis M, Kallen B (2010) Delivery outcome after maternal use of antidepressant drugs in pregnancy: an update using Swedish data. Psychol Med 40: 1723–1733.
6. Berard A, Ramos E, Rey E, Blais L, St-Andre M, et al. (2007) First trimester exposure to paroxetine and risk of cardiac malformations in infants: the importance of dosage. Birth Defects Res B Dev Reprod Toxicol 80: 18–27.
7. Moses-Kolko EL, Bogen D, Perel J, Bregar A, Uhl K, et al. (2005) Neonatal signs after late in utero exposure to serotonin reuptake inhibitors: literature review and implications for clinical applications. JAMA 293: 2372–2383.
8. Laine K, Heikkinen T, Ekblad U, Kero P (2003) Effects of exposure to selective serotonin reuptake inhibitors during pregnancy on serotonergic symptoms in newborns and cord blood monoamine and prolactin concentrations. Arch Gen Psychiatry 60: 720–726.
9. Kieler H, Artama M, Engeland A, Ericsson O, Furu K, et al. (2012) Selective serotonin reuptake inhibitors during pregnancy and risk of persistent pulmonary hypertension in the newborn: population based cohort study from the five Nordic countries. BMJ 344: d8012.
10. Bonari L, Pinto N, Ahn E, Einarson A, Steiner M, et al. (2004) Perinatal risks of untreated depression during pregnancy. Can J Psychiatry 49: 726–735.
11. Finnegan LP, Connaughton JF, Jr., Kron RE, Emich JP (1975) Neonatal abstinence syndrome: assessment and management. Addict Dis 2: 141–158.
12. Levinson-Castiel R, Merlob P, Linder N, Sirota L, Klinger G (2006) Neonatal abstinence syndrome after in utero exposure to selective serotonin reuptake inhibitors in term infants. Arch Pediatr Adolesc Med 160: 173–176.
13. Sarman I (2000) [Methadone treatment during pregnancy and its effect on the child. Better than continuing drug abuse, should be monitored by a specialized antenatal care center]. Lakartidningen 97: 2182–2184, 2187–2188, 2190.
14. Socialstyrelsen (2013) Statistikdatabasen. In: Socialstyrelsen, editor. wwwsocialstyrelsense. www.socialstyrelsen.se.
15. Rampono J, Simmer K, Ilett KF, Hackett LP, Doherty DA, et al. (2009) Placental transfer of SSRI and SNRI antidepressants and effects on the neonate. Pharmacopsychiatry 42: 95–100.
16. Oberlander TF, Misri S, Fitzgerald CE, Kostaras X, Rurak D, et al. (2004) Pharmacologic factors associated with transient neonatal symptoms following prenatal psychotropic medication exposure. J Clin Psychiatry 65: 230–237.
17. Kallen B (2004) Neonate characteristics after maternal use of antidepressants in late pregnancy. Arch Pediatr Adolesc Med 158: 312–316.
18. Hawdon JM, Ward Platt MP, Aynsley-Green A (1992) Patterns of metabolic adaptation for preterm and term infants in the first neonatal week. Arch Dis Child 67: 357–365.
19. Boardman JP, Wusthoff CJ, Cowan FM (2013) Hypoglycaemia and neonatal brain injury. Arch Dis Child Educ Pract Ed 98: 2–6.
20. Duvanel CB, Fawer CL, Cotting J, Hohlfeld P, Matthieu JM (1999) Long-term effects of neonatal hypoglycemia on brain growth and psychomotor development in small-for-gestational-age preterm infants. J Pediatr 134: 492–498.
21. Winklbaur B, Baewert A, Jagsch R, Rohrmeister K, Metz V, et al. (2009) Association between prenatal tobacco exposure and outcome of neonates born to opioid-maintained mothers. Implications for treatment. Eur Addict Res 15: 150–156.
22. Leibovitch L, Rymer-Haskel N, Schushan-Eisen I, Kuint J, Strauss T, et al. (2013) Short-Term Neonatal Outcome among Term Infants after in utero Exposure to Serotonin Reuptake Inhibitors. Neonatology 104: 65–70.
23. Warburton W, Hertzman C, Oberlander TF (2010) A register study of the impact of stopping third trimester selective serotonin reuptake inhibitor exposure on neonatal health. Acta Psychiatr Scand 121: 471–479.
24. Hilli J, Heikkinen T, Rontu R, Lehtimaki T, Kishida I, et al. (2009) MAO-A and COMT genotypes as possible regulators of perinatal serotonergic symptoms after in utero exposure to SSRIs. Eur Neuropsychopharmacol 19: 363–370.
25. Oberlander TF, Bonaguro RJ, Misri S, Papsdorf M, Ross CJ, et al. (2008) Infant serotonin transporter (SLC6A4) promoter genotype is associated with adverse neonatal outcomes after prenatal exposure to serotonin reuptake inhibitor medications. Mol Psychiatry 13: 65–73.
26. Ter Horst PG, Jansman FG, van Lingen RA, Smit JP, de Jong-van den Berg LT, et al. (2008) Pharmacological aspects of neonatal antidepressant withdrawal. Obstet Gynecol Surv 63: 267–279.

Coverage and Quality of Antenatal Care Provided at Primary Health Care Facilities in the 'Punjab' Province of 'Pakistan'

Muhammad Ashraf Majrooh[1]*, Seema Hasnain[1], Javaid Akram[1], Arif Siddiqui[1], Zahid Ali Memon[2]

1 Allama Iqbal Medical College, Lahore, Pakistan, **2** Population Survives International – Greenstar, Karachi, Pakistan

Abstract

Background: Antenatal care is a very important component of maternal health services. It provides the opportunity to learn about risks associated with pregnancy and guides to plan the place of deliveries thereby preventing maternal and infant morbidity and mortality. In 'Pakistan' antenatal services to rural population are being provided through a network of primary health care facilities designated as 'Basic Health Units and Rural Health Centers. Pakistan is a developing country, consisting of four provinces and federally administered areas. Each province is administratively subdivided in to 'Divisions' and 'Districts'. By population 'Punjab' is the largest province of Pakistan having 36 districts. This study was conducted to assess the coverage and quality antenatal care in the primary health care facilities in 'Punjab' province of 'Pakistan'.

Methods: Quantitative and Qualitative methods were used to collect data. Using multistage sampling technique nine out of thirty six districts were selected and 19 primary health care facilities of public sector (seventeen Basic Health Units and two Rural Health Centers were randomly selected from each district. Focus group discussions and in-depth interviews were conducted with clients, providers and health managers.

Results: The overall enrollment for antenatal checkup was 55.9% and drop out was 32.9% in subsequent visits. The quality of services regarding assessment, treatment and counseling was extremely poor. The reasons for low coverage and quality were the distant location of facilities, deficiency of facility resources, indifferent attitude and non availability of the staff. Moreover, lack of client awareness about importance of antenatal care and self empowerment for decision making to seek care were also responsible for low coverage.

Conclusion: The coverage and quality of the antenatal care services in 'Punjab' are extremely compromised. Only half of the expected pregnancies are enrolled and out of those 1/3 drop out in follow-up visits.

Editor: Zulfiqar A. Bhutta, The Hospital for Sick Children, Pakistan

Funding: This manuscript is an output from a research funded by Maternal and Newborn Health Programme – Research and Advocacy Fund (RAF) and conducted by Research Society Allama Iqbal Medical College Lahore, Pakistan. The views expressed and the information contained is not necessarily endorsed by funding agencies DFID/AusAID. The funders had no role in study design, data collection and analysis, decision to publish, or preparation of the manuscript.

Competing Interests: The author have declared that no competing interests exist.

* Email: majrooh58@yahoo.com

Introduction

Low up take of Antenatal care (ANC) is an important determinant of high maternal mortality rate in developing countries and is one of the basic components of maternal care on which the life of mothers and babies depend [1]. According to WHO, 536000 women die every year in the world from causes relating to pregnancy, childbirth or postpartum. Ninety nine percent of these deaths occur in the developing countries. The majority of these deaths could be avoided if women had access to quality medical care during pregnancy, childbirth and postpartum [2]. ANC services help pregnant women by identifying complications associated with pregnancy or diseases that might adversely affect the pregnancy [3]. The ANC coverage in the Punjab province of Pakistan is only 53% and there isinequity in provision of ANC services to rural population as depicted by some studies which is 50% in comparison to 71% of urban women. About 25% of women in rural and urban areas of Punjab consulted health care providers at a public sector health care facility [4]. Multiple reasons have been reported for low coverage of ANC services that includes the weak health systems, inadequate training [5] and inaccessibility of health facilities and ANC services in Pakistan are widely cited as being responsible for a high proportion of maternal and infant deaths [6]. However, in recent decades certain low income countries have witnessed dramatic improvements in publically funded health care delivery system. For instance in Sri Lanka maternal health care is provided free of charge to all women and in 2000, 94.5% of expected mothers had visited an antenatal care clinic at least once [7]. Social developmental factors like education markedly influence the ANC coverage in low income countries for instance in a study in Ethiopia ANC utilization increases by skilled care providers as the level of education of woman increases. Only 25% of women who had no education used skilled ANC attendants compared with 90% of those who had higher than secondary level education [8]. Introduction of group ANC sessions at public health centers in Iran showed a significant improvement in patient satisfaction and mean patient satisfaction score increased for women participating in group sessions compared to individual care. Significant improvements were seen in number of women receiving full number of ANC visits. Further, increase in birth weight and use of supplements was observed among the ladies receiving group ANC sessions [9]. An intervention in India for improvement of ANC through ensuring staff had necessary equipment, increased monitoring and supervision, focused training, re-organisation of outreach clinics and scheduling Quality of care increased as more than 60% of women received all ANC components. Significant increase in blood pressure and urine testing increased significantly. Attendance at clinics also increased by 30% [10].

In a study of expectant mothers in an urban squatter settlement of Karachi, indicated that 49% received no antenatal care, even in the presence of no cost and low cost public health sector ANC services [11]. A cross-sectional community-based study in Sudan reported that out of 900 pregnant women, 811 (90%) had at least one visit. Only 11% of the women had ≥ four antenatal visits [12]. In another study conducted in North West of Pakistan about the utilization of prenatal care services by the rural women, it was reported that only 28.1% (34/121) pregnant women of Sarbund village utilized prenatal care service in either private (6/121; 0.5%) or public sectors 28/121; 23.1%) [13]. Pakistan Demographic and Health Survey confirms that maternal deaths are not merely a result of treatment failure; rather they are the final outcome of a complex interplay between a myraid of social, cultural and economic factors [14].

Client satisfaction is the litmus test that enables health programs to assess the impact of their service; hence it is an integral part of the quality assurance process of health delivery. In recent years, there has been an increasing demand of accountability and productivity by consumers. It is now a global trend in health care development towards integrating subjective user satisfaction into the evaluation of medical service quality [15]. Patients' voice must begin to play a greater role in the design of health care service delivery process in the developing countries [16]. The satisfaction of female clients of ANC has been studied in the past in other countries [17]. A study in India reported that the overall summative index for clinical quality using a scale of 0–5 was 2.1% in the North and 4.1 in the South [18]. Similarly in another studyin Oman the overall satisfaction for antenatal care was excellent in 49 (CI 48.5–69.6) respondents. Out of 89 women, 67 (81%) were satisfied with the services because of the attitude of the doctors and nurses. The main causes of dissatisfaction were the laboratory services and overcrowding in the morning hours [19]. However in a study conducted at a Hyderabad, Sindh, half of the women in study sample were satisfied with the overall care provided to them. The routine antenatal investigations were provided to majority of women like urine, blood, antenatal examination and blood pressure. About 86.2% women said that they have to wait for more than two hours for checkups. Regarding satisfaction with getting medicine 63% were found dissatisfied, 75% of women did not have complete tetanus vaccine. Only 31% received instructions about perinatal care, 46% received information about exercise and 36% were reassured about discussing fear and anxiety [20].

In 'Punjab' province of Pakistan, there is network of PHC health facilities named as Rural Health Centers (RHCs) and Basic Health Units (BHUs). RHCs are relatively larger PHC facilities serving 10–50 thousands rural population while BHUs are relatively smaller health facilities providing PHC services to 5000 to 10,000 rural populations. One BHU is available up to almost each 'Union Council' level. There is uniform package of health services, infrastructure, physical and human resources. Medical Officers are in-charge of RHCs/BHUs and ANC services are supposed to be provided by the Lady Health Visitors (LHVs) at these facilities. This study is an attempt to evaluate the coverage and quality of antenatal care being provided to the rural population of this province. Although the study was focused on antenatal care but it will reflect the overall gaps in the health system of Pakistan to be bridged through appropriate interventions. The objectives of the study were:

1. To assess the proportion of expected pregnancies enrolled for ANC services in the catchment areas of PHC health facilities.
2. To assess the proportion of the enrolled clients coming for follow-up ANC visits.
3. To assess the quality ANC services delivery process in terms of assessment, treatment and counseling of the clients.
4. To explore and identify the causes of low coverage and quality of services at managerial, provider and client level.

Methods

A cross-sectional study was conducted to assess the coverage and quality of ANC services in first-level health care facilities. Both quantitative and qualitative research methods were used to undertake this study. The study proposal was approved by National Bioethics Committee (NBC) Pakistan vide Ref No.4-87/09/NBC-36/RDC/7451 and the inception of the study was undertaken after the approval. A multi-stage sampling procedure was adopted to select the districts and primary level health facilities from each district. In first stage all the districts of Punjab were ranked from 1 to 36 on the basis of a composite indicator which was developed from eight socio-demographic indicators [21]. Total nine out of thirty six districts were selected from the Punjab province so that three district from each high, medium and low social stratum could be included in the study. In the second stage of sampling, 19 health facilities (17 BHUs and 2 RHCs) were randomly selected from each district. Initially a total 171 health facilities BHUs/RHCs were accessed for completion of facility performance data. Approval for health facility assessment and interviews for health care providers was taken from Punjab Health Department. A consent form was developed in the local language that was approved by National Bioethics Committee (NBC) Pakistan. Informed verbal consent was taken from the clients and health care providers for interviews. The Consent form for each interview was filled and signed by a witness at health facilities and its record was maintained along with other data forms. Written consent was not possible for the reason that majority of the clients were illiterate (unable to read or write). During the survey in the first attempt, data collection from 151 health care facilities was completed and an additional 20 alternate health facilities were visited by teams in second attempt due to non-availability of providers or clients to complete the target sample. Client exit interviews were conducted after each client-provider interaction to assess the client satisfaction. The client exit interviews included the questions about the behavior of provider, ANC examination, time spent and the overall perception of satisfaction for the services provided.

Focal Group Discussions (FGDs) and in-depth interviews were conducted in qualitative part of assessment. Nine FGDs for clients and nine for providers were conducted in each of the nine sampled districts. The criteria for the selection of the clients was pregnant women who had already experienced at least one pregnancy and birth process, belonged to lower or middle social class and these clients came from the catchment area of health facility. There were 12 clients in each FGD session who were identified by the 'Lady Health Workers (LHW) in the catchment areas of the health facilities. LHWs enroll the pregnant ladies keep the records and refer them to the BHUs and RHCs for ANC services. The selection criterion for health care providers (Lady Health Visitor) was that their duration of working in these facilities was more than six months. The participation of health care providers was voluntary and the invitations were extended to them with permission of management of provincial health department. A total of 12 LHVs were included in each FGD. One FGD was conducted for Medical Officers/Women Medical Officers at the provincial level. In-depth interviews were conducted with district health managers (Executive District Officers for Health/District Officers for Health) and the provincial managers (Director General Health, Director MNCH Program and Director MIS Cell.

The data was collected on objectively developed semi-structured questionnaire from October-November 2010. Total eight teams were engaged for data collection and each team consisted of one team leader/supervisor and two surveyors/interviewers. A qualitative assessment team comprised of two sociologists and one public health consultant. All teams were provided extensive training in two separate 3-day workshops, one for qualitative and other for quantitative assessment teams. Field monitoring was carried out by two Regional Coordinators, a Public Health Consultant and the Principal investigator. Qualitative data was collected from December 2010 to February 2011.

Univariate analysis was done to describe the frequency and percentage by type of facility and by districts. ANC coverage was evaluated by examining the record of services provided to ANC clients at health facilities. For this purpose, annual ANC first enrolment and ANC follow-up visits were used as indictors. The percentage of the annual expected [22] pregnancies in the catchment area of health facility who reported first time for ANC services during the year before survey (2010) was operationally defined as ANC Enrollment. Percentage of the annual expected pregnancies in the catchment area of health facility reported for follow-up ANC services during the year before survey (2010) was defined as ANC-follow-up visits [19]. It was not possible to calculate the number of visits of a particular client from this data source. The revisits reported from this column are also termed as revisits in the reporting tools of Punjab MIS. The quality of ANC services was based on the steps followed by the health care-providers. A standard check list of steps to be followed health care provider, was developed by consultation of WHO criteria and Minimum Service Delivery Standards (MSDS) adopted by Maternal and Newborn and Child Health Program (MNCH) of the Punjab. This check list was used to observe the client provider interaction during ANC service provision. The providers that follow more than 80% of the steps enlisted in the checklist of assessment, treatment and counseling of the clients were ranked as good, between 60–80% as average and less than 60% as poor to measure the quality of ANC.

The qualitative data processing was initiated in the field with development of field transcripts by the interviewers/facilitator. A qualitative analysis framework was prepared for each target group e.g. clients, providers, facility in-charges, district health managers and provincial stakeholders. The findings were categorized under the main titles of the themes included in qualitative tools relevant to specific participants in FGDs. Findings were analyzed by inductive reasoning approach and qualitative assessment report was compiled under the supervision of a senior sociologist by consulting the individual session reports, transcripts/notes of FGDs and transcripts/notes of all in-depth interviews. Broadly, the analysis of data was arranged by the objectives of the study as stipulated in the research proposal.

Results

ANC coverage

The overall enrollment was 51.6% in sampled districts of the Punjab province including the 17 redundant health facilities where no services being provided. Wide range of variations was observed among districts in ANC enrollment. Maximum coverage was observed in district Gujranwala at 79.6% followed by district Toba Tek Singh with 79.1% ANC-1 coverage annually. Minimum coverage was reported from district Sahiwal as 24.9% followed by district Multan as 33.8%. Out of the whole sample, five districts – Multan, Vehari, Bahawalnagar, Sahiwal and Sargodha – had coverage below overall mean and four districts – Gujranwala, Rawalpindi, Toba Tek Singh and Kasur – had ANC coverage above overall mean. (Fig. 1) The regression analysis indicates that there was 1.347% decrease in ANC coverage with one digit rise in ranking of the districts with constant value at base line of 71.7%. The Pearson Product Correlation coefficient, r = 0.64 and r2 = 0.41. All the districts in the Punjab were ranked from 1 to 36 according to a composite indicator based on adult literacy, primary school enrolment, under-five mortality, prevalence of under-nutrition, adequate water and sanitation, the percentage of deliveries with a skilled birth attendant, and use of contraceptive. The rank 1 mean most developed district and rank 36 mean least developed district. The higher ranks number are indicating lower social developmental index and low coverage. In other words with one degree increase rank mean decrease in social development and there is decrease in 1.347% ANC coverage and 71.7% is the highest base line coverage on the line of best fit of regression line. (Fig. 2).

ANC-enrollment percentage was increased from 51.6% to 55.9% when the data from 17 alternative non-redundant facilities was added to the analysis. The overall dropout was 32.8% in subsequent visits after the ANC visit in the health facilities. The drop was observed in all the districts except 'Rawalpindi' where there was a 29.1% increase in the number of follow-up visits. The reason for increase follow-up visits in this district was the availability of WMOs, free ultrasound services and accessible locations of some of the RHC health facilities.

Health facilities were ranked according to monthly percentage of expected pregnancies enrolled for ANC in the catchment area of health facilities. Health facilities enrolling more than 80% of expected pregnancies were ranked as good, 60–80% as average and less than 60% as poor. ANC coverage facility ranking revealed that overall only 24% facilities achieved a good ranking, 13.5% had average and 62.6% facilities had poor ranking in monthly ANC-1 coverage. ANC-follow-up/revisits followed a similar trend. (See Table 1).

The inferential analysis shows that <80% coverage was observed in 76% of facilities with 95% confidence limits from 69% to 82%. In comparison by type of facility, 56% of RHCs were providing good coverage compared to only 20% of BHUs. Thus more than half of RHCs had a good ranking for coverage while 80% BHUs had poor or average ranking.

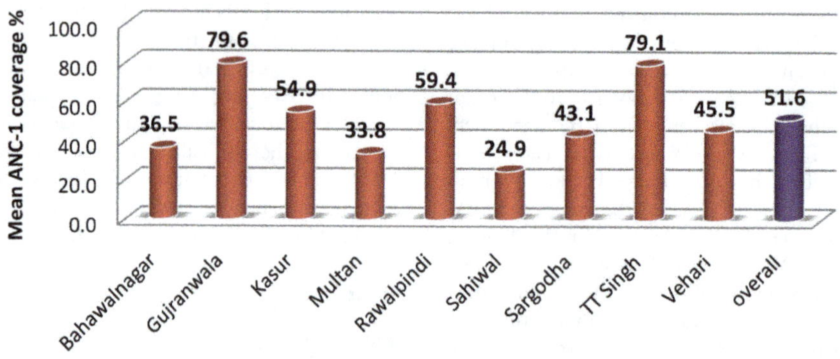

Figure 1. District-wise and overall mean annual ANC-1 coverage in PHC health facilities.

Service quality

The appropriate history taking was followed by less 30% of providers in the context of asking about previous still births, bleeding, assisted deliveries, abortions, headache/blurring of vision, swelling and fever. Feeling of baby movement was enquired from only 9% of the clients. Most of the history steps were falling less than 50% range. The standard protocols for clinical examination were not being fulfilled in most of the cases. The breast examination was practiced in 10%, looked for edema 25%, test advised 21%, heard fetal heart sound in 51%, abdomen was palpated in 76% and BP was recorded in 74% of the services provided. The overall ranking of quality of clinical assessment was poor in 72%, average in 23% and good in only 5% of the services provided. (Fig. 3, Table 2).

The standard protocol steps for counseling were at lowest level that extremely compromised the quality of the ANC services. Counseling for breast feeding was 6%, talked about contraception 6%, asked about place of delivery 31%, transport arrangement 20% and discussed about cost of delivery by 5% providers. TT was advised by 57% and next date of visits was advised by the 80% of the health care providers. The overall ranking of quality of counseling was poor in 92%, average in 6% and good in only 2% of the services provided.

Service delivery protocols practice for the treatment were relatively better than assessment and counseling but the large gaps were identified in treatment practices of the health care providers that includes Tetanus Toxoide (TT) vaccination, prescription for antimalarials, iron and folic acid tablets. Iron and folic acid and TT were prescribed by 69, 64 and 62% respectively but anti-malarial was advised by only by 2% of the health care providers in suspected malaria cases. The overall ranking of quality of treatment was poor in 32%, average in 23% and good in 44% of the services provided. Inferential statistical analysis showed that the overall gap to achieve above 80% level of counseling quality was 48 to 63% at 95% confidence limits. In response to questions in the client exit interview overall 46% clients perceived that they were satisfied with the provided ANC services. The proportion of clients who were satisfied with the services was almost similar in RHCs (50%) and BHUs (46%). (See detail in Table 2).

Qualitative findings

The underlying factors for low coverage and quality explored from the clients, providers and managers. The translated views of each stakeholder are given in the Box-1. Distant location of facilities and lack of functional equipment, medicines and supplies was perceived by the clients, providers as well as health managers. Indifferent attitude and uncertainty in availability of the staff was complained by most of the clients. Community based indigenous ANC providers (Dais) are negatively influencing the ANC services enrollment due to affordability, availability 24/7 at door steps, providing massage, helping for household work and attending the deliveries at home. All these services can't be taken as substitute of the ANC services that needs examination from skilled persons and needs some lab diagnostic services from the health facility set-up.

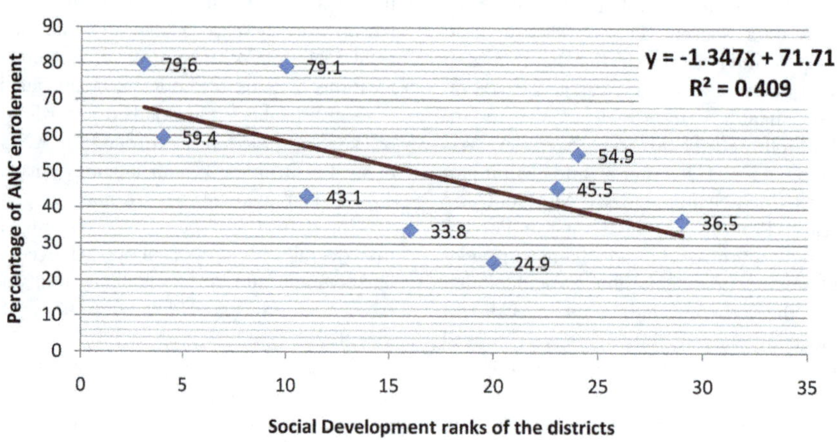

Figure 2. Association of Social Development Ranking with the District ANC coverage.

Table 1. Ranking of health facility by ANC-enrolment and follow-up visits in the catchment areas.

	Overall		RHCs		BHUs	
Number of facilities	**171**		**18**		**153**	
	n	**%**	**n**	**%**	**n**	**%**
Ranking of facilities by monthly ANC enrolment						
Good coverage >80%	41	24	10	56	31	20
Average coverage ≥60% ≤80%	23	13	3	17	20	13
Poor coverage <60	107	63	5	28	102	67
Ranking of facilities by monthly ANC-follow-up/revisits						
Good coverage >80%	27	16	6	33	21	14
Average coverage ≥60% ≤80%	19	11	3	17	16	10
Poor coverage <60	125	73	9	50	116	76

Lack of awareness and self decision power to visit the health facilities are also contributory factors for low coverage of ANC services in the rural area. Most of clients are visiting health facilities with expectation of being examined by ultrasound machine (USG) with hope to determine the sex of the fetus. The specific problems pointed out by providers were lack of guidance and supervision from the WMOs and facility in-charges and managers pointed out the deficiencies in district target setting, periodic monitoring systems, cumbersome purchase process and lack of training and skills.

Discussion

Antenatal care is a very important component of maternal health services. It gives women and their families an opportunity to learn about the risks associated with pregnancy and guides their health seeking practices and decision making thereby preventing maternal and infant morbidity and mortality. Counseling during ANC provides a critical opportunity for women to learn when to seek help and where to give birth. It also helps prepare women for the mental and physical challenges they may face during pregnancy and childbirth. This study was focused on the current situation of coverage and quality of ANC services being provided to the rural mothers in the Punjab. ANC services are being offered by the government in rural areas of the Punjab through a network of PHC health facilities designated as 'RHCs' and 'BHUs'. The private clinics/maternity homes and community health care providers are mainly providing delivery services because they are unable to provide the essential laboratory services package included in the standard ANC protocol. The rural women are mainly dependent on government's PHC health facilities for ANC services. The study finding revealed that overall 51.6% of the expected pregnancies first time reported for the ANC and out of those 33% didn't return back for follow-up. These findings straight way revealed that there is a gap of about 50% in the coverage of ANC services in the Punjab. The dropout in follow-up indicates the poor quality of the services that are annoying the clients not to return back for follow-up services. The overall coverage indicated in this study is very closer to that (57%) claimed by the HMIS cell Punjab [19] in DHIS report of 2010 and MICS 2007–2008, that is about (53%) [23]. This study was focused on rural areas and there was no opportunity for urban comparison but inequity in provision of ANC services to rural population have been reported in the literature [4]. The variation in coverage is associated with the number of standard ANC visits in assessment criteria e.g. in a study conducted in Alwar district of Rajasthan state, India, the practices of 3 or more ANC visits were lower in rural (36.1%) as compared to (71.4%) in urban areas [24].

Fifty percent ANC-1 registration of clients does not mean that the services are fulfilling quality of ANC services. It is just a registration figures. Although WHO recommends four ANC visits for every pregnant woman but the facility register contains only two columns one for the first visit and the other for revisits. Since all revisits are recorded in the same column, it is impossible to know how many of the registered cases completed four ANC visits. On the other hand, revisit/follow-up data indicates that about one third of the clients dropped out after the first visit, which means that a majority of the clients did not even complete two visits. Generally there were dropouts in revisits, in majority of the districts but in Rawalpindi there was an increase in revisits after

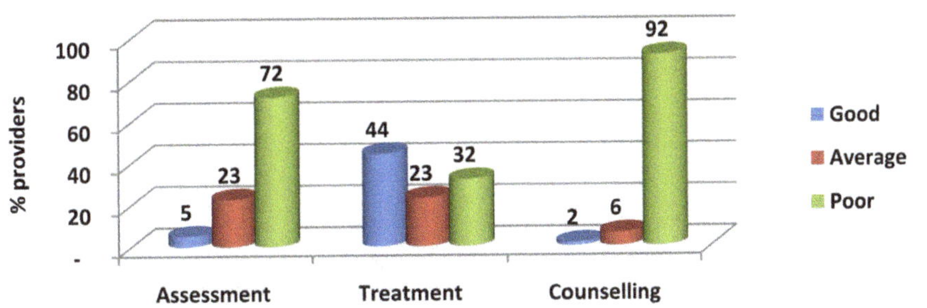

Figure 3. Ranking of ANC Services for Assessment Treatment and Counselling.

Table 2. Quality of ANC services and client satisfaction (Overall and by types of facilities).

	Overall		RHCs		BHUs	
Number of facilities	**171**		**18**		**153**	
	n	**%**	**n**	**%**	**n**	**%**
Areas of client assessment by history						
Age of client	139	81	15	83	124	81
Use of medication by client	77	45	8	44	69	45
Date of LMP asked	103	60	10	56	93	61
Previous pregnancies	111	65	11	61	100	65
Previous still births/neonatal deaths	45	26	6	33	39	25
Heavy bleeding	23	13	5	28	18	12
Assisted deliveries	30	18	4	22	26	17
Abortions	42	25	5	28	37	24
Asked about bleeding	47	27	6	33	41	27
Fever	57	33	6	33	51	33
Headache/blurred vision	45	26	5	28	40	26
Swelling	59	35	6	33	53	35
Tiredness/breathlessness	56	33	6	33	50	33
Felt fetal movement	105	61	12	67	93	61
Mentioned bleeding	16	9	4	22	12	8
Mentioned fever	35	20	4	22	31	20
Mentioned headache/blurred vision	30	18	3	17	27	18
Mentioned swelling	36	21	5	28	31	20
Mentioned tiredness/breathlessness	52	30	6	33	46	30
Mentioned Fetal Movements	79	46	9	50	70	46
Areas of client assessment by examination						
Record BP	127	74	9	50	118	77
Recorded weight	102	60	7	39	95	62
Palpated abdomen	130	76	16	89	114	75
Foetal heart sounds heard	88	51	12	67	76	50
Looked for oedema	42	25	5	28	37	24
Breast exam done	17	10	3	17	14	9
Tests advised	36	21	9	50	27	18
ANC card filled	73	43	10	56	63	41
Talked about TT	109	64	11	61	98	64
Areas of client counselling						
Advice about food	108	63	10	56	98	64
Importance of TT vaccination told	48	28	6	33	42	27
Advised TT	97	57	7	39	90	59
Talked about Contraception	10	6	2	11	8	5
Talked about breast feeding	10	6	2	11	8	5
Place of delivery	53	31	7	39	46	30
Arrangement for transport	35	20	4	22	31	20
Who will accompany her	9	5	1	6	8	5
Time to reach place of delivery	9	5	1	6	8	5
Cost of delivery	11	6	1	6	10	7
Give next visit date	136	80	12	67	124	81
Ranking of client counselling						
Adequate counselling practices >80%	3	2	1	6	2	1
Average counselling practices ≥60% ≤80%	11	6	2	11	9	6
Poor counselling practices <60%	157	92	15	83	142	93

Table 2. Cont.

	Overall		RHCs		BHUs	
Number of facilities	**171**		**18**		**153**	
	n	**%**	**n**	**%**	**n**	**%**
Areas of client treatment						
Iron pills prescribed	118	69	12	67	106	69
Folic acid tablets prescribed	109	64	10	56	99	65
TT injection prescribed	106	62	11	61	95	62
Anti-malarial prescribed	4	2		–	4	3
Ranking of client treatment						
Good quality of treatment >80%	76	44	9	50	67	44
Average quality of treatment ≥60% ≤80%	40	23	2	11	38	25
Poor quality of treatment <60%	55	32	7	39	48	31
Areas of client satisfaction						
Respectful behavior	113	66	13	72	100	65
Physical examination done	166	97	18	100	148	97
Satisfied with exam time	94	55	11	61	83	54
Satisfied with answers	155	91	16	89	139	91
Respectful behaviour of the facility staff	98	57	11	61	87	57
Client was satisfied	79	46	9	50	70	46

the first visit. The reasons for this increase in revisits were the availability of Women Medical Officers, free facility of ultrasound, accessible locations, and availability of resources and awareness of the clients in these areas.

The ANC coverage was linearly increasing with better social developmental ranking a. composite proxy indicator [18]. The social factors have 'push' factor and quality of services have 'pull' factor for availing ANC services by the clients. Regarding quality of services the healthcare providers are not following the standard services delivery protocols during the history taking, clinical examination, treatment and counseling of the clients. Although about half of the clients were satisfied but that was their subjective perception that does not mean that quality services are being provided. Normative quality needs were not being met in more than 90% of the services being provided. The ultimate outcome of poor quality was reflected in the form of loss of follow-up for ANC. The loss of follow-up in about one 3rd of the enrolled clients raised a serious question on the quality of the services being provided. The evidence from another study supported that there was a significant association between satisfaction (outcome) and type of care, attitude of care provider, assessment of weight of women and waiting time [25]. The reasons identified for dissatisfaction among pregnant women in a public sector hospital of Hyderabad, Sindh were long waiting time, inadequate medicine supply and incomplete tetanus vaccination which were reported by 50% clients [19]. It is evident from a study conducted in Oman that short waiting time and positive behavior providers were the most satisfying aspects of the services [26]. Another study in India revealed that, the quality is a more significant predictor of utilization antenatal care services [17].

Reasons for low coverage at managerial level were distant location of health facilities, lack of functional equipment, medicine and supplies. Although government is providing services free or on nominal user charges, but the cost become unaffordable to marginralized clients due to unauthorized over changing for services in the PHC health facilities. Social factor effecting the coverage and drop-out at client level were lack of awareness and self decision power to visit the health facilities. The decisions about availing of ANC culturally endowed to the mother in law or husband. One of the factors responsible for the drop outs were indifferent attitude and uncertainty in availability of the staff.

Community based indigenous maternal care providers (Dais) are negatively influencing the ANC services enrolment due to affordability and availability 24/7 at door steps. The objective of ANC is to detect the high risk pregnancies and deliveries and if any services fail to do so can't be labeled as ANC whether provided at health facility or at home.

Conclusion

The study revealed that both coverage and quality of the ANC services in Punjab are extremely inadequate. For coverage, only half of the expected pregnancies in the catchment areas of PHC health facilities are enrolled for ANC and out of those 1/3 never returned for follow-up visits. The quality of ANC is extremely compromised as perceived by clients and observed during the study. More than 50% of the clients are not satisfied with the ANC services they receive.

The major factors contributing for low coverage and quality at managerial and provider levels were distant location of health facilities, lack of functional equipment, insufficient supplies, inconvenient facility working hours and uncertainty in availability of staff. The social factors include lack of awareness, self decision power for seeking ANC, indifferent attitude of facility staff, affordability and availability of transport services. The miscellaneous home services provided by indigenous birth attendants are mistakenly considered as substitute of quality ANC, able to detect high risk pregnancies and deliveries.

Interventions are recommended to address the both coverage and quality issues depicted in the study findings. Health mangers can address the quality issues training, motivation and monitoring of health facility staff for client friendly behavior. Facility working hours must be extended and adjusted according to the convenience of clients in PHC health facilities. Removing transport barriers through sustainable public private partnerships or community development programs and retention of health care providers through incentivized package and facilities. Client awareness and self empowerment should be improved through involvement of local NGOs and social workers. For ANC client referral, the community based service health workers such as LHWs and CMWs must be targeted for advocacy and motivation for referring the clients to the public health facilities for ANC services.

To improve the quality of services health care providers should be trained to improve their technical skills for assessment, treatment and counseling of clients. Providers should get motivation and training to encourage them to follow the standard protocols for provision of quality ANC services.

Acknowledgments

We acknowledge the efforts of Research and Advocacy Fund (RAF) team members for their financial assistance in logistic and field work of both quantitative and qualitative data collection and provision of technical assistance. We are grateful for the cooperation of Director General Health Punjab Dr. Muhammad Aslam, Director MNCH programme Dr. Sabiha Khurshid and Director MIS Dr. Muhammad Anwar Janjua. We also acknowledge with thanks the efforts of consultants, Dr. Muhammad Anwar, Head of Sociology Department, University of Central Punjab, Irum Bukhari, Saima Aslam and Sabahat Mushtaq for their contributions in the qualitative and quantitative interviews. We appreciate the efforts of the regional Coordinators Inam-ul-Haq and Fayyaz Ahmed Butt, team supervisors and field enumerators (both male and female) made it possible to complete this assignment on schedule. Particular gratitude is due to the entire field team. All district health managers (EDOH/DOH, district coordinators for MNCH programme) provided valuable support by contributing the services of their staff. Special thanks are owed to the communities, local leadership and clients of sampled districts who devoted their time and resources to enable the survey teams to complete their assignment and focus group discussions.

Author Contributions

Conceived and designed the experiments: AM SH. Performed the experiments: AM SH JA AS. Analyzed the data: AM SH ZM. Contributed reagents/materials/analysis tools: JA AS ZM. Wrote the paper: AM SH JA AS ZM. Developed proposal and supervised all the steps from development of data collection tools to completion of draft of the manuscript: AM. Remained actively involved in pre-testing, review of tools and monitoring the quality of data collection, entry and analysis: AM. Involved in the preparation of manuscript: AM SH JA AS. Involved in the process development of study proposal, qualitative themes, qualitative data collection: SH JA AS. Provided technical assistance in analysis and interpretation of focal group discussions and in depth interviews: SH JA AS. Drafted qualitative findings, discussion, field monitoring and involved in data entry and analysis: ZM.

References

1. McCarthy J, Maine D (1992) A framework for analyzing the determinants of maternal mortality. Stud FamPlann 23(1): 23–33.
2. World Health Organization (2008) Maternal mortality in 2005: estimates developed by WHO, UNICEF, UNFPA, and the World Bank. Geneva: World Health Organization: 48.
3. Abou-Zahr CL, Wardlaw TM (2003) *Antenatal care in developing countries: promise, achievements and missed opportunity: an analysis of trends, levels and differentials, 1990–2001*. Geneva: World Health Organization.
4. Pakistan Statistical Year Book (2007) Federal Bureau of Statistic Government of Pakistan.
5. Raisa BG, Paul P, Oslon JK (2009) Strengths and challenges of the first pre-licensure Baccalaureate of Science in Nursing Program of Pakistan. Journal of Professional Nursing 25(4): 240–248.
6. Jabeen M, Gul F, Rehman M (2005) Maternal Mortality ratio and its causes in a District Headquarter Hospital of NWFP. Journal of Postgraduate Medical Institute 19(4): 377–381.
7. Millenium Development Goals Country Report Sri Lanka (2005) Improve Maternal Health. NewYork: United Nations Development Programme: 1–6.
8. Tarekegn SM, Lieberman LS, Giedraitis V (2014) Determinants of maternal health service utilization in Ethiopia: analysis of the 2011 Ethiopian Demographic and Health Survey. BMC Pregnancy and Childbirth. 2014; 14: 161.
9. Jafari F, Eftekhar H, Fotouhi A, Mohammad K, Hantoushzadeh S (2010) Comparison of maternal and neonatal outcomes of group versus individual prenatal care: a new experience in Iran. Health Care for Women International 31: 571–584.
10. Barua A, Waghmare R, Venkiteswaran S (2003) Implementing reproductive and child health services in rural Maharashtra, India: a pragmatic approach. Reproductive Health Matters 11: 140–149.
11. Nisar N, White F (2003) Factors affecting utilization of Antenatal Care among reproductive age group (15–49years) in an urban squatter settlement of Karachi. JPMA 53(2): 1–10.
12. Ali AA, Osman MM, Abbaker AO, Adam I (2010) Use of antenatal care services in Kassala, eastern Sudan. BMC Pregnancy and Childbirth 10: 67 doi:10.1186/1471-2393-10-67.
13. Hasan Z, Zia S, Maracy M (2007) Prenatal care service uptake by rural women in North West of Pakistan. JPMI vol 21(1): 29–35.
14. National Institute of Population Sciences (NIPS), Macro International Ltd. (2008) Pakistan. Demographic and Health Survey 2006–2007. Islamabad: National Institute of Population Studies & Macro International Ltd.
15. Hudak PL, Wright JG (2000) The characteristics of patient satisfaction measures. Spine 25: 3167–3177.
16. Andaleeb SS (2001) Service quality perceptions and patient satisfaction: a study of hospitals in developing countries. Social Science and Medicine 52(90): 1359–1370.
17. Luyben AG, Fleming VE (2005) Women needs from ANC in three European countries. Midwifery 21: 212–223.
18. Rani M, BonuSekhar, Harvey S (2008) Differentials in the quality of antenatal care in India. International Journal for Quality in Health Care 20(1): 62–71.
19. Ghobashi M, Khandekar R (2008) Satisfaction among expectant mothers with antenatal care services in the Musandam region of Oman. Sultan QaboosUniv Med J 8(3): 325–332.
20. Nisar N, Amjad R (2007) Pattern of antenatal care provided at a public sector hospital Hyderabad Sindh. J Ayub Med Coll Abbottabad 19(4): 11–13.
21. District –Based Multiple Indicators Cluster Survey 2003–2004. Lahore: Government of Punjab. Planning & Development. Department: 12–13.
22. District Health Information System (DHIS) Repot 2010. Lahore. Health Department, Government of Punjab.
23. Multiple Indicator Cluster Survey (MICS) Punjab 2007–2008. Provincial Report. Government of the Punjab Planning and Development Bureau of Statistics.
24. Gupta RS, Gupta A, Gupta HO, Venkatesh S, Shiv Lal (2006). Mother and Child Service Coverage: Reproductive and Child Health Prgramme in Alwar District, Rajasthan state. J. Commun. Dis 38(1): 79–87.
25. Zeidan ZA, Idris AM, Bhairy M (2011) Satisfaction among pregnant women towards antenatal care in public and private care clinics in Khartoum. Khartoum Medical Journal Vol. 04, No. 02, 590–595.
26. Ghobashi M, Khandekar R (2008) Satisfaction among expectant mothers with antenatal care services in the Musandam Region of Oman. Sultan QaboosUniv Med J 8(3): 325–332.

13

Multidisciplinary Predialysis Education Reduced the Inpatient and Total Medical Costs of the First 6 Months of Dialysis in Incident Hemodialysis Patients

Yu-Jen Yu[1,2]⁹, I-Wen Wu[1,2]⁹, Chun-Yu Huang[3], Kuang-Hung Hsu[3], Chin-Chan Lee[1,2], Chio-Yin Sun[1,2], Heng-Jung Hsu[1,2], Mai-Szu Wu[1,4,5]*

1 Department of Nephrology, Chang Gung Memorial Hospital, Keelung, Taiwan, **2** College of Medicine, Chang Gung University, Tao-Yuan, Taiwan, **3** Laboratory for Epidemiology, Department of Health Care Management, Chang Gung University, Tao-Yuan, Taiwan, **4** Division of Nephrology, Taipei Medical University Hospital, Taipei, Taiwan, **5** School of Medicine, Taipei Medical University, Taipei, Taiwan

Abstract

Background: The multidisciplinary pre-dialysis education (MPE) retards renal progression, reduce incidence of dialysis and mortality of CKD patients. However, the financial benefit of this intervention on patients starting hemodialysis has not yet been evaluated in prospective and randomized trial.

Methods: We studied the medical expenditure and utilization incurred in the first 6 months of dialysis initiation in 425 incident hemodialysis patients who were randomized into MPE and non-MPE groups before reaching end-stage renal disease. The content of the MPE was standardized in accordance with the National Kidney Foundation Dialysis Outcomes Quality Initiative guidelines.

Results: The mean age of study patients was 63.8±13.2 years, and 221 (49.7%) of them were men. The mean serum creatinine level and estimated glomerular filtration rate was 6.1±4.0 mg/dL and 7.6±2.9 $mL \cdot min^{-1} \cdot 1.73\ m^{-2}$, respectively, at dialysis initiation. MPE patients tended to have lower total medical cost in the first 6 months after hemodialysis initiation (9147.6±0.1 USD/patient vs. 11190.6±0.1 USD/patient, $p = 0.003$), fewer in numbers [0 (1) vs. 1 (2), $p < 0.001$] and length of hospitalization [0 (15) vs. 8 (27) days, $p < 0.001$], and also lower inpatient cost [0 (2617.4) vs. 1559,4 (5019.6) USD/patient, $p < 0.001$] than non-MPE patients, principally owing to reduced cardiovascular hospitalization and vascular access–related surgeries. The decreased inpatient and total medical cost associated with MPE were independent of patients' demographic characteristics, concomitant disease, baseline biochemistry and use of double-lumen catheter at initiation of hemodialysis.

Conclusions: Participation of multidisciplinary education in pre-dialysis period was independently associated with reduction in the inpatient and total medical expenditures of the first 6 months post-dialysis owing to decreased inpatient service utilization secondary to cardiovascular causes and vascular access–related surgeries.

Trial Registration: ClinicalTrials.gov NCT00644046

Editor: Emmanuel A. Burdmann, University of Sao Paulo Medical School, Brazil

Funding: Chang Gung Memorial Hospital at Keelung provided grant support for this research (CMRPG260323/CMRPG2A0422). The funder had no role in study design, data collection and analysis, decision to publish, or preparation of the manuscript.

Competing Interests: The authors have declared that no competing interests exist.

* Email: maiszuwu@gmail.com

⁹ These authors contributed equally to this work.

Introduction

The number of patients worldwide with chronic kidney disease (CKD) and end-stage renal disease (ESRD) being treated with renal replacement therapy has been continuously increasing in recent years, with a 7% rate of increase per year [1]. Aging and type 2 diabetes mellitus are the two most important factors [2]. Taiwan is the leading country in terms of ESRD prevalence, with a rate of 2447 per million population [3]. The implementation of National Health Insurance (NHI) has helped drive the growth of the ESRD populations in Taiwan [4]. However, the official prohibition of the use of aristolochic acid–containing herbs and the introduction of the nationwide CKD Preventive Project with a multidisciplinary care program have proved their effectiveness in decreasing the incidence of dialysis, and mortality and medical costs of CKD patients [5]. However, the financial benefit of this intervention has not yet been evaluated in prospective and randomized manner on patients starting hemodialysis.

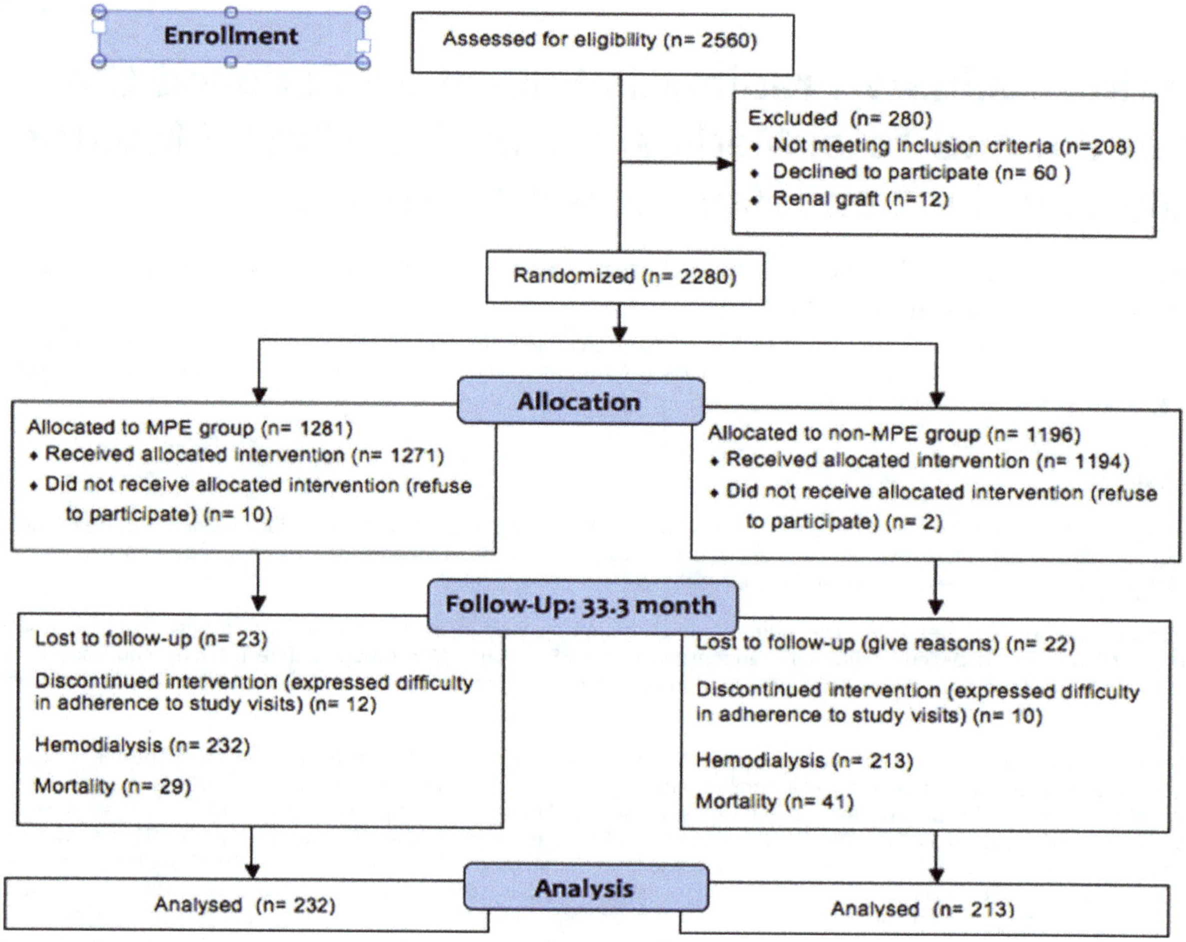

Figure 1. Enrolment scheme and patient status. MPE: multidisciplinary predialysis education.

High ESRD prevalence constitutes a large economic burden for the patient, society, and the country. Renal insufficiency represents a status of increased cardiovascular disease risk, comorbidities, and mortality [6], demanding high medical expenditures and health-care utilization [1]. The cost for ESRD has increased to $34.3 billion, accounting for 6.3% of the total Medicare budget according to the 2013 US Renal Data System Annual Data Report [7]. Similarly, in Taiwan, the annual dialysis costs have accounted for 5.0–7.52% of the total budget of the NHI in recent years [8]. Optimal and efficient treatment strategies to combat the high prevalence of ESRD and its high cost of care are thus urgently needed.

Predialysis education can decrease the ESRD incidence and mortality in the first year of dialysis [9,10]. Nephrology-based care has also significantly improved the clinical outcomes of CKD patients in both the predialysis and postdialysis periods [11,12], especially in type 2 diabetes patients [13,14]. It has been associated with better biochemical variables, shorter hospitalization length, a higher percentage of elective construction of the arteriovenous fistula, and the availability of alternative dialysis modality [15]. Our previous controlled cohort study has confirmed that multidisciplinary predialysis education (MPE) based on the National Kidney Foundation Dialysis Outcomes Quality Initiative (NKF/DOQI) guidelines provides a better outcome with a significantly reduced incidence of ESRD and all-cause mortality [16]. The MPE program has effectively improved the quality of pre-ESRD care, increased patients' self-care ability, and has retarded renal progression and reduced morbidities in late-stage CKD patients [17]. Multidisciplinary predialysis team care was found to decreased service utilization and saved medical costs in the 6 months before dialysis initiation and at dialysis initiation, being secondary to the early preparation of vascular access and the lack of hospitalization at dialysis initiation [18]. Predialysis nephrology-based care has been associated with reduced costs in elderly patients after the initiation of dialysis [19]. Most of these controlled or randomized trials have used the renal or patient outcome as their endpoints. However, randomized studies to evaluate the cost-saving effect of MPE in the post-dialysis period have been seldom reported to date.

Most of the medical costs associated with caring for CKD patients are incurred for the treatment of comorbidities, hospitalization, and transition into ESRD [20]. After dialysis initiation, most of the adverse outcomes occurred within the first year of hemodialysis. The all-cause mortality and mortality due to cardiovascular disease or other causes is found to peaked in the second month after initiation, and then decreased [20]. It is unclear whether the MPE program could extend the financial benefit to after the initiation of dialysis and reduces the medical costs during the first 6 months of hemodialysis initiation. We hypothesize that knowledge acquisition from MPE in the predialysis period may have a "legacy effect" during the postdialysis period. This beneficial effect of MPE may result in differences in disease patterns, reduced medical expenditure and utilization, and reduced medical costs in the immediate post-dialysis period. To further clarify this issue, we studied the medical expenditure and utilization incurred during the first 6 months of dialysis initiation in 425 incident hemodialysis patients who were randomized into MPE and non-MPE groups before reaching ESRD.

Materials and Methods

Patient cohort and settings The protocol for this trial and supporting CONSORT checklist are available as supporting information; see Checklist S1 and Protocol S1. This is an analysis of a subset population from our previously reported randomized cohort (Clinical Trials.gov NCT00644046) [16]. Briefly, the cohort includes predialysis CKD patients with an estimated glomerular filtration rate (eGFR) of $<60\ mL\cdot min^{-1}\cdot 1.73\ m^{-2}$ (determined by using the Modification of Diet in Renal Disease equation) who visited the nephrology outpatient clinics of the Department of Nephrology, Chang Gung Memorial Hospital, Keelung, from July 2007 and followed up to June 30, 2011. Patients aged 18–80 years and without renal graft failure were included in the study after obtaining informed consent from them. A total of 2280 patients were enrolled in the study and were randomly divided into the MPE group and the non-MPE group by using a random table at study entry. Four hundred and five patients reached ESRD needing hemodialysis after a mean follow-up of 33±2.6 months (232 patients in the MPE group and 213 patients in the non-MPE group, as shown in Figure 1). The medical expenditure and utilization in the first 6 months of initiation of hemodialysis in these 425 patients were accurately recorded and compared between MPE and non-MPE patients. Medical service utilization was calculated as the frequency of outpatient visits and the frequency and length of hospitalization. Outpatient visits were categorized as outpatient services, preventive care (e.g., influenza vaccination and dietary counseling), and emergency services. Medical service expenditures included outpatient expenditures (all costs including physicians' and nursing fees, examinations, surgery, and medication) and inpatient expenditures (all costs including laboratory testing, imaging testing, medications, surgery and consulting, ward and administrative, nasogastric tube feeding, and hemodialysis fees). The expenditures for each participant were totaled to compute the sum of ambulatory and inpatient medical service utilization costs and expenditures. The analysis of costs in this study only included those medical costs for which our hospitals made reimbursement claims to the NHI. The salaries, overheads, and administrative costs of the care team were not included. This study was approved by the ethics committee of

Table 1. baseline characteristics of study patients.

Parameter	MPE group (n = 232)	Non-MPE group (n = 213)	p
Age, years	67.5±11.4	61.8±15.0	<0.001
Male, n (%)	116 (50.0%)	105 (49.3%)	0.882
Diabetes, n (%)	153 (65.9%)	127 (59.6%)	0.168
Hypertension, n (%)	202 (87.1%)	171 (80.3%)	0.052
Coronary artery disease, n (%)	30 (12.9%)	41 (19.2%)	0.069
Cerebrovascular disease, n (%)	30 (12.9%)	29 (13.6%)	0.832
Gout, n (%)	61 (26.3%)	44 (20.7%)	0.162
eGFR, ml/min	7.49±3.1	7.87±3.6	0.228
Serum albumin, mg/dL	3.1±0.7	3.2±0.8	0.062
Hemoglobin, g/dL	9.4±1.6	9.0±2.7	0.100
Urea reduction rate, %	0.74±0.7	0.76±0.8	0.464
Kt/V, Daugirdas	1.66±0.36	1.71±0.38	0.509
nPCR, g/Kg/day	1.13±0.37	1.20±0.32	0.371
Systolic blood pressure, mmHg	144.3±22.7	147.2±25.9	0.221
Primary renal disease			0.135
Diabetes, n (%)	139 (59.9%)	118 (55.4%)	
Hypertension, n (%)	6 (2.6%)	5 (2.3%)	
Chronic glomerulonephritis, n %	16 (6.9%)	13 (6.1%)	
Others, n %	71 (30.6%)	77 (36.2%)	
Education levels			0.650
Below elementary	42 (18.1%)	3 (1.4%)	
Elementary	151 (65.1%)	207 (97.2%)	
High school	31 (13.4%)	3 (1.4%)	
University	8 (3.4%)	0 (0%)	
Vascular access at initiation of dialysis			
Patients with vascular access created, n (%)	143 (61.6%)	100 (46.9%)	0.002
Patients without insertion of double-lumen catheter, n (%)	129 (55.6%)	96 (45.1%)	0.029

Abbreviation: eGFR, estimated glomerular filtration rate; nPCR, normalized protein catabolic rate.

the institutional review board of Chang Gung Memorial Hospital (Number: 100-0040A3, 96-0408B) and was conducted according to the principles expressed in the Declaration of Helsinki. All patients provided written informed consent. The registration of our cohort at Clinical Trials.gov was delayed by administrative issues (set up of Core Lab, employment of research assistance). The authors confirm that all ongoing and related trials for this drug/intervention were registered.

MPE

The MPE program was implemented in May 2006 at the Keelung Center. The team comprised a nurse for case management, social workers, dietitians, hemodialysis, peritoneal dialysis patient volunteers and 10 nephrologists. The program consisted of an integrated course involving individual lectures on renal health, delivered by the case-management nurse, according to the guidelines given in a standardized instruction booklet. The lectures focused on nutrition, lifestyle, nephrotoxin avoidance, dietary principles, and pharmacological regimens. Furthermore, the case-management nurse contacted the patients to ensure timely follow-up. Standardized interactive educational sessions were periodically conducted wherein all patients were interviewed depending on their CKD stage, determined earlier by using the NKF/DOQI guideline. Stage III or IV CKD patients were followed up every 3 months, and stage V CKD patients were followed up on a monthly basis. For stage III CKD patients, the program consisted of lectures on healthy renal function, the clinical presentation of uremia, risk factors and complications associated with renal progression, and an introduction to the various renal replacement therapies (i.e., hemodialysis, peritoneal dialysis, and renal transplantation). For stage IV CKD patients, the program included discussions on the management of complications associated with CKD, indications of renal replacement therapy, and the evaluation of vascular or peritoneal access. Patients with stage V CKD were monitored for timely initiation of renal replacement therapies, the care of vascular or peritoneal access, dialysis-associated complications, and registration for inclusion in the renal transplantation waiting list. All patients received dietary counseling biannually from a dietitian. In addition, the case-management nurse often contacted the participants by telephone to encourage them to inform their nephrologists of their symptoms and to reinforce the importance of medical visits. The MPE program was discontinued once renal replacement therapies were initiated for these patients.

Customary care

The same group of nephrologists instructed all participants about renal function, the evaluation of laboratory data, and clinical indicators of chronic renal failure, as well as about the strategies for its management and treatment. Furthermore, the nephrologists explained the general principles of hemodialysis and peritoneal dialysis when the patients exhibited an eGFR of < 30 $mL{\cdot}min^{-1}{\cdot}1.73\ m^{-2}$ (stage IV CKD). All patients were provided with written instructions. The nephrologists evaluated the comorbidity factors influencing each patient's condition before referral to a nurse specializing in hemodialysis or peritoneal dialysis. The nursing staff provided instructions for daily living and explained the criteria used for hemodialysis and peritoneal dialysis selection, and the difference between the two modalities.

Statistical analysis

Descriptive statistics were expressed as the mean (standard deviation) or median (interquartile range). Discrete variables were presented in terms of frequencies and percentages. The normality of numerical variables was tested using the Kolmogorov-Smirnov method, and an appropriate transformation was considered before statistical testing. The Student t-test or Mann-Whitney U-test was applied to compare mean or median values among the groups. The association between categorical variables was analyzed by using the χ^2 test. Multiple linear regression analysis was applied to calculate the unstandardized coefficients associated with MPE in both inpatient and total medical cost. All statistical tests were two-tailed, and a p value <0.05 was considered to be statistically significant. Data were analyzed by using SPSS 17.0 for Windows XP (SPSS Inc., Chicago, IL, USA).

Results

The mean age of study patients was 63.8±13.2 years, and 221 (49.7%) of them were men. The mean serum creatinine level and eGFR was 6.1±4.0 mg/dL and 7.6±$mL{\cdot}min^{-1}{\cdot}1.73\ m^{-2}$, respectively, at dialysis initiation. Diabetes mellitus was identified as the leading cause of renal disease in both groups, followed by chronic glomerulonephritis. Table 1 shows the demographic and clinical characteristics of the patients in the MPE and non-MPE

Table 2. Medical utilization and expenditure between groups.

Parameter	MPE group (n = 232)	Non-MPE group (n = 213)	p
No. outpatient visits, times/patient	15.1±11.6	17.9±11.1	0.009
No. of hospitalization, times/patient	0.00 (1.00)	1.00 (2.00)	<0.001*
Frequency of hospitalization, n (%)			<0.001
Never	144 (62.1%)	86 (40.4%)	
1 time	47 (20.2%)	73 (34.2%)	
2 times	31 (13.4%)	30 (14.1%)	
≥3 times	10 (4.3%)	24 (11.3%)	
Length of hospitalization, days/patient	0.00 (15.00)	8.00 (27.00)	<0.001*
Cost of outpatient service, mean, USD/patient	6885.7±5201.2	7491.8±4200.2	0.175
Log cost of inpatient service, mean, USD/patient	3.09±4.02	4.95±4.15	<0.001
Log total cost of medical service, mean, USD/patient	6.75±4.21	8.58±2.43	<0.001

*p value using Mann-Whitney U test.

Table 3. Costs of outpatient service between groups.

Variables	MPE group (n = 232)	Non-MPE group (n = 213)	p
Hemodialysis, laboratory and imagen	6258.8±4647.2	6841.5±3883.1	0.154
Physician fee	94.4±80.1	116.9±93.4	0.007
Medication fee	512.6±120.1	510.8±75.4	0.985
Pharmacist, nursing and administrative fee	19.9±16.4	22.5±17.4	0.107

Costs were expressed in mean ± SD, USD/patient.

groups at the initiation of hemodialysis. These patients received 4 hours of hemodialysis 3 times weekly. Hemodialysis for these patients used single-use hollow-fiber dialyzers equipped with modified cellulose-based, polyamide, or polysulfone membranes. The dialysate used in all patients was a standard ionic composition and bicarbonate-based buffer. Many indices of dialysis adequacy (Urea reduction rate, Kt/V and normalized protein catabolic rate) were similar at baseline for the two groups of patients. However, the MPE group patients were more likely to have permanent vascular access created (61.6% vs. 46.9%, p = 0.002) and less insertion of double-lumen catheter at initiation of hemodialysis (55.6% vs. 45.1%, p = 0.029, Table 1).

MPE patients tended to have lower total medical cost in the first 6 months after hemodialysis initiation (9147.6±0.1 USD/patient vs. 11190.6±0.1 USD/patient, p = 0.003, Table 2). Despite the fewer outpatient visits of MPE patients, the cost of outpatient service did not differ between the groups. Most of the costs of outpatient service were spent for treatment (including hemodialysis, laboratory, and image study; Table 3). However, MPE patients were significantly fewer in numbers [mean (SD) 0.61±0.9 vs. 1.0±1.2, p<0.001; median (IQR) 0 (1) vs. 1 (2), p<0.001] and had shorter lengths [mean (SD) 10.6±21.9 days vs. 19.3±29.3 days, p<0.001; median (IQR) 0 (15) vs. 8 (27) days, p<0.001] of hospitalization than non-MPE patients. Therefore, the medical cost of inpatient service was significantly lower in MPE patients [median 0 (2617.4) or (mean 2261.8±5635.8) USD/patient in MPE patients vs. median 1559, 4 (5019.6) or (mean 3698.8±5540.9) USD/patient in non-MPE patients, respectively, p<0.001, Table 2]. The reduced cost of inpatient service observed in MPE patients was attributed to the reduction in the costs of physicians, wards, nasogastric feeding, radiology examination, nursing, blood transfusion, hemodialysis, medication, and pharmacist service fees. Most of the costs of inpatient service were spent on hemodialysis treatment in both groups of patients (Table 4). Eighty-eight (37.9%) patients in the MPE group had at least one hospitalization, compared with 127 patients (59.6%) in the non-MPE group (p<0.001). In all first hospitalizations, 66 (75%) patients in the MPE group were admitted to the nephrology ward. Similarly, 94 (74%) of the non-MPE patients were admitted to the nephrology ward at their first hospitalization. Table 5 lists the main causes of the first hospitalization and surgery in both groups of patients. Cardiovascular disease (including uncontrolled hypertension, coronary artery disease, stroke, heart failure, and peripheral artery occlusive disease) was the main cause of first hospitalization in all patients. Participation in the MPE program reduced cardiovascular hospitalization during the first 6 months postdialysis (18.53% vs. 29.58%, p = 0.007). Among all patients, those in the MPE group were more likely to have fewer vascular access related surgeries during the first admission [35 patients (15.09%) vs. 55 (25.82%), p = 0.005]. Most first surgeries were performed for Hickman catheter–related intervention (implantation, exchange, and removal) and arteriovenous fistula/graft–related intervention (creation, thrombectomy, repair, and excision; Table 5).

Participation in MPE was independently associated with reduced inpatient cost and total medical cost in the first 6 months of dialysis initiation by using various adjustment strategies, including demographic characteristics (age and gender) in model 2, concomitant disease (diabetes mellitus and number of comorbidities) in model 3, baseline biochemistry at entry to hemodialysis

Table 4. Log-transformed costs of inpatient service between groups.

Variables	MPE group (n = 232)	Non-MPE group (n = 213)	p*
Physician fee	2.03±2.67	3.28±2.79	<0.001
Ward fee	2.49±3.26	3.99±3.38	<0.001
Laboratory examination fee	5.22±1.32	5.52±1.15	0.126
Nasogastric tube feeding fee	0.56±1.61	1.40±2.36	<0.001
Radiology examination fee	1.17±2.05	1.84±2.29	<0.001
Nursing fee	1.78±2.69	2.83±2.91	<0.001
Surgery fee	1.89±3.82	3.31±4.58	<0.001
Blood transfusion fee	1.04±1.93	1.89±2.39	<0.001
Hemodialysis fee	2.65±3.46	4.13±3.58	<0.001
Medication fee	2.16±2.94	3.45±3.08	<0.001
Pharmacist service fee	1.48±1.98	2.32±2.04	<0.001

Costs were expressed in mean ± SD, USD/patient.

Table 5. Main cause of first hospitalization and surgery.

	MPE group	Non-MPE group
Cause of first hospitalization, n		
Renal-related disease	12 (5.17%)	26 (12.21%)
Cardiovascular disease	43 (18.53%)	63 (29.58%)
Vascular access infection	9 (3.88%)	11 (5.16%)
Acute pulmonary edema	3 (1.29%)	4 (1.88%)
Other	21 (9.05%)	23 (10.8%)
No hospitalization	144 (62.07%)	86 (40.38%)
Cause of first surgery, n		
Hickman catheter related	25 (10.78%)	36 (16.9%)
Arteriovenous fistula/graft related	24 (10.34%)	39 (18.31%)
Limb amputation	2 (0.86%)	3 (1.41%)
Hemothorax/pneumothorax	1 (0.43%)	6 (2.82%)
Other	15 (6.47%)	4 (1.88%)
No surgery	165 (71.12%)	125 (58.69%)

Cardiovascular disease includes uncontrolled hypertension, coronary artery disease, stroke, heart failure, and peripheral artery occlusive disease.

(eGFR, hemoglobin, and serum albumin levels) in model 4 and status of use of double-lumen catheter at initiation of hemodialysis (model 5, Table 6).

Discussion

In this prospective study, we examined the medical expenditure and utilization incurred in the first 6 months of dialysis initiation in 425 incident hemodialysis patients who were randomized into MPE and non-MPE groups before reaching ESRD. We found that participation in a multidisciplinary education program at the predialysis period was associated with reduced inpatient service utilization, reduced inpatient cost, and reduced total medical cost in the first 6 months of hemodialysis. The reduction of cost in inpatient service was attributed to the reduction in cardiovascular disease and vascular access–related surgery during hospitalization. The decreased inpatient cost and total medical cost of service associated with MPE were independent of patients' demographic characteristics, concomitant disease, baseline biochemistry at entry to hemodialysis and use of double-lumen catheter at initiation of hemodialysis. The findings of the present study provide evidence supporting the implementation of MPE as part of integrative CKD care to combat the high economic burden and financial impact of hemodialysis on patients.

A previous prospective controlled study demonstrated that MPE based on the NKF/DOQI guidelines effectively reduced the incidence of ESRD and all-cause mortality with a significantly reduced overall hospitalization rate among MPE patients [16]. In our study, the delivery of MPE was stopped once the patient started hemodialysis therapy. After the initiation of hemodialysis, all patients received dietary counseling in the hemodialysis room on a monthly basis. On the basis of these assumptions, knowledge acquisition from a multidisciplinary education program in the predialysis period might be one of the factors that influence the disease pattern and health-care utilization in the postdialysis period. The positive effect of MPE in the postdialysis period could be the result of many factors, such as increased knowledge about self-care [17], better diet and fluid control, medication compliance, better preparation of vascular access, the adoption of a healthier lifestyle, and greater awareness about the use of

Table 6. Multiple linear regression analysis of effect of MPE on inpatient and total medical cost.

	Inpatient cost		Total cost	
	Unstandardized Coefficients	p	Unstandardized Coefficients	p
Model 1	−43109.74	0.007	−61289.80	0.003
Model 2	−46226.19	0.005	−60200.11	0.005
Model 3	−44575.46	0.005	−62959.92	0.003
Model 4	−44447.13	0.001	−54490.22	0.013
Model 5	−33826.85	0.029	−52241.43	0.011

Both of the two dependent variables in these models were the log transformation of inpatient costs and total costs.
Model 1: crude.
Model 2: adjusted for age and gender.
Model 3: adjusted for diabetes status and number of comorbidities.
Model 4: adjusted for eGFR, hemoglobin and serum albumin levels at initation of hemodialysis.
Model 5: adjusted for insertion of double-lumen catheter at initiation of hemodialysis.

nephrotoxin. The transition period into ESRD and the first year of dialysis therapy represented the most vulnerable point that demands the highest health-care expenditure and utility in CKD patients [20]. The cost-saving effect of MPE in terms of inpatient and total medical service in this immediate postdialysis period was confirmed by the regression models with the adjustment of different covariates. The total medical cost of the first 6 months of hemodialysis in MPE participants was 18% less than that of nonparticipants (9147.6 USD/patient vs. 11190.6 USD/patient). For a total of 8000 incident hemodialysis patients each year in Taiwan [3], the crude estimation of cost-saving could be up to 16.3 million USD per 6 months if each incident patient was to be provided with the MPE program before reaching ESRD.

MPE is certainly beneficial in lowering the enormous cost for the care of hemodialysis patients. Although the long-term economic impact of MPE has not been studied, the findings of the present study suggest the need for a universal and efficient delivery of multidisciplinary education to all CKD patients as early as possible.

Several studies have reported on the cost-saving effect of MPE in the hospitalization of CKD patients; however, only a few retrospective studies have addressed the financial benefits of MPE in the postdialysis period [18,19]. From this prospective study, we have found that hemodialysis and the diseases associated with this treatment (cardiovascular disease and noninfectious vascular access complication) were responsible for most of the health-care cost incurred in both inpatient and outpatient services (Tables 3 and 4). Taking into account the beneficial effect of MPE in reducing renal progression [17], the incidence of ESRD [16], and cardiovascular hospitalization and vascular access surgery in the postdialysis period in our study, the implementation of MPE could result in an overall reduction in the medical utilization and expenditure of CKD patients. Similarly, Wei et al., in their retrospective observational study, found that participants in the CKD care program had lower medical costs at dialysis initiation and lower medical cost for the total period of observation than nonparticipants because of the early preparation of vascular access and the lack of hospitalization at dialysis initiation [18]. A retrospective observational study described fewer hospital days and lower total health-care costs during the year after dialysis initiation in patients receiving predialysis nephrology care [19]. We have reported a reduction in the 1-year hospitalization rate (2.8% vs. 16.4%) in recipients of MPE in a controlled prospective cohort. However, the reason for hospitalization for these patients did not differ significantly between them [16]. In a 3-year prospective study, participation in multidisciplinary care was associated with a 40% reduction in the risk of infection-related hospitalization in the predialysis period [21]. A propensity score matched cohort study found that MPE participants had less unplanned urgent dialysis, shorter hospital days, and a lower incidence of cardiovascular events than non-MPE patients during the observation period [22]. A novel finding of our study was that patients with MPE had reduced cardiovascular-related hospitalization in their postdialysis period. This finding could possibly be attributed to better control of cardiovascular risk factors, better medical adherence, fluid control, and compliance with dietary restriction in the postdialysis period with a prior acquisition of renal knowledge.

Our study included a comprehensive analysis of medical service utilization and expenditures with detailed information about outpatient and inpatient costs in patients with comparable baseline characteristics derived from a randomized cohort. The delivery of MPE was standardized according to the NKF/DOQI guidelines. A single nurse conducted the MPE program for all patients to limit interpersonal variability. This single-center study has been conducted in a university-afflicted teaching hospital. All enrolled participants were patients who visited the nephrology outpatient clinics of Chang Gung Memorial Hospital at Keelung and underwent dialysis treatment at the hemodialysis unit of the same hospital. This hospital is a group practice institution comprised 10 nephrologists and only one hemodialysis unit. Furthermore, variation within dialysis units did not exist, because the single hemodialysis unit setting. In this group practice setting, all nephrologists followed the same institutional regulation. All nephrologists were subject to the same criteria of reimbursement under a single NHI system of government of Taiwan. These 10 nephrologists took care of all renal patients at outpatient and inpatient departments. The same group of 10 nephrologists instructed the MPE and non-MPE patients at their predialysis education and also continuous their medical care in the post-dialysis period at our hemodialysis unit. For these reasons, confounding effects by practice pattern of individual nephrologists might be neglected. Despite the several advantages of MPE presented in our investigation, several limitations should be addressed. First, the study represented a secondary cost analysis of a subset of patients who started hemodialysis and were randomized into MPE and non-MPE groups before reaching ESRD. Second, patients who had died before reaching ESRD were excluded. It was unclear how MPE could influence the postdialysis health-care expenditure and utility costs of these critically ill patients. Third, the age of patients in the two groups was not comparable at the baseline. However, despite the older age of the MPE patients, the outcome of interest was consistently better than that of the non-MPE patients. In addition, the adjustment for age in the regression model has indicated no significance of this factor in our outcome. Finally, although this study examined the economic impact of MPE for the first 6 months of dialysis, its long-term effect remains unclear. Further investigations with a large-scale population, including other treatment modalities (peritoneal dialysis or renal transplantation) and a longer duration would be needed to demonstrate the cost benefit of MPE for an extended period.

In conclusion, in this prospective study, we demonstrated the lowered inpatient and total medical costs in the first 6 months postdialysis in patients receiving the MPE program. This cost reduction was attributed to decreased inpatient service utilization, and principally concerning services used because of cardiovascular causes and vascular access–related surgeries. This reduction in cost was independent of the patients' demographic characteristics, concomitant disease, baseline biochemistry and status of use of double-lumen catheter at entry to hemodialysis. This valuable information confirmed the legacy effect of the MPE program on the economic outcome in the postdialysis period. Although the optimal dose and duration of MPE remains debated, an efficient and universal delivery of multidisciplinary education should be considered as part of the integrative care of CKD patients. This simple strategy could be an ideal resolution to the problem of the increasing financial burden of renal failure worldwide.

Author Contributions

Conceived and designed the experiments: YJU IWW MSW. Performed the experiments: YJU IWW. Analyzed the data: IWW CYH KHH. Contributed reagents/materials/analysis tools: YJU IWW CCL CYS HJH. Wrote the paper: YJU IWW.

References

1. Lysaght MJ (2002) Maintenance dialysis population dynamics: current trends and long-term implications. J Am Soc Nephrol 13 Suppl 1: S37–40.
2. Meguid El Nahas A, Bello AK (2005) Chronic kidney disease: the global challenge. Lancet 365: 331–340.
3. Wu MS, Wu IW, Shih CP, Hsu KH (2011) Establishing a platform for battling end-stage renal disease and continuing quality improvement in dialysis therapy in Taiwan - Taiwan Renal Registry Data System (TWRDS). Acta Nephrologica 25: 148–153.
4. Yang WC, Hwang SJ, Taiwan Society of Nephrology (2008) Incidence, prevalence and mortality trends of dialysis end-stage renal disease in Taiwan from 1990 to 2001: the impact of national health insurance. Nephrol Dial Transplant 23: 3977–3982.
5. Hwang SJ, Tsai JC, Chen HC (2010) Epidemiology, impact and preventive care of chronic kidney disease in Taiwan. Nephrology (Carlton) 15 Suppl 2: 3–9.
6. Muntner P, He J, Hamm L, Loria C, Whelton PK (2002) Renal insufficiency and subsequent death resulting from cardiovascular disease in the United States. J Am Soc Nephrol 13: 745–753.
7. Collins AJ, Foley RN, Chavers B, Gilbertson D, Herzog C, et al. (2014) US Renal Data System 2013 Annual Data Report. Am J Kidney Dis 63: A7.
8. Department of Health. National Health Insurance Annual Statistical Report 2012. Taiwan: Department of Health, 2014. Available: http://www.nhi.gov.tw. Accessed 2014 September 2.
9. Goldstein M, Yassa T, Dacouris N, McFarlane P (2004) Multidisciplinary predialysis care and morbidity and mortality of patients on dialysis. Am J Kidney Dis 44: 706–714.
10. Devins GM, Mendelssohn DC, Barre PE, Taub K, Binik YM (2005) Predialysis psychoeducational intervention extends survival in CKD: a 20-year follow-up. Am J Kidney Dis 46: 1088–1098.
11. Bradbury BD, Fissell RB, Albert JM, Anthony MS, Critchlow CW, et al. (2007) Predictors of early mortality among incident US hemodialysis patients in the Dialysis Outcomes and Practice Patterns Study (DOPPS). Clin J Am Soc Nephrol 2: 89–99.
12. Jungers P, Massy ZA, Nguyen-Khoa T, Choukroun G, Robino C, et al. (2001) Longer duration of predialysis nephrological care is associated with improved long-term survival of dialysis patients. Nephrol Dial Transplant 16: 2357–2364.
13. Wu MS, Lin CL, Chang CT, Wu CH, Huang JY, et al. (2003) Improvement in clinical outcome by early nephrology referral in type II diabetics on maintenance peritoneal dialysis. Perit Dial Int 23: 39–45.
14. Tseng CL, Kern EF, Miller DR, Tiwari A, Maney M, et al. (2008) Survival benefit of nephrologic care in patients with diabetes mellitus and chronic kidney disease. Arch Intern Med 168: 55–62.
15. Dogan E, Erkoc R, Sayarlioglu H, Durmus A, Topal C (2005) Effects of late referral to a nephrologist in patients with chronic renal failure. Nephrology (Carlton) 10: 516–519.
16. Wu IW, Wang SY, Hsu KH, Lee CC, Sun CY, et al. (2009) Multidisciplinary predialysis education decreases the incidence of dialysis and reduces mortality–a controlled cohort study based on the NKF/DOQI guidelines. Nephrol Dial Transplant 24: 3426–3433.
17. Chen SH, Tsai YF, Sun CY, Wu IW, Lee CC, et al. (2011) The impact of self-management support on the progression of chronic kidney disease–a prospective randomized controlled trial. Nephrol Dial Transplant 26: 3560–3566.
18. Wei SY, Chang YY, Mau LW, Lin MY, Chiu HC, et al. (2010) Chronic kidney disease care program improves quality of pre-end-stage renal disease care and reduces medical costs. Nephrology (Carlton) 15: 108–115.
19. Stroupe KT, Fischer MJ, Kaufman JS, O'Hare AM, Sohn MW, et al. (2011) Predialysis nephrology care and costs in elderly patients initiating dialysis. Med Care 49: 248–256.
20. U.S. Renal Data System, USRDS 2013. Annual Data Report: Atlas of Chronic Kidney Disease and End-Stage Renal Disease in the United States, National Institutes of Health, National Institute of Diabetes and Digestive and Kidney Diseases, Bethesda, MD, 2013.
21. Chen YR, Yang Y, Wang SC, Chiu PF, Chou WY, et al. (2013) Effectiveness of multidisciplinary care for chronic kidney disease in Taiwan: a 3-year prospective cohort study. Nephrol Dial Transplant 28: 671–682.
22. Cho EJ, Park HC, Yoon HB, Ju KD, Kim H, et al. (2012) Effect of multidisciplinary pre-dialysis education in advanced chronic kidney disease: Propensity score matched cohort analysis. Nephrology (Carlton) 17: 472–479.

14

A Comparison between the EQ-5D and the SF-6D in Patients with Chronic Obstructive Pulmonary Disease (COPD)

Jing Chen[1]*, Carlos K. H. Wong[2], Sarah M. McGhee[1], Polly K. P. Pang[3], Wai-Cho Yu[3]

1 School of Public Health, The University of Hong Kong, Hong Kong, China, **2** Department of Family Medicine and Primary Care, The University of Hong Kong, Hong Kong, China, **3** Department of Medicine and Geriatrics, Princess Margaret Hospital, Hong Kong, China

Abstract

Background: The appropriate use of generic preference-based measures determines the accuracy of disease assessment and further decision on healthcare policy using quality adjusted life years. The discriminative capacity of different instruments would differ across disease groups. Our study was to examine the difference in utility scores for COPD patients measured by EQ-5D and SF-6D and to assist the choice of a proper instrument in this disease group.

Methods: Differences of mean utility scores of EQ-5D and SF-6D in groups defined by socio-demographic characteristics, comorbidities, health service utilisation and severity of illness were tested using Mann-Whitney test, t-test, Kruskal-Wallis test, Pearson's correlation coefficient and ANOVA, as appropriate. The discriminative properties of the two instruments were compared against indicators of quality of life using receiver operating characteristic curves. The statistical significance of the area under the curves (AUC) was tested by ANOVA and F-statistics used to compare the efficiency with which each instrument discriminated between disease severity groups.

Results: Mean utility scores of EQ-5D and SF-6D were 0.644 and 0.629 respectively in the 154 subjects included in the analysis. EQ-5D scores were significantly higher than SF-6D in groups less severe and these differences corresponded to a minimally important difference of greater than 0.03 ($p<0.001$). EQ-5D and SF-6D scores were strongly correlated across the whole sample ($r=0.677$, $p<0.001$) and in pre-defined groups ($r>0.5$ and $p<0.05$ for all correlation coefficients). AUCs were above 0.5 against the indicators of health-related quality of life for both instruments. F-ratios suggested SF-6D was more efficient in discriminating cases of different disease severity than EQ-5D.

Conclusions: Both EQ-5D and SF-6D appeared to be valid preference-based measures in Chinese COPD patients. SF-6D was more efficient in detecting differences among subgroups with differing health status. EQ-5D and SF-6D measured different things and might not be used interchangeably in COPD patients.

Editor: Delphine Sophie Courvoisier, University of Geneva, Switzerland

Funding: This work was supported by the University of Hong Kong Technology and Innovation seed funding. The funders had no role in study design, data collection and analysis, decision to publish, or preparation of the manuscript.

Competing Interests: The authors have declared that no competing interests exist.

* Email: pianogal@hku.hk

Background

There is an increasing need to express effectiveness of interventions in terms of quality-adjusted life years (QALYs) in health economic evaluations. The QALY accounts for both length of life and health-related quality of life (HRQoL) in a single outcome measure. Preference-based measures of health are designed to construct QALYs. They consist of two parts, one a standardized descriptive system for people to describe their own health state, the other an algorithm for assigning values to each state. The algorithm is usually based on valuations from a general population sample of adults which are derived using techniques such as standard gamble (SG) or time trade off (TTO). Preference-based measures score health states on a scale of 0 to 1 equivalent to death and full health respectively [1].

There are several preference-based measures including the EQ-5D [2], the 15D [3], Health utility index (HUI) [4], Quality of Well-Being (QWB) [5] and most recent of all, the SF-6D [6]. The EQ-5D is currently the most popular preference-based instrument, used in about half of published studies [7]. It is a two part instrument, with the first part describing problems in five dimensions with three response levels for each. The second part consists of a vertical visual analogue scale (VAS) with zero at the bottom referring to the worst health state and 100 at the top referring to the best health state. The participant pointed to the level on the scale indicating their overall health on the day of the interview. The five dimensions (mobility, self-care, usual activities, pain/discomfort, anxiety/depression) each with three levels (no problems, some problems, extreme problems) can thus define 243 (3^5) different health states [1]. Using the TTO technique, country specific scoring algorithms have been developed for the EQ-5D in

UK [8], Norway [9], and Japan [10]. The EQ-5D has been translated into Chinese and used in China, Taiwan, Hong Kong, Singapore and Malaysia [11]. The SF-6D, which is increasingly used, was developed from the SF-36 [6]. Six dimensions (physical functioning, role limitation, social functioning, pain, mental health, vitality) were retained from the original SF-36, each with 4 to 6 levels and it can define 18 000 (6*6*5*5*5*4) different health states. Using the standard gamble (SG) technique, a scoring algorithm for the SF-6D was developed for the UK [6,12].

The EQ-5D and the SF-6D differ from one another in terms of their valuation techniques, classification systems, dimensions and items covered. There is therefore a possibility that they will generate a different utility score for a specific health state. Several studies have directly compared these two instruments in different populations, and these generally show disparities in the utility scores derived from the EQ-5D and the SF-6D [12–20]. The EQ-5D tends to generate higher scores than the SF-6D in healthy population or patients with mild conditions and vice versa in less healthy populations or among patients with severe conditions [13,17,19], leading to variation in the estimation of utility scores and QALYs which could influence decisions taken on resource use [21–23].

Harper *et al* showed that the SF-36 performed better in detecting changes in HRQoL in patients with mild COPD in outpatient settings than did the EQ-5D [24]. However, no study to our knowledge has directly compared the performance of EQ-5D and SF-6D for those with more severe stages of COPD. In order to assist clinicians and researchers in choosing the most appropriate instrument for discriminative and evaluative purposes we performed a head-to-head comparison of the EQ-5D and the SF-6D in a group of severe and very severe COPD patients. COPD was chosen because it is known to have a significant adverse impact on HRQoL [25–30]. The burden of the disease in terms of morbidity and mortality is projected to increase in the next few decades in East Asia and elsewhere making the ability to determine QALY loss important [31,32], thus a precise measure is required in estimate of QALYs and to better inform the healthcare policy using quality-adjusted life years as outcome.

Methods

Sample and data collection

The study was conducted between September 2010 and May 2011 in a respiratory specialist out-patient clinic (SOPC) in a public hospital (Princess Margret Hospital) in Hong Kong. All the patients with COPD who regularly attended the SOPC were screened by their medical records for the study. Patients who had severe (post-bronchodilator FEV_1 30–49% of predicted) or very severe (post-bronchodilator $FEV_1\% < 30\%$ of predicted) COPD according to the Global Obstructive Lung Disease (GOLD) standard [33] during the past one year were included. Those who had significant comorbidities which prevented their participation, such as dementia or Parkinson's disease, who did not have a pulmonary function test result within the past one year or who did not speak Cantonese were excluded and all the eligible patients were invited to participate in the study. From 166 patients approached, 2 patients were incommunicable (one was deaf and one was unable to speak), 5 refused to participate, and 159 (95.8%) provided written consent to participate and were interviewed by trained interviewers. Five of the interviewed participants were excluded from the analysis because their post FEV_1 was 50% of predicted which classified their severity stage as moderate. Thus, 154 patients were included in the final data analysis.

Subjects completed the respiratory disease specific Saint George's Respiratory Questionnaire (SGRQ), the SF-6D and the EQ-5D. They also answered questions on socio-demographic information (sex, age, education, housing type and income), self-rated health status ("Compared with past 12 months, what do you think about your present health condition? Better, The same, Worse") and life style information (e.g. smoking). The SF-6D and the EQ-5D were asked in a random sequence to avoid possible order effects. Utilization of health services (hospital admissions in the past 12 month) and presence of comorbidities (i.e. other than COPD, whether being diagnosed with hypertension, heart diseases, pneumonia, diabetes, asthma, rheumatoid arthritis, liver disease, cancers and other chronic diseases) were extracted directly from patients' medical records by one research nurse in the SOPC.

The study was approved by the Kowloon West Cluster Clinical Research Ethics Committee, Hong Kong. All participants provided written informed consent to participate in this study.

HRQoL Measures

The Cantonese Chinese version of the EQ-5D and the Chinese (Hong Kong) SF-6D questionnaire were used to measure the Health Related Quality of Life (HRQoL) of the sample patients [34]. Because a Hong Kong specific scoring algorithm was not available for the EQ-5D, the UK one was used for which direct valuations of 43 health states had been elicited from a sample of the general population using TTO and the theoretic utility scores ranged from -0.59 to 1 [35].

Direct valuations for 196 health states from the SF-6D HK had been valued by a representative sample of the Hong Kong population ($n = 582$) using SG and the theoretic utility scores ranged from 0.315 to 1 [36]. This algorithm was employed in the present study to generate utility scores but, in order to compare with scores from the EQ-5D, the UK scoring algorithm for the SF-6D [6] was also used.

The Hong Kong Chinese version of the St. George's Respiratory Questionnaire (SGRQ) was included as a measure of disease specific quality of life. The SGRQ contains 76 weighted responses divided into three sections covering distress due to respiratory symptoms, disturbance of physical activity and overall impact on daily life and well-being. A total score from 0 to 100 is summed from weighted positive responses and a higher score indicates worse HRQoL [37]. The Chinese version of the SGRQ had already been validated in patients with COPD in Hong Kong [38] and, although the weights applied to the responses have not been developed in Hong Kong, they appear to be similar in different countries and in different languages [39] so cultural or linguistic factors may not greatly affect responses to this questionnaire [40].

Statistical analysis

Utility scores for the EQ-5D and the SF-6D were both estimated using UK-derived scoring algorithms for direct comparison and a SGRQ total summary score was calculated. Possible ceiling and floor effects, represented by the proportion of participants with the best and worst theoretical scores respectively, were identified. Correlation between the SGRQ scores and EQ-5D or SF-6D or EQ-VAS scores were tested using Pearson's correlation coefficient.

The EQ-5D, SF-6D and SGRQ mean scores were compared for different groups defined by levels of socio-demographic variables, comorbidities or health service utilisation. Where the relevant variable had two levels, this between-group comparison used the Mann-Whitney test for the EQ-5D or t-test for the SF-6D

Table 1. Characteristics of the study sample (n = 154).

	Severe COPD		Very severe COPD		Total	
	n	%	n	%	n	%
Number of patients	100	65.0	54	35.0	154	100.0
Age (yrs, mean ±, sd)[¶]	74.8±7.9		69.4±7.4		72.9±8.1	
Gender (male)	98	98	54	100	152	98.7
COPD duration						
(yrs, mean ± sd)	6.8±4.2		7.9±4.8		7.2±4.4	
Lung function: post FEV_1% (mean ± sd)[¶]	38.1±5.7		22.6±5.1		32.7±9.2	
Education						
No/pre-primary	30	30.0	7	13.0	37	24.0
Primary	49	49.0	31	57.4	80	52.0
Secondary	20	20.0	15	27.8	35	22.7
Post-secondary	1	1.0	1	1.9	2	1.3
Monthly family income (HK$)						
No income	73	73.0	33	61.1	106	68.8
<$10,000	26	26.0	20	37.0	46	29.9
>$10,000	1	1.0	1	1.9	2	1.3
Housing						
Public or aided	76	76.0	47	87.0	123	79.9
Private or Old people's home	24	24.0	7	13.0	31	20.1
Smoking[‡]						
Current smoker	16	16.0	3	5.6	19	12.3
Ex-smoker	83	83.0	47	87.0	130	84.4
Never smoker	1	1.0	4	7.4	5	3.3
Comorbidity[II]						
No	35	35.0	15	27.8	50	32.5
Yes	65	65.0	39	72.2	104	67.5
Hospital admission in the past 12 month						
No	33	33.0	10	18.5	43	27.9
Yes	67	67.0	44	81.5	111	72.1
Perceived health (compared to previous year)						
Better	11	11.0	4	7.4	15	9.7
Same	18	18.0	7	13.0	25	16.2
Worse	71	71.0	43	79.6	114	74.0

[II]Presence with any following disease: hypertension, heart diseases, pneumonia, diabetes, asthma, rheumatoid arthritis, liver disease, cancers and other chronic diseases.
[¶]$p<0.001$, significance was tested by t-test.
[‡]$p<0.05$, significance was tested by chi-square test.
Note: COPD = Chronic Obstructive Pulmonary Disease.

and SGRQ. Where the relevant variable had three or more levels, this comparison used the Kruskal-Wallis test for the EQ-5D scores or the one way analysis of variance (ANOVA) for SF-6D scores and SGRQ. Association between the EQ-5D and SF-6D mean scores of each level of each variable was identified using Pearson's correlation coefficient and statistical significance of the difference was assessed by paired-sample t-test. A minimally important difference (MID) was defined as a difference of at least 0.03 between the EQ-5D and the SF-6D mean scores [20,41,42].

To determine whether the mean utility scores of the EQ-5D and SF-6D followed the pattern that less severe patients had higher scores on the EQ-5D and more severe patients scored higher on SF-6D, the correlations between EQ-5D and SGRQ as well as SF-6D and SGRQ were tested by simple linear regression. The difference between the SF-6D and EQ-5D scores was regressed to SGRQ scores to further explore whether the two utility scores vary with severity differently. SGRQ was used as an external indicator of disease severity in COPD patients.

The discriminative properties of the EQ-5D and SF-6D were compared using receiver operating characteristic (ROC) curves. The area under the ROC curve (AUC) indicates the possibility of correctly discriminating between dichotomized groups (e.g. "severe" vs. "very severe"). In our analysis, the performance of the EQ-5D and SF-6D was evaluated against a couple of commonly used external indicators of HRQoL: the EQ-VAS scores and the SGRQ summary scores. These indicators were dichotomized using different cut-off points. EQ-VAS scores and SGRQ scores was grouped according to the percentiles of the

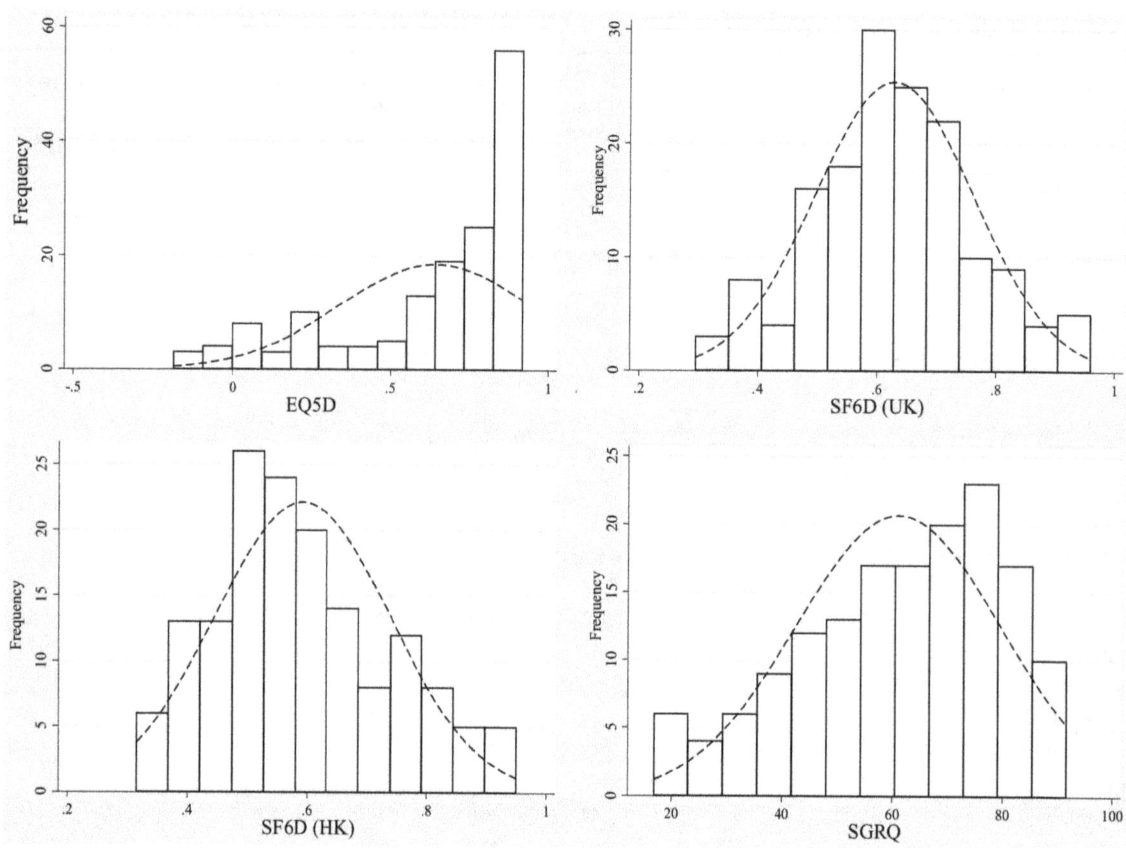

Figure 1. Distribution of EQ-5D, SF-6D (UK), SF-6D (HK) and SGRQ scores.

score distribution. The statistical significance of the AUC (F-statistic) was tested by ANOVA for each instrument. F-statistics for the SF-6D and EQ-5D were compared by dividing the F-statistic of the SF-6D by that of the EQ-5D (F-ratio). A value greater than one indicates that the SF-6D is more efficient than the EQ-5D at detecting differences in quality of life. The significance level was set as $p<0.05$ and all analyses were performed using STATA (StataCorp. 2013. Stata Statistical Software: Release 13. College Station, TX: StataCorp LP).

Results

Almost all the patients were male (98.7%), 65.0% were in the severe COPD stage and, on average, had been diagnosed with COPD for 7 years (SD 4.4) (Table 1). More than 80% were ex-smokers while 12% were current smokers. Fewer than 30% had secondary education or higher and 68.8% had no family income while 67.5% of them were with comorbid conditions and 72.1% had been admitted to hospital at least once in the past 12 months. Around three-quarters of the group (74.0%) reported their health to be worse compared with the previous year.

The mean scores on the EQ-5D and the SF-6D (UK) were 0.644 and 0.629 respectively. The distribution of EQ-5D, SF-6D (UK and HK) and SGRQ scores were generally skewed, particularly noticeable for the EQ-5D (Figure 1). The EQ-5D showed a ceiling effect with 22.1% of patients reporting the highest possible scores. No ceiling effect was observed in the SF-6D or SGRQ. Both EQ-5D and SF-6D scores were negatively associated with SGRQ since high scores indicated good HRQoL on EQ-5D and SF-6D but poor HRQoL on the SGRQ. Correlation was

Table 2. Distribution of EQ-5D, SF-6D (UK & HK), EQ-VAS and SGRQ scores in the sample subjects and their correlations with SGRQ.

Measures	Theoretical range	Observed range	Mean ± sd	Ceiling effect (%)	Floor effect (%)	Pearson correlation¶
EQ-5D	−0.590, 0.919	−0.184, 0.919	0.644±0.306	34 (22.1)	0	−0.583
SF-6D (HK)	0.315, 1	0.315, 0.950	0.591±0.147	0	2 (1.3)	−0.745
SF-6D (UK)	0.296, 1	0.296, 0.960	0.629±0.133	0	1 (0.6)	−0.728
EQ-VAS	0, 100	0, 100	55.28±20.42	4 (2.6)	5 (3.2)	−0.437
SGRQ	100, 0	91.62, 16.84	61.07±18.53	0	0	–

¶EQ-5D, SF-6D and EQ-VAS correlated with SGRQ; $p<0.001$ for all Pearson's correlation coefficient.
Note: SGRQ = Saint George's Respiratory Questionnaire.

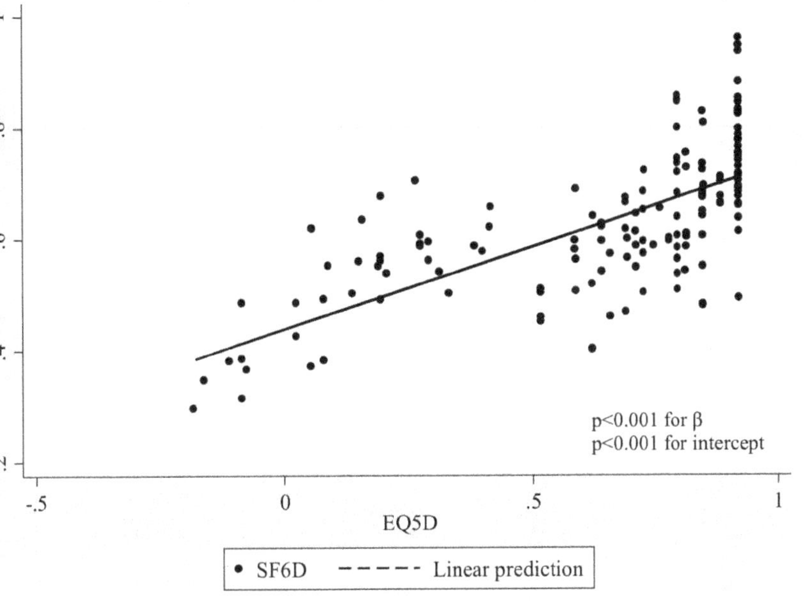

Figure 2. Scatter plot of EQ-5D and SF-6D.

higher between SF-6D (HK and UK) and SGRQ ($r = -0.745$ and -0.728, $p<0.001$) than between EQ-5D and SGRQ ($r = -0.583$, $p<0.001$) (Table 2).

The EQ-5D and SF-6D mean scores were strongly correlated across the whole sample ($r = 0.677$, $p<0.001$) and a scatter plot further showed this when regressing EQ-5D to SF-6D (the coefficient $\beta = 0.30$, $p<0.001$, and the constant = 0.44, $p<0.001$) (Figure 2). In subgroups defined by disease severity, socio-demographic characteristics and utilization of health services, the EQ-5D and SF-6D mean scores were strongly correlated as well (Table 3). Both measures were sensitive to differences within subgroups in disease severity, hospital admission and presence or not of comorbidities and differences detected were statistically significant.

Direct comparison of the EQ-5D and SF-6D showed that in the less severe cases indicated by lower SGRQ scores, the EQ-5D scores were higher than SF-6D (Figure 3 above). On the contrary, the SF-6D scores were higher than EQ-5D in more severe cases indicated by a higher SGRQ scores. There appeared a cross-over of these two utility scores. The correlation between the difference of the SF-6D and EQ-5D (SF-6D – EQ-5D) and SGRQ score was positive ($\beta = 0.004$, $p<0.001$) (Figure 3 below). The difference in most cases (88.3%) were greater than the MID of 0.03.

The AUC showed the discriminative ability of the EQ-5D and SF-6D to distinguish between very severe and severe COPD as defined by EQ-VAS and SGRQ summary scores. Against both indicators of HRQoL, the AUC scores for both instruments were above 0.5 suggesting that they can detect the difference between severe and very severe cases (Table 4). For most of the comparisons, the SF-6D generated a larger AUC than the EQ-5D. Most of the F-ratios was greater than 1 which showed SF-6D to be more efficient in discriminating cases of differed disease severity than EQ-5D.

Discussion

It is important to compare the available preference-based measures of health because the choice of instrument can greatly influence the eventual decision-making based on the results. Different instruments can have differing sensitivity to disease-related quality of life impacts and can display ceiling or floor effects in some populations. This comparative study of the EQ-5D and the SF-6D in people with severe or very severe COPD confirmed the ceiling effect of the EQ-5D, that is, a substantial group of subjects scored the highest possible score, even though all had COPD classed as severe by lung function tests. This ceiling effect of the EQ-5D has been noted in other studies [12,13,16]. Both of the instruments demonstrated a moderate capacity to distinguish between previously defined groups in terms of disease severity as assessed by lung function, by whether they had a recent hospital admission and by whether they had any comorbidities. Neither instrument was found to be clearly superior. When compared with the SGRQ, the SF-6D showed stronger correlation coefficients and generated a larger AUC than EQ-5D implying that SF-6D may be better at reflecting the health status of those with severe COPD.

Both the EQ-5D and the SF-6D discriminated well between pre-defined subgroups with mainly significant differences between mean scores for groups defined by disease severity, hospital admissions and presence of comorbidities. Thus there is evidence of construct validity for each measure in identifying HRQoL of people with severe and very severe COPD. The EQ-5D and SF-6D were strongly positively correlated (Pearson's correlation coefficient >0.5 and statistically significant) throughout the entire sample and pre-defined subgroups. Despite this, the difference in mean scores on the two measures in pre-defined subgroups often constituted a MID.

Even though the EQ-5D and SF-6D generated similar mean scores in our sample, the distributions were very different. The SF-6D utility scores followed a relative normal distribution, unlike the EQ-5D scores which were negatively skewed with a clustering at the maximum score of one. It was clear from the analysis that the EQ-5D appeared with larger ceiling effect (22.1%) compared with the SF-6D (UK and HK) in our sample. Previous studies in populations with chronic diseases have also reported ceiling effects for the EQ-5D [43–45]. It suggested that the EQ-5D, in which

Table 3. EQ-5D and SF-6D (UK) mean scores, mean score difference between EQ-5D and SF-6D, and correlation between EQ-5D and SF-6D scores by group.

		Mean scores			Mean score difference (EQ-5D – SF-6D)		Pearson correlation between EQ-5D and SF-6D	
Variables	**n (%)**	**SGRQ**	**EQ-5D**	**SF-6D**	**Estimate**	**p value for md[#]**	**Estimate**	**p value for pcc**
Total sample	154	61.07	0.644	0.629	0.015	0.21	0.677	<0.001
Stage of COPD								
Severe	100 (64.9)	57.76	0.686	0.646	0.041	0.03	0.688	<0.001
Very severe	54 (35.1)	67.19	0.565	0.597	−0.032	0.19	0.633	<0.001
p value[§]		0.001	0.007	0.015				
Age								
50–59	12 (7.8)	58.27	0.808	0.650	0.158	<0.001	0.684	0.014
60–69	39 (25.3)	61.69	0.655	0.611	0.044	0.12	0.652	<0.001
70–79	75 (48.7)	61.43	0.611	0.629	−0.018	0.27	0.716	<0.001
80+	28 (18.2)	60.43	0.646	0.643	0.002	0.48	0.701	<0.001
p value[Π]		0.98	0.54	0.72				
Education								
No/pre-primary	37 (24.0)	62.32	0.618	0.610	0.008	0.42	0.784	<0.001
Primary	80 (52.0)	62.72	0.657	0.634	0.022	0.19	0.657	<0.001
Secondary	35 (22.7)	56.76	0.630	0.630	0.0003	0.50	0.604	<0.001
Post-sec/degree	2 (1.3)	47.20	0.833	0.708	0.125	0.08	1.0000	<0.001
p value[Π]		0.28	0.82	0.67				
Hospital admission								
No	43 (27.9)	52.07	0.772	0.688	0.084	<0.001	0.533	<0.001
Yes	111 (72.1)	64.55	0.594	0.605	−0.011	0.32	0.689	<0.001
p value[§]		<0.001	0.002	<0.001				
Comorbidities								
No	50 (32.5)	59.77	0.706	0.650	0.056	0.03	0.745	<0.001
Yes	104 (67.5)	61.69	0.614	0.618	−0.004	0.43	0.642	<0.001
p value[§]		0.27	0.04	0.04				

[#]Significance test by paired-samples t-test.
[§]P value for between-group comparison, significance test by t-test for SF-6D and SGRQ; Mann-Whitney test for EQ-5D.
[Π]P value for between-group comparison, significance test by ANOVA for SF-6D and SGRQ; Kruskal-Wallis test for EQ-5D.
Note: COPD = Chronic Obstructive Pulmonary Disease; SGRQ = Saint George's Respiratory Questionnaire.

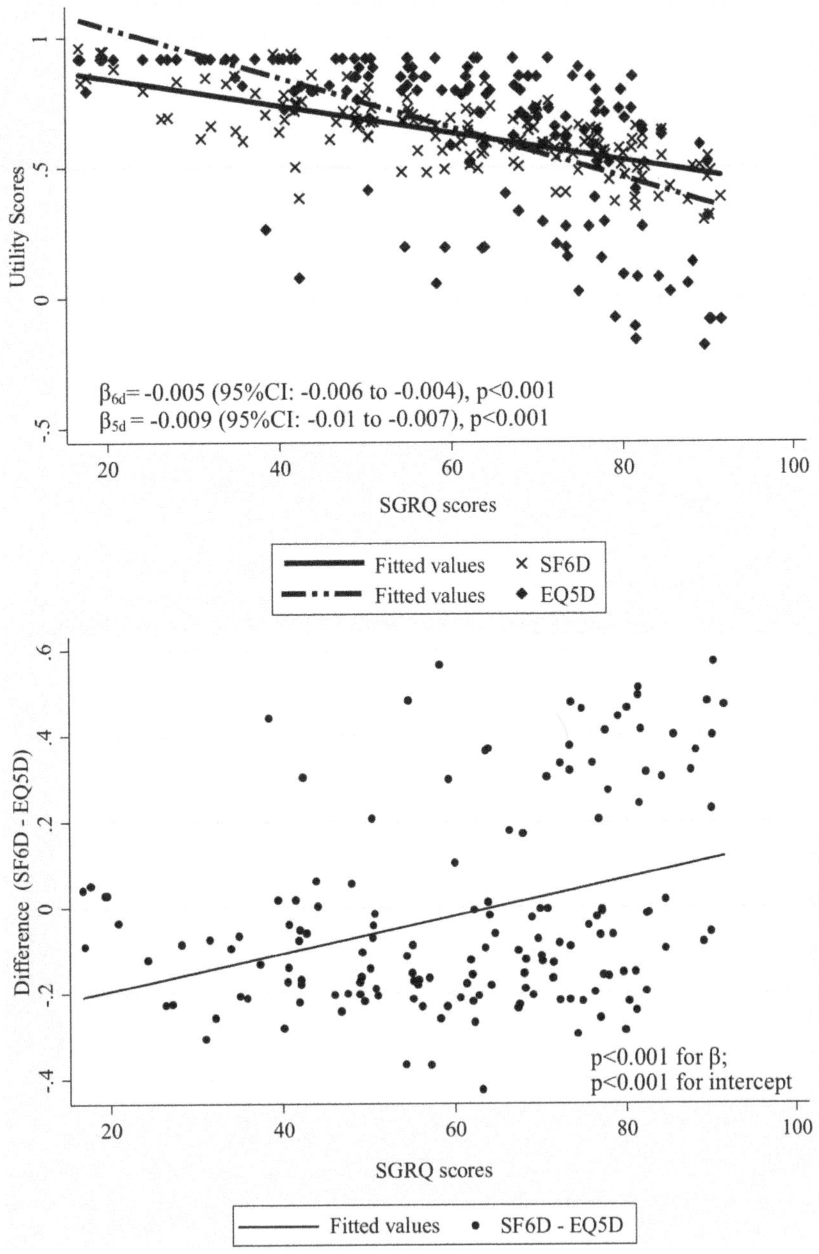

Figure 3. Scatter plots of SF-6D vs. SGRQ, EQ-5D vs. SGRQ (above) and difference (SF-6D – EQ-5D) vs. SGRQ (below).

22.1% of our sample patients scored the highest possible score, may not be as efficient as SF-6D in reflecting the disease severity. Further direct comparison of the EQ-5D and the SF-6D scores against disease severity indicated by SGRQ scores also confirmed this. The relationship observed between the SF-6D and SGRQ differed from that between the EQ-5D and SGRQ, where the SF-6D scored higher in more severe cases and the EQ-5D scored higher in less severe cases. This may be due to valuation techniques, which is TTO for the EQ-5D, as well as scaling properties. Others have found that SG generally produces higher values than TTO for the same condition [35,46] but TTO usually gives higher values than SG for milder health states [47]. This suggests that there might be a "cross-over" point for TTO and SG scores along the axis of illness severity and hence, also, for EQ-5D and SF-6D values. We did indeed see this crossover point in our study.

Moreover, consistent with other studies [19,21,45], the SF-6D was more efficient in detecting HRQoL differences between subgroups than the EQ-5D with the SF-6D generating larger AUCs and the F-ratio of SF-6D to EQ-5D being greater than 1 in most cases in our study. Specifically, Harper *et al* had already shown that SF-36 was better than EQ5D in detecting minor changes in HRQoL for those with mild COPD in outpatient settings [24] and our study adds evidence that in severe and very severe stages of COPD, the EQ-5D and the SF-6D show different discriminative capacities with SF-6D being more efficient in detecting changes in HRQoL. However, some studies have still preferred to use the EQ-5D for chronic disease in clinic settings and for comparing HRQoL pre and post-intervention [43]. Stel *et*

Table 4. Area under receiver operating characteristic curves (AUC) for EQ-5D and SF-6D with different cut-off points in external indicators.

	SF-6D				EQ-5D				
	AUC	95%CI		F statistics	AUC	95%CI		F statistics	F ratio
EQ-VAS scores									
>=50 vs. <50	0.718	0.631	0.804	18.37	0.724	0.629	0.818	24.13	0.76
>=60 vs. <60	0.672	0.587	0.756	16.21	0.649	0.562	0.735	14.11	1.15
>=70 vs. <70	0.695	0.602	0.788	18.02	0.652	0.559	0.746	8.15	2.21
>=80 vs. <80	0.733	0.610	0.856	13.11	0.687	0.563	0.812	5.32	2.46
>=90 vs. <90	0.763	0.592	0.934	6.41	0.755	0.610	0.899	4.13	1.55
SGRQ scores									
>49 vs. <=49	0.864	0.789	0.938	67.26	0.826	0.749	0.902	23.88	2.82
>64 vs. <=64	0.835	0.769	0.900	66.30	0.850	0.788	0.911	54.97	1.21
>77 vs. <=77	0.867	0.809	0.925	60.02	0.846	0.784	0.908	54.34	1.10

Note: AUC = Area under receiver operating characteristics curves; CI = Confidence interval; SGRQ = Saint George's Respiratory Questionnaire.

al found that the EQ-5D had a substantially lower percentage of missing data than the SF-6D both at baseline and post-intervention assessments when assessing the impact of different surgical interventions on patients with coronary heart disease. Our study did not find such a difference in completeness. Thus along with Harper *et al* [24], the SF-6D would be a more precise measurement in estimate of QALYs in patients with COPD than the EQ-5D. It is evident that the EQ-5D and the SF-6D yield different utility values and measured different things in COPD patients. There two instruments might not be used interchangeably, so a careful choice needs to be made. It is therefore important for clinical and health technology assessment authorities to choose the most appropriate measurement to better inform the healthcare policy using QALYs as outcome. More comparative studies would be useful.

Strengths and limitations

To our knowledge, our study was the first head to head comparison of the SF-6D and the EQ-5D among Chinese subjects with a severe chronic disease. Classifying health status using SGRQ and EQ-VAS scores could capture the underlying disease severity and provide reliable and validated external measures of HRQoL. Existing clinical conditions and related health care utilization data were extracted directly from medical records which minimized errors and bias in recall.

However, there were several potential limitations in our study. Firstly, the UK-derived scoring algorithms were used for comparing the EQ-5D and the SF-6D since there was no local algorithm available for the EQ-5D. This may fail to reflect the true preference in a Chinese population. Secondly, our sample was mainly male (98%) which may limit the external validity of our results. However, evidence on any gender difference in HRQoL is not conclusive with many studies showed non-significant differences [25,27,29,48,49]. A local study did not find any difference in the HRQoL of males and females with COPD who were attending community health centers (unpublished data). Finally, the cross-sectional nature of this study renders it unable to test the ability of the instruments to detect changes in HRQoL.

Conclusions

Both the EQ-5D and the SF-6D appeared to be valid and discriminative preference-based measures of health in Chinese patients with severe and very severe COPD. Our study added evidence that the SF-6D was more efficient in detecting differences among subgroups with differing disease severity of COPD. The EQ-5D and the SF-6D measured different things and might not be used interchangeably in COPD patients. Further research would be needed to determine other psychometric properties of the EQ-5D and the SF-6D such as responsiveness to assess ability to detect longitudinal changes.

Acknowledgments

We are grateful to Ms. Tam Wai Ying and Mr. Wong Wa Keung for their help with data collection in PMH and to Mr. Jason So for assistance in statistical analysis.

Author Contributions

Conceived and designed the experiments: JC SMM WCY. Performed the experiments: JC SMM WCY PP. Analyzed the data: JC CW SMM. Wrote the paper: JC CW SMM PP WCY.

References

1. Brazier J (2007) Measuring and valuing health benefits for economic evaluation. Oxford; New York: Oxford University Press. xi, 344 p.
2. Rabin R, de Charro F (2001) EQ-5D: a measure of health status from the EuroQol Group. Ann Med 33: 337–343.
3. Sintonen H (2001) The 15D instrument of health-related quality of life: properties and applications. Ann Med 33: 328–336.
4. Horsman J, Furlong W, Feeny D, Torrance G (2003) The Health Utilities Index (HUI): concepts, measurement properties and applications. Health Qual Life Outcomes 1: 54.
5. Kaplan RM, Anderson JP (1988) A general health policy model: update and applications. Health Serv Res 23: 203–235.
6. Brazier J, Roberts J, Deverill M (2002) The estimation of a preference-based measure of health from the SF-36. J Health Econ 21: 271–292.
7. Rasanen P, Roine E, Sintonen H, Semberg-Konttinen V, Ryynanen OP, et al. (2006) Use of quality-adjusted life years for the estimation of effectiveness of health care: A systematic literature review. Int J Technol Assess Health Care 22: 235–241.
8. Dolan P, Gudex C, Kind P, William A (1995) A social tariff for EuroQol: Results from a UK general population study. Discussion paper 138. York: The University of York.
9. Nord E (1991) EuroQol: health-related quality of life measurement. Valuations of health states by the general public in Norway. Health Policy 18: 25–36.
10. Tsuchiya A, Ikeda S, Ikegami N, Nishimura S, Sakai I, et al. (2002) Estimating an EQ-5D population value set: the case of Japan. Health Econ 11: 341–353.
11. EuroQol Group (2013) About EQ-5D Rotterdam. Available: http://www.euroqol.org/about-eq-5d.html
12. Brazier J, Roberts J, Tsuchiya A, Busschbach J (2004) A comparison of the EQ-5D and SF-6D across seven patient groups. Health Econ 13: 873–884.
13. Cunillera O, Tresserras R, Rajmil L, Vilagut G, Brugulat P, et al. (2010) Discriminative capacity of the EQ-5D, SF-6D, and SF-12 as measures of health status in population health survey. Qual Life Res 19: 853–864.
14. Gerard K, Nicholson T, Mullee M, Mehta R, Roderick P (2004) EQ-5D versus SF-6D in an older, chronically Ill patient group. Appl Health Econ Health Policy 3: 91–102.
15. Kontodimopoulos N, Argiriou M, Theakos N, Niakas D (2011) The impact of disease severity on EQ-5D and SF-6D utility discrepancies in chronic heart failure. Eur J Health Econ 12: 383–391.
16. Kontodimopoulos N, Pappa E, Papadopoulos AA, Tountas Y, Niakas D (2009) Comparing SF-6D and EQ-5D utilities across groups differing in health status. Qual Life Res 18: 87–97.
17. Lamers LM, Bouwmans CA, van Straten A, Donker MC, Hakkaart L (2006) Comparison of EQ-5D and SF-6D utilities in mental health patients. Health Econ 15: 1229–1236.
18. Longworth L, Bryan S (2003) An empirical comparison of EQ-5D and SF-6D in liver transplant patients. Health Econ 12: 1061–1067.
19. Szende A, Leidy NK, Stahl E, Svensson K (2009) Estimating health utilities in patients with asthma and COPD: evidence on the performance of EQ-5D and SF-6D. Qual Life Res 18: 267–272.
20. Walters SJ, Brazier JE (2005) Comparison of the minimally important difference for two health state utility measures: EQ-5D and SF-6D. Qual Life Res 14: 1523–1532.
21. Grieve R, Grishchenko M, Cairns J (2009) SF-6D versus EQ-5D: reasons for differences in utility scores and impact on reported cost-utility. Eur J Health Econ 10: 15–23.
22. Joore M, Brunenberg D, Nelemans P, Wouters E, Kuijpers P, et al. (2010) The impact of differences in EQ-5D and SF-6D utility scores on the acceptability of cost-utility ratios: results across five trial-based cost-utility studies. Value Health 13: 222–229.
23. Scott NW, Fayers PM, Aaronson NK, Bottomley A, de Graeff A, et al. (2009) The practical impact of differential item functioning analyses in a health-related quality of life instrument. Qual Life Res 18: 1125–1130.
24. Harper R, Brazier JE, Waterhouse JC, Walters SJ, Jones NM, et al. (1997) Comparison of outcome measures for patients with chronic obstructive pulmonary disease (COPD) in an outpatient setting. Thorax 52: 879–887.
25. Engstrom CP, Persson LO, Larsson S, Ryden A, Sullivan M (1996) Functional status and well being in chronic obstructive pulmonary disease with regard to clinical parameters and smoking: a descriptive and comparative study. Thorax 51: 825–830.
26. Ferrer M, Alonso J, Morera J, Marrades RM, Khalaf A, et al. (1997) Chronic obstructive pulmonary disease stage and health-related quality of life. The Quality of Life of Chronic Obstructive Pulmonary Disease Study Group. Ann Intern Med 127: 1072–1079.
27. Ketelaars CA, Schlosser MA, Mostert R, Huyer Abu-Saad H, Halfens RJ, et al. (1996) Determinants of health-related quality of life in patients with chronic obstructive pulmonary disease. Thorax 51: 39–43.
28. Lam CL, Lauder IJ (2000) The impact of chronic diseases on the health-related quality of life (HRQOL) of Chinese patients in primary care. Fam Pract 17: 159–166.
29. Stahl E, Lindberg A, Jansson SA, Ronmark E, Svensson K, et al. (2005) Health-related quality of life is related to COPD disease severity. Health Qual Life Outcomes 3: 56.
30. Voll-Aanerud M, Eagan TM, Wentzel-Larsen T, Gulsvik A, Bakke PS (2008) Respiratory symptoms, COPD severity, and health related quality of life in a general population sample. Respir Med 102: 399–406.
31. Buist AS, Vollmer WM, McBurnie MA (2008) Worldwide burden of COPD in high- and low-income countries. Part I. The burden of obstructive lung disease (BOLD) initiative. Int J Tuberc Lung Dis 12: 703–708.
32. World Health Organization Quick COPD facts. Available: http://www.who.int/respiratory/copd/en/.
33. GOLD Executive Committee (2011) Global initiative for Chronic Obstructive Lung Disease: Global strategy for the diagnosis, management, and prevention of Chronic Obstructive Pulmonary Disease. USA.
34. Lam CL, Brazier J, McGhee SM (2008) Valuation of the SF-6D Health States Is Feasible, Acceptable, Reliable, and Valid in a Chinese Population. Value Health 11: 295–303.
35. Dolan P, Gudex C, Kind P, Williams A (1996) Valuing health states: a comparison of methods. J Health Econ 15: 209–231.
36. McGhee SM, Brazier J, Lam CL, Wong LC, Chau J, et al. (2011) Quality adjusted life years: Population specific measurement of the quality component. Hong Kong Med J 17: 17–21.
37. Jones PW, Quirk FH, Baveystock CM, Littlejohns P (1992) A self-complete measure of health status for chronic airflow limitation. The St. George's Respiratory Questionnaire. Am Rev Respir Dis 145: 1321–1327.
38. Yu TW, Scudds RJ, Scudds RA (2004) Reliability and Validity of a Hong Kong Chinese Version of the St George's Respiratory Questionnaire in Patients with COPD. 22: 33–39.
39. Quirk FH, Baveystock CM, Wilson R, Jones PW (1991) Influence of demographic and disease related factors on the degree of distress associated with symptoms and restrictions on daily living due to asthma in six countries. Eur Respir J 4: 167–171.
40. Jones PW (1994) Quality of life, symptoms and pulmonary function in asthma: long-term treatment with nedocromil sodium examined in a controlled multicentre trial. Nedocromil Sodium Quality of Life Study Group. Eur Respir J 7: 55–62.
41. Sullivan PW, Lawrence WF, Ghushchyan V (2005) A national catalog of preference-based scores for chronic conditions in the United States. Med Care 43: 736–749.
42. Walters SJ, Brazier JE (2003) What is the relationship between the minimally important difference and health state utility values? The case of the SF-6D. Health Qual Life Outcomes 1: 4.
43. van Stel HF, Buskens E (2006) Comparison of the SF-6D and the EQ-5D in patients with coronary heart disease. Health Qual Life Outcomes 4: 20.
44. McCrone P, Patel A, Knapp M, Schene A, Koeter M, et al. (2009) A comparison of SF-6D and EQ-5D utility scores in a study of patients with schizophrenia. J Ment Health Policy Econ 12: 27–31.
45. Zhao FL, Yue M, Yang H, Wang T, Wu JH, et al. (2010) Validation and comparison of EuroQol and short form 6D in chronic prostatitis patients. Value Health 13: 649–656.
46. Green C, Brazier J, Deverill M (2000) Valuing health-related quality of life. A review of health state valuation techniques. Pharmacoeconomics 17: 151–165.
47. Dolan P, Sutton M (1997) Mapping visual analogue scale health state valuations onto standard gamble and time trade-off values. Soc Sci Med 44: 1519–1530.
48. Renwick DS, Connolly MJ (1996) Impact of obstructive airways disease on quality of life in older adults. Thorax 51: 520–525.
49. Shoup R, Dalsky G, Warner S, Davies M, Connors M, et al. (1997) Body composition and health-related quality of life in patients with obstructive airways disease. Eur Respir J 10: 1576–1580.

15

Moving to and Dying in a Nursing Home Depends Not Only on Health – An Analysis of Socio-Demographic Determinants of Place of Death in Switzerland

Damian Hedinger[1], Julia Braun[1], Ueli Zellweger[1], Vladimir Kaplan[2], Matthias Bopp[1]*, for the Swiss National Cohort Study Group[¶]

1 Epidemiology, Biostatistics and Prevention Institute, University of Zurich, Zurich, Switzerland, 2 District Hospital Freiamt Muri, Muri, Switzerland

Abstract

Background: In developed countries generally about 7 out of 10 deaths occur in institutions such as acute care hospitals or nursing homes. However, less is known about the influence of non-medical determinants of place of death. This study examines the influence of socio-demographic and regional factors on place of death in Switzerland.

Data and Methods: We linked individual data from hospitals and nursing homes with census and mortality records of the Swiss general population. We differentiated between those who died in a hospital after a length of stay ≤2 days or ≥3 days, those who died in nursing homes, and those who died at home. In gender-specific multinomial logistic regression models we analysed N = 85,129 individuals, born before 1942 (i.e., ≥65 years old) and deceased in 2007 or 2008.

Results: Almost 70% of all men and 80% of all women died in a hospital or nursing home. Regional density of nursing home beds, being single, divorced or widowed, or living in a single-person household were predictive of death in an institution, especially among women. Conversely, homeownership, high educational level and having children were associated with dying at home.

Conclusion: Place of death substantially depends on socio-demographic determinants such as household characteristics and living conditions as well as on regional factors. Individuals with a lower socio-economic position, living alone or having no children are more prone to die in a nursing home. Health policy should empower these vulnerable groups to choose their place of death in accordance to needs and wishes.

Editor: Erik von Elm, University Hospital Lausanne, Switzerland

Funding: The project is funded by the Swiss National Science Foundation (SNSF, grants 3347CO-108806, 33CS30-134273 and 406740-139331), project 67 "end-of-life". Persons who received fundings from the SNSF: DH JB. Website with detail information about the financing situation: http://p3.snf.ch/Project-139331. The funders had no role in study design, data collection and analysis, decision to publish, or preparation of the manuscript.

Competing Interests: The authors have declared that no competing interests exist.

* Email: matthias.bopp@uzh.ch

¶ Membership of the Swiss National Cohort Study Group is provided in the Acknowledgments.

Background

The place of death is often considered as an important indicator of life quality in end-of-life care. [1,2] In the early 20th century, most people died at home, but since the mid-20th century, the majority of people in industrialized countries die in health care institutions. [3] In spite of overwhelming individual preference for dying at home [4,5] about two thirds of all deaths occur in acute care hospitals or long-term care facilities. [2,3,6] This "hospitalization of death" [7] or "medicalization of dying" [1] is often considered as undesirable. [8] The divergence between preferences and reality makes place of death and the organization of end-of life care an important issue in medical and social research. Nevertheless, some researchers dispute the advantage of death at home compared to death in an institution. Dying at home can be very stressful in some situations for those involved, [9] especially when people need a lot of care. However, most authors agree that a "good death" should be a death that is - regardless of the place - in accordance with the patient's and his or her family's wishes. [3,7,10] Therefore, it is important to gain a better understanding of the reasons why people die where they do.

There is evidence that health care expenditure is highest at the end-of-life, and even increasing during the last months of life. [11,12] Estimates show that 27% of Medicare's annual budget is spent for the care of patients in their last year of life. [13] However, this "proximity to death" hypothesis is challenged by

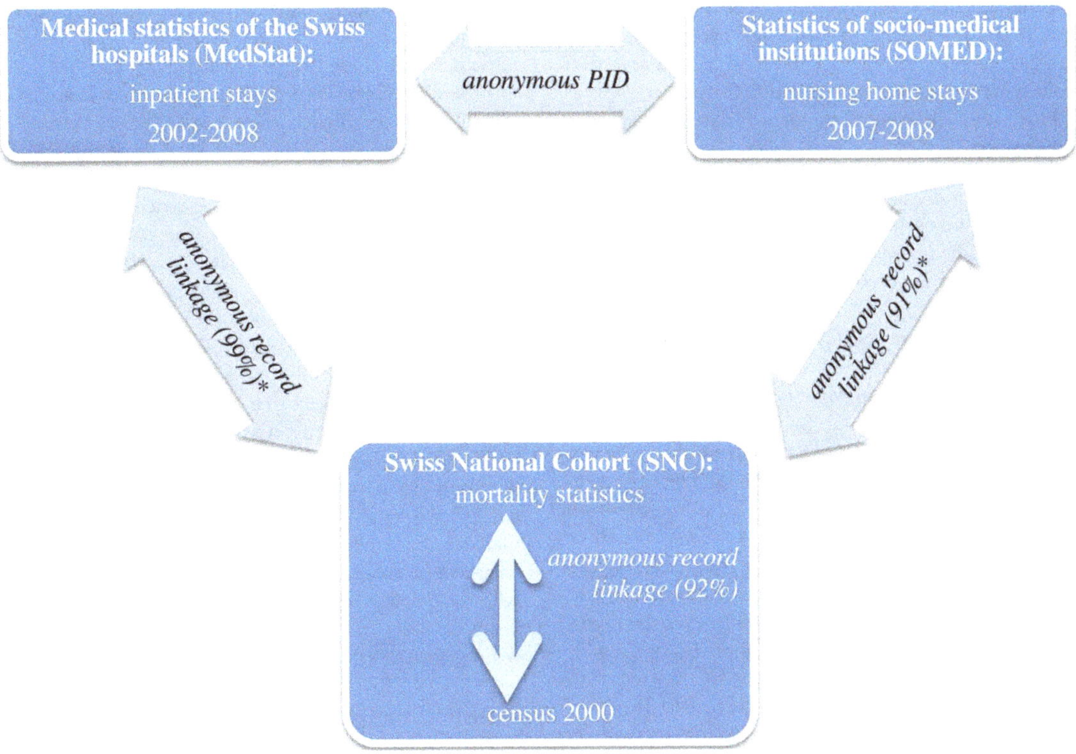

Figure 1. Three data sources and linkage. *using exact date of birth and death, sex, place of residence. Linkage success in brackets.

many confounders such as age, functional impairment, accumulation of chronic medical conditions and socio-economic characteristics of the deceased individuals. [14,15] Indeed, place of death has a considerable impact on health care costs, with end-of-life care being more expensive in hospitals than in nursing homes or at private settings [16].

In some European countries, different models of palliative care have been developed. Their effectiveness and their impact on care at the end-of-life varies substantially. [17] It seems that home-based palliative care models increase the quality of end-of-life care. [18] Unfortunately, the situation of palliative care in Switzerland is difficult to assess because of regional variation and lack of representative data. [19] Specific hospices with in-patient facilities are scarce in Switzerland and cannot be reliably identified from the available data sources. Regional differences related to place of death have been described in few studies. The proportion of deaths occuring in hospitals in 1979/80 varied widely between 27% and 81%, [20] and that of deaths occurring at home 2007–11 between 22% and 33%. [16] It was argued that the proportion of deaths in hospital beds decreased when the access to primary care providers and nursing home beds increased. [16,20] However, without information about socio-demographic characteristics a proper adjustment was not possible. Previous studies from other countries suggest that individual characteristics including old age, poor health status, living alone, female gender and low socio-economic status increase the risk for dying in an institution [21–23].

In our study, we extracted a variety of socio-demographic characteristics from the Swiss National Cohort, and explored their association with place of death adjusting for health related factors. In addition to socio-economic position (SEP) and age, we included other socio-demographic and several family and housing variables. [22,23] Given the substantial regional variation in health care use and health-related outcomes in Switzerland, [20,24] we also adjusted for regional characteristics. We hypothesized that people with a low SEP or poor living and household conditions have a higher probability to die in a nursing home.

Data and Methods

Data

We extracted data from three different sources covering all individuals living in Switzerland:

(1) The Swiss National Cohort (SNC, www.swissnationalcohort.ch) is an anonymous linkage of census, mortality and emigration records. [25] Decennial censuses were conducted between 1850 and 2000 and registered sex, age, date of birth, nationality, marital status, religious affiliation, educational level and living arrangements. In addition, a variety of information about housing was registered. The 1990 census included for the first time the exact date of birth, which allowed linking census and mortality data.

(2) The medical statistics of the Swiss hospitals (MedStat), administered by the Swiss Federal Statistical Office, register all hospital discharges since 1998. [26] Data collection is mandatory for all Swiss hospitals. Since 2002, the data source is more or less complete for the entire country. Besides medical information like diagnoses and treatments, [27] age, sex, place of residence, admission and discharge date and administration information like medical-insurance specifications are available.

(3) The statistics of socio-medical institutions (SOMED) encompass nursing homes, homes for disabled, institutions for

addiction patients and institutions for people with social problems. It is administered by the Swiss Federal Statistical Office and mandatory for all socio-medical institutions. [28] The institutions report limited patient information such as year of birth, sex, ZIP-code of residence, date of admission and discharge.

All three data sources are fully anonymized. For the purpose of privacy protection there is no common personal identification number that would allow to directly link the three data sources on an individual level. A common person identifier is only available for two of the three data sources (MedStat and SOMED). The linkage with the third source (SNC) had to rely on common identification variables such as place of residence, date of birth and date of death (see also Figure 1). In MedStat, the full date of death and date of birth are only available for those who died during their hospital stay. In SOMED, the full date of death and the year of birth are available for those who deceased. [29,30] The linkage to the SNC was therefore only possible for those who died in an institution. [25] Figure 1 shows the linkage process of the three data sources.

The first step was MedStat data cleaning (e.g. correct bad encoding, duplicate records) from 2002 to 2008 of persons born before the 2000 census (N hospitalizations before: 12,629,525, N after: 12,234,964). Linkage of MedStat and SNC started with hospital deaths between 2002 and 2008 (N = 165,843 deceased patients). Of these, N = 163,971 (98.9%) could be successfully linked to a record in the mortality statistics. 95.1% of the links were totally concordant and 3.8% partially concordant (e.g., a record in MedStat and SNC with identical sex, birth date, and region of residence [around 600 regions in Switzerland] but some minor discordance regarding date of death, was assumed to belong to the same person). The data quality of MedStat was comparable for the time period from 2002 to 2008. The linkage of mortality statistics with SOMED started with data cleaning of the inpatient stays from 2006 to 2008. Because there were records from previous years and missing codes (mainly for 2006 cases), the number of retained cases dropped by more than 50%: From N = 486,681 to N = 229,367 cases. For a lot of the 2006 cases, which had also a 2007 record from the same institution, the anonymous person number from 2007 could be used. The linkage rate with the mortality records for the years 2007 and 2008 was about 91% [30] (N total: 44,124, N with successful link: 40,168). 65.1% of SOMED cases could be linked with totally concordant criteria and additional 25.9% with partially discordant criteria. Finally, 92% of the mortality records could be linked to a 2000 census record.

We restricted the study population to elderly people born before 1942 (≥65 years) and who had died in 2007 and 2008. We excluded people who already lived in a collective household (mostly nursing homes) during the 2000 census. Thereafter, we cleaned the data again (e.g. clean-up of duplicate records), leading to a final study population of N = 85,129 people (N = 39,798 men, N = 45,331 women).

Study design

We categorized the outcome variable place of death as nursing home, hospital long (length of stay ≥3 days), hospital short (length of stay ≤2 days) and private home. The latter encompassed all deaths that could not be linked to a hospital or a nursing home record. We stratified our analysis by gender because there are fundamental differences between men and women regarding the place of death [2,16,21,23,31].

The independent variables were grouped into individual, familial/housing and structural/regional attributes. As control variables we included age and nationality (Swiss or foreign) as well as important causes of death: malignant neoplasms (ICD 10: C00-C99), coronary heart disease (I20-I25), chronic obstructive pulmonary disease (COPD, J40-J47), dementia (F01, F03, G30), stroke (I60-I69) and all other causes. Marital status was assessed at the time of death (never married, married, widowed and divorced). From the 2000 census we derived the educational level according to the International Standard Classification of Education (ISCED), version 1997: no secondary education completed (ISCED 0-1), lower secondary ("low", ISCED 2), post-secondary non-tertiary ("medium", ISCED 3-4), and tertiary education ("high", ISCED 5). Also from the 2000 census we extracted information on homeownership (owner-occupier household yes vs. no), number of children (independently assessed for men and women), living arrangement (single-person- vs. multi-person- household), number of rooms per person in the flat or house. Place of residence was categorized into the three main Swiss language areas, namely German, French and Italian. In order to account for geographical variation in nursing home bed availability, we included a variable with the density of nursing home beds per 100 inhabitants aged 65 years or older in 2010 for small and homogenous regions (106 regions for the whole country).

Statistical methods

For descriptive analysis, we calculated means, frequencies and proportions of the respective variables. Separate multinomial logistic regression models for both men and women, yielding estimated relative risk ratios (RRR), [32] were used to assess the impact of several independent variables on the relative risks for dying at different places of death. For better understanding of the interpretation of RRRs, we give an easy example using a hypothetical estimated RRR of 1.5 for a person in category B of some categorical variable: This would mean that in comparison to somebody in category A (reference category) of that variable, the relative risk of dying in an institution compared to dying at home is 1.5 times higher. As the interpretation of the results is not always easy, especially for categorical variables, we additionally provide graphical representations of the predicted probabilities of dying at different locations for a selection of the independent variables.

The variables age, nationality and language region were included in the model, because we felt them to be definite confounders. Age was modelled as restricted cubic spline with five knots (at 69, 78, 84, 89, 96 years). The remaining variables cause of death, educational level, home-ownership, number of children, marital status, single versus multi-person-household, rooms per person and average number of nursing home beds per region were included because of their particular connection with the place of death. To choose the form of the continuous variables of interest, the Bayesian information criterion (BIC) was used, comparing several forms of these variables (linear, square root transformation, categorization). Based on the BIC and for the sake of easy interpretation, we decided to include the number of children in four categories (0, 1–2, 3 or more and an unknown number), the number of rooms in the household per person in three categories (0–<=1.5, >1.5–<=2.5 and more than 2.5 rooms) and the number of available beds in a nursing home as a continuous variable. We also tested if interaction terms improved the model which was not the case. Global p-values for each covariate in the final model were obtained using a likelihood ratio test. The level of significance was chosen to be $\alpha = 0.05$ (two sided tests). Note that no correction for multiple testing was introduced to the model

Table 1. Study population characteristics, men.

	Total N	at home	hospital short	hospital long	nursing home
Deaths	(39,798)	(11,008)	(4,634)	(13,723)	(10,433)
%		*27.7*	*11.6*	*34.5*	*26.2*
Age (mean)		80.3	80.0	79.7	85.5
Nationality*: Swiss nationals (%)	36,874	*28.0*	*11.5*	*33.5*	*27.0*
Nationality*: Non-Swiss (%)	2,924	*24.1*	*13.4*	*46.4*	*16.1*
Cause of death: cancer (%)	11,886	*26.1*	*10.0*	*47.9*	*16.0*
Cause of death: coronary heart disease (%)	6,954	*41.1*	*13.2*	*22.1*	*23.6*
Cause of death: COPD (%)	1,678	*28.1*	*11.7*	*30.2*	*30.0*
Cause of death: dementia (%)	2,136	*15.5*	*0.8*	*9.8*	*73.8*
Cause of death: stroke (%)	2,514	*14.8*	*13.8*	*34.7*	*36.6*
Cause of death: other (%)	14,630	*26.5*	*13.4*	*33.5*	*26.5*
Educational level*: no (%)	1,221	*26.1*	*12.1*	*34.5*	*27.3*
Educational level*: low (%)	10,264	*27.7*	*11.3*	*33.7*	*27.2*
Educational level*: medium (%)	15,744	*28.0*	*12.2*	*35.1*	*24.7*
Educational level*: high (%)	6,814	*30.1*	*11.4*	*36.0*	*22.5*
Educational level*: unknown (%)	5,755	*23.9*	*11.0*	*32.2*	*32.9*
Home-ownership*: Owner-occupiers (%)	18,472	*31.2*	*11.7*	*33.3*	*23.8*
Home-ownership*: Tenants (%)	21,326	*24.6*	*11.6*	*35.5*	*28.3*
Number of children*: 0 (%)	5,861	*25.9*	*11.2*	*34.1*	*28.8*
Number of children*: 1–2 (%)	16,499	*26.7*	*12.1*	*36.8*	*24.4*
Number of children*: >3 (%)	15,018	*29.8*	*11.5*	*32.6*	*26.1*
Number of children*: unknown (%)	2,420	*25.0*	*10.5*	*30.9*	*33.6*
Marital status: never married (%)	2,735	*28.6*	*10.7*	*28.5*	*32.2*
Marital status: married (%)	25,694	*29.5*	*12.6*	*37.7*	*20.2*
Marital status: widowed (%)	9,082	*22.4*	*9.5*	*26.7*	*41.4*
Marital status: divorced (%)	2,287	*26.3*	*11.2*	*36.6*	*25.9*
Single-person-household* (%)	8,205	*24.4*	*9.7*	*29.3*	*36.5*
Multi-person-household* (%)	31,593	*28.5*	*12.1*	*35.8*	*23.5*
Rooms per person*: 0–<=1.5 (%)	14,653	*26.3*	*12.0*	*35.7*	*26.0*
Rooms per person*: >1.5–<=2.5 (%)	16,247	*28.9*	*11.9*	*35.3*	*23.9*
Rooms per person*: >2.5 (%)	8,898	*27.6*	*10.5*	*30.9*	*31.0*
Language region*: german (%)	28,747	*29.7*	*11.4*	*31.2*	*27.7*
Language region*: french (%)	9,270	*22.3*	*12.2*	*43.4*	*22.2*
Language region*: italian (%)	1,781	*23.1*	*12.5*	*41.2*	*23.2*
Average number of nursing home beds per 100 inhabitants above 65 years per (per 106 regions)		6.8	6.7	6.6	7.1

Percentages in italic.
Data source: Swiss Federal Statistical Office, MedStat/SOMED/SNC.
*2000 census data.

coefficients. All analyses were performed using STATA version 12.1 (StataCorp LP, College Station, Texas, 2011).

Results

Descriptive analysis

Tables 1 and 2 present the gender-specific characteristics of our study population.

Table 1 and table 2 depict the characteristics of the study population stratified by the location of death for men and women, separately. 72% of all men and 80% of all women died in an institution. Almost half of all women (44.5%) and slightly more than one out of four men (26.2%) died in a nursing home. Persons with dementia had the highest percentage of death in nursing homes (74% for men and 81% for women). A higher educational level was associated with a higher proportion of deaths at private homes. Homeowners died more often at home than tenants and so

Table 2. Study population characteristics, women.

	Total N	at home	hospital short	hospital long	nursing home
Deaths	(45,331)	(9,267)	(3,900)	(11,992)	(20,172)
%		*20.4*	*8.6*	*26.5*	*44.5*
Age (mean)		83.9	82.7	81.6	88.0
Nationality*: Swiss nationals (%)	43,317	*20.4*	*8.6*	*25.9*	*45.1*
Nationality*: Non-Swiss (%)	2,014	*20.8*	*10.0*	*37.9*	*31.3*
Cause of death: cancer (%)	9,351	*20.1*	*6.9*	*47.6*	*25.4*
Cause of death: coronary heart disease (%)	6,865	*27.8*	*9.5*	*16.6*	*46.1*
Cause of death: COPD (%)	1,132	*22.7*	*11.4*	*25.4*	*40.5*
Cause of death: dementia (%)	4,309	*13.4*	*0.6*	*4.7*	*81.3*
Cause of death: stroke (%)	3,979	*13.0*	*11.1*	*26.9*	*49.0*
Cause of death: other (%)	19,695	*21.0*	*10.2*	*24.6*	*44.3*
Educational level*: no (%)	2,159	*20.0*	*7.8*	*25.5*	*46.7*
Educational level*: low (%)	20,569	*19.8*	*8.6*	*25.9*	*45.6*
Educational level*: medium (%)	12,539	*21.7*	*8.8*	*28.0*	*41.5*
Educational level*: high (%)	1,676	*23.4*	*8.7*	*33.0*	*35.0*
Educational level*: unknown (%)	8,388	*19.7*	*8.5*	*24.4*	*47.5*
Home-ownership*: Owner-occupiers (%)	16,839	*24.1*	*9.0*	*27.0*	*39.9*
Home-ownership*: Tenants (%)	28,492	*18.3*	*8.4*	*26.1*	*47.2*
Number of children*: 0 (%)	7,815	*19.3*	*7.9*	*25.8*	*47.0*
Number of children*: 1–2 (%)	18,144	*19.5*	*8.8*	*28.4*	*43.3*
Number of children*: >3 (%)	15,836	*22.2*	*8.7*	*25.6*	*43.5*
Number of children*: unknown (%)	3,536	*19.5*	*8.7*	*21.9*	*49.9*
Marital status: never married (%)	4,489	*20.3*	*7.7*	*23.8*	*48.3*
Marital status: married (%)	9,469	*23.9*	*11.7*	*38.4*	*26.1*
Marital status: widowed (%)	28,109	*19.3*	*7.7*	*22.4*	*50.6*
Marital status: divorced (%)	3,264	*20.5*	*8.8*	*30.6*	*40.2*
Single-person-household* (%)	25,855	*18.7*	*7.5*	*22.8*	*50.9*
Multi-person-household* (%)	19,476	*22.7*	*10.0*	*31.3*	*36.0*
Rooms per person*: 0–<=1.5 (%)	10,737	*20.4*	*9.0*	*29.1*	*41.5*
Rooms per person*: >1.5–<=2.5 (%)	14,787	*20.6*	*9.4*	*27.6*	*42.4*
Rooms per person*: >2.5 (%)	19,807	*20.3*	*7.8*	*24.2*	*47.7*
Language region*: german (%)	32,699	*21.7*	*8.5*	*24.7*	*45.1*
Language region*: french (%)	10,545	*17.5*	*8.7*	*31.2*	*42.6*
Language region*: italian (%)	2,087	*15.8*	*9.6*	*30.0*	*44.7*
Average number of nursing home beds per 100 inhabitants above 65 years (per 106 regions)		6.9	6.8	6.6	7.0

Percentages in italic.
Data source: Swiss Federal Statistical Office, MedStat/SOMED/SNC.
*2000 census data.

did married men and women compared to never married, divorced and widowed individuals. Furthermore, individuals living in a single-person household were more likely to die in an institution compared to those living in a multi-person household.

Multivariate analysis

The estimated relative risk ratios (RRR) of men and women to die at the three different places of death are presented in Table 3 with death at home as reference category, along with 95% confidence intervals and a joint p-value for each variable from a likelihood ratio test. Note that the p-values were of the same magnitude in men and women, for which reason we only provide one p-value for each variable. For better understanding of the estimated relative risk ratios, Figure 2 presents a series of predicted probability plots for selected variables for both, men and women. Other variables in the model are kept constant at their mean value or their reference category, respectively.

Table 3. Results of the multinomial logistic regression analysis for four different places of death (reference value: death at home), Switzerland, 2007 & 2008, individuals born before 1942.

	hospital short				hospital long				nursing home			
	men		women		men		women		men		women	
	RRR	conf. Int	RRR	conf. Int	RRR	conf. Int	RRR	conf. Int	RRR	conf. Int	RRR	conf. Int
Cause of death (p<0.001)												
Cancer condition (reference)	1.00		1.00		1.00		1.00		1.00		1.00	
coronary heart disease	0.87	0.78–0.96	1.13	0.99–1.29	0.30	0.28–0.33	0.29	0.26–0.32	0.64	0.59–0.70	0.81	0.74–0.88
COPD	1.10	0.92–1.31	1.48	1.17–1.86	0.59	0.51–0.67	0.47	0.39–0.56	1.27	1.10–1.47	1.09	0.92–1.29
dementia	0.13	0.08–0.22	0.14	0.09–0.21	0.33	0.28–0.40	0.16	0.13–0.19	5.26	4.59–6.03	3.04	2.72–3.40
stroke	2.49	2.12–2.93	2.73	2.33–3.20	1.30	1.14–1.48	0.97	0.86–1.09	2.72	2.37–3.12	1.91	1.70–2.16
other	1.35	1.23–1.47	1.59	1.42–1.77	0.69	0.65–0.74	0.55	0.51–0.59	1.09	1.01–1.18	1.05	0.98–1.14
Educational level (p<0.001)												
medium (ref.)	1.00		1.00		1.00		1.00		1.00		1.00	
unknown	1.02	0.90–1.14	1.00	0.88–1.12	1.02	0.94–1.11	1.01	0.92–1.10	1.22	1.11–1.34	1.05	0.97–1.14
no	1.00	0.81–1.22	0.92	0.76–1.12	0.99	0.85–1.16	0.99	0.86–1.14	1.16	0.97–1.37	1.16	1.02–1.32
low	0.92	0.84–1.01	1.05	0.95–1.15	0.95	0.89–1.02	1.04	0.98–1.12	1.05	0.98–1.13	1.11	1.04–1.18
high	0.88	0.80–0.98	0.89	0.73–1.10	0.95	0.88–1.02	0.99	0.86–1.14	0.85	0.78–0.93	0.81	0.70–0.93
House or flat owner (p<0.001)												
tenant (ref.)	1.00		1.00		1.00		1.00		1.00		1.00	
owner-occupier	0.82	0.76–0.88	0.80	0.74–0.88	0.76	0.72–0.80	0.77	0.73–0.82	0.73	0.69–0.78	0.72	0.68–0.77
Children (p<0.001)												
0 (ref.)	1.00		1.00		1.00		1.00		1.00		1.00	
1–2	0.98	0.87–1.11	1.05	0.92–1.19	0.91	0.83–0.99	1.00	0.92–1.10	0.89	0.81–0.99	0.96	0.88–1.04
>3	0.88	0.78–1.00	0.92	0.81–1.05	0.79	0.72–0.87	0.85	0.77–0.94	0.84	0.76–0.93	0.86	0.79–0.94
unknown	0.94	0.78–1.12	1.08	0.91–1.29	0.90	0.78–1.03	0.86	0.75–0.98	0.96	0.83–1.10	0.94	0.84–1.06
Marital status (p<0.001)												
married (ref.)	1.00		1.00		1.00		1.00		1.00		1.00	
never married	0.84	0.70–1.01	0.74	0.62–0.89	0.71	0.62–0.81	0.74	0.65–0.85	1.55	1.34–1.79	1.28	1.13–1.44
widowed	1.07	0.96–1.19	0.86	0.77–0.96	1.04	0.96–1.13	0.87	0.80–0.95	1.84	1.69–1.99	1.38	1.27–1.50
divorced	0.97	0.81–1.15	0.81	0.68–0.96	1.04	0.91–1.18	0.87	0.77–0.99	1.74	1.51–2.01	1.31	1.15–1.48
Living condition (p<0.001)												
Single-person household (ref.)	1.00		1.00		1.00		1.00		1.00		1.00	
Multi-person household	1.11	0.97–1.27	0.97	0.86–1.10	1.04	0.94–1.15	0.94	0.86–1.03	0.87	0.79–0.97	0.81	0.75–0.88
Rooms per person (p<0.05)												
0–<=1.5 (ref.)	1.00		1.00		1.00		1.00		1.00		1.00	
>1.5–<=2.5	0.98	0.91–1.07	1.11	1.00–1.23	1.02	0.96–1.08	1.00	0.92–1.08	0.93	0.87–1.00	0.97	0.90–1.05

Table 3. Cont.

	hospital short				hospital long				nursing home			
	men		women		men		women		men		women	
	RRR	*conf. Int*	RRR	*conf. Int*	RRR	*conf. Int*	RRR	*conf. Int*	RRR	*conf. Int*	RRR	*conf. Int*
>2.5	0.98	*0.87–1.11*	0.99	*0.87–1.13*	1.00	*0.91–1.09*	0.97	0.88–1.07	0.86	0.78–0.95	0.86	0.79–0.94
Language region (p<0.001)												
german (ref.)	*1.00*		*1.00*		*1.00*		*1.00*		*1.00*		*1.00*	
french	1.37	*1.25–1.50*	1.28	*1.16–1.42*	1.69	*1.58–1.81*	1.47	1.36–1.58	1.06	0.98–1.15	1.14	1.06–1.22
italian	1.38	*1.16–1.64*	1.65	*1.37–1.99*	1.53	*1.35–1.75*	1.54	1.33–1.77	1.28	1.10–1.49	1.40	1.22–1.60
NH beds density* (p<0.001)	0.99	*0.97–1.01*	1.00	*0.98–1.03*	0.98	*0.97–0.99*	0.97	0.96–0.99	1.07	1.05–1.09	1.04	1.03–1.06

RRR = relative risk ratios, conf. interval = 95% conf. interval, p-values from likelihood ratio tests.
model also included control variablHes nationality and age as cubic spline, results not shown.
* = average number of nursing home beds per 100 habitants above 65 years (per 106 regions).
Data source: Swiss Federal Statistical Office, MedStat/SOMED/SNC.

Older persons of both sexes were more likely to die in nursing homes than comparatively younger people within the age group over 65 years. We found significant differences between causes of death. In comparison to patients with malignant neoplasms (reference category), persons with dementia had a significantly higher risk of dying in a nursing home than dying at home (men: RRR 5.26, CI 4.59–6.03; women RRR 3.04, CI 2.72–3.40). In contrast, persons with coronary heart disease had a significantly lower relative risk for dying in any institution than for dying at home. The estimated coefficients and graphs show that a higher educational level slightly reduced the relative risk to die in nursing homes compared to a medium educational level (men: RRR 0.85, CI 0.78–0.93; women: RRR 0.81, CI 0.70–0.93). Homeowners died more often at home than in an institution.

Having many children prevents dying in an institution: Having at least three children compared to no children, for instance, decreased the risk ratio for dying in a nursing home compared to death at home significantly (men: RRR 0.84, CI 0.76–0.93; women: RRR 0.86, CI 0.79–0.94). Being never married increased the relative risk of dying in a nursing home in compared to dying at home (men: RRR 1.55, CI 1.34–1.79; women: RRR 1.28, CI 1.13–1.44), and decreases the relative risk of dying in a hospital after a long stay (men: RRR 0.71, CI 0.62–0.81; women: RRR 0.74, CI 0.65–0.85). Being widowed or divorced had different effects for men and women: Compared to being married, it significantly increases the relative risk ratios of dying in a nursing for both men and women, but the respective relative risk ratio for death in a hospital was only significant for women. Living in a multi-person household compared to living alone decreased the relative risks for dying in a nursing home (men: RRR 0.87, CI 0.79–0.97; women: RRR 0.81, CI 0.75–0.88). The higher the number of rooms in a household per person, the higher the relative risk of dying at home compared to dying in a nursing home. We found for instance a significance effect for 2.5 rooms or more per person compared to 0–1.5 rooms per person (men: RRR 0.86, CI 0.78–0.95; women: RRR 0.86, CI 0.79–0.94).

In both the French and the Italian speaking part of Switzerland, the relative risks of dying in an institution rather than at home were significantly higher than in the German speaking part. We found, for instance, higher relative risks of hospital deaths after a longer stay in the French speaking part (men RRR 1.69, CI 1.58–1.81; women: RRR 1.47, CI 1.36–1.58) and Italian speaking part (men RRR 1.53, CI 1.35–1.75; women RRR 1.54, CI 1.33–1.77) compared to the German speaking part, which is also illustrated in Figure 2. The availability of nursing home beds showed the expected effect: the higher the density of beds, the higher the relative risk of dying in a nursing home (men: RRR 1.07, CI 1.05–1.09; women: RRR 1.04, CI 1.03–1.06).

Discussion

We found substantial socio-demographic variation concerning the place of death. The place of death was not determined by underlying somatic diseases alone, but also by a variety of socio-demographic and familial/housing determinants, with a different impact on men and women. While hospital deaths appeared to be mostly due to medical reasons, dying in a nursing home was mainly determined by socio-demographic, familial and regional characteristics. Persons with a low SEP had higher relative risks of dying in a nursing home compared to dying at home. This is in line with a study from Belgium. [2] Considering homeownership and the number of rooms per person as other proxies for SEP confirmed this pattern. One explanation for this may be that people with a higher SEP have generally a better health status and

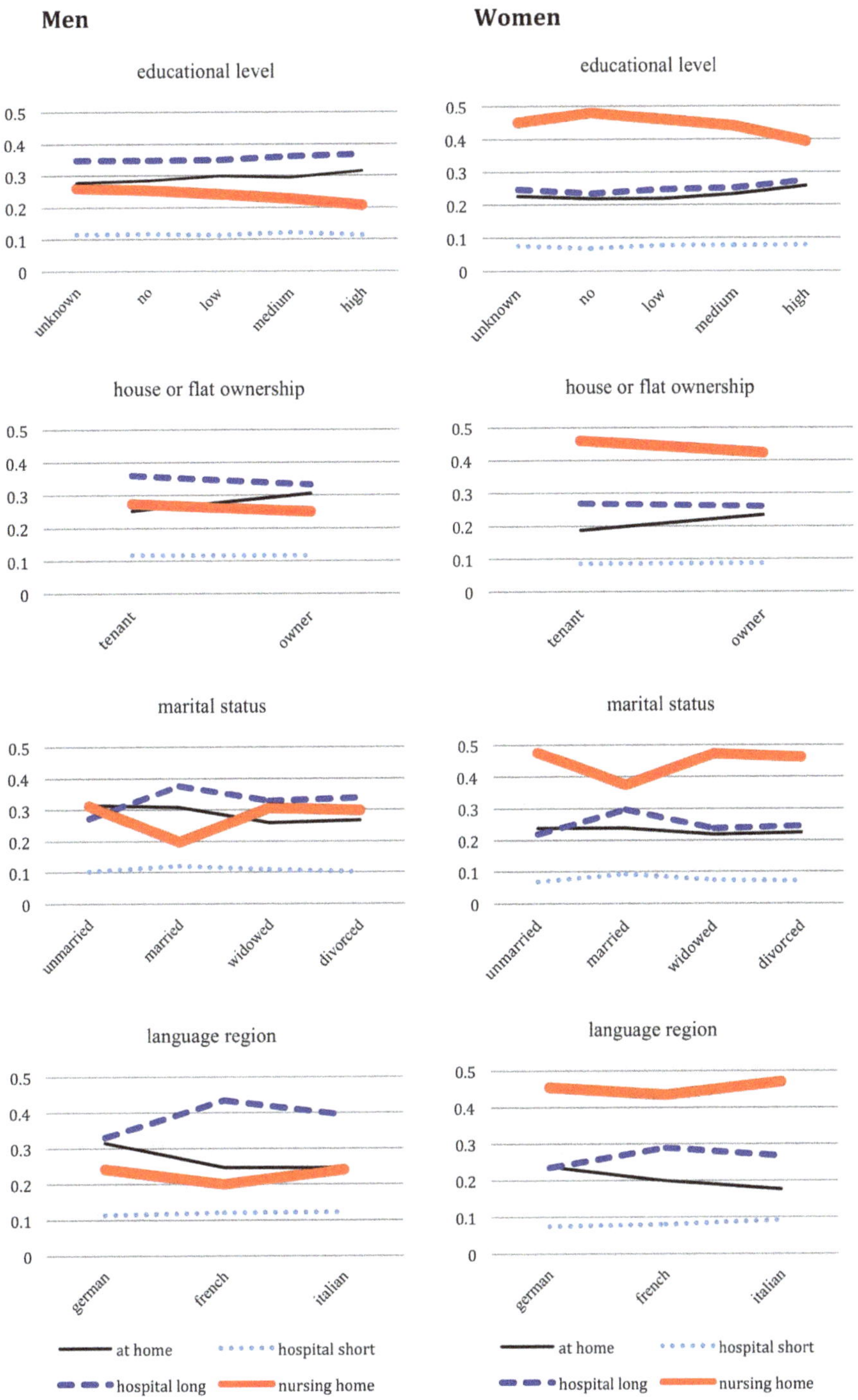

Figure 2. Predicted probabilities to die in one of four types of places of death for selected independent variables. Legend: The probabilities add up to 1 per category of the independent variable which means they can be interpreted as percent. One example: the probability to die in a nursing home compared to other places of death for women is higher for all educational levels compared to other places of death, but it is highest for those with no formal education. Data source: Swiss Federal Statistical Office, MedStat/SOMED/SNC.

need therefore less nursing care than people with a lower SEP. Another explanation could be that people with higher SEP can afford home nursing care more frequently. More empirical research is needed to explore this issue.

In our study population, nearly 45% of women died in a nursing home compared to 26% of men. In spite of a general wish to die at home, [4] only around 28% of men and 20% of women died at home. These results are in line with precedent studies from Switzerland following another approach [16] and comparable with studies from other countries. [2,21–23,33,34] The gender difference is most likely due to the longer life expectancy of women. Men live more often in a multi-person household, possibly together with a younger female partner. In contrast, women more often survive their spouses or stay divorced. We therefore hypothesize that men often continue to live in their private home, even when their health status is getting worse and health care is needed, whereas single women with similar health status are placed in a nursing home.

Among those dying in a hospital, there were noticeable differences between persons with longer and short (≤2 days) stays preceding death. Relative to cancer deaths, individuals deceased due to stroke or respiratory diseases were more likely to have died after a short hospitalisation than at home, whereas the corresponding effect was not significant or reversed for long-term hospitalisations for stroke and COPD, respectively. We suppose that short hospital stays preceding deaths are often due to acute exacerbation of a pre-existing disease. Familial factors were also important: Having children, being married and living with a spouse or any other person increased the relative risks of dying at home, which is probably more in accordance with the patient's and his relatives' wishes, [3,7] unless it becomes too stressful for the caregivers. [9] On the other hand, being never married, widowed or divorced and living alone increases the relative risks to die in a nursing home. Dying in nursing homes could become even more frequent in the future due to the aging of the population: the older the people, the higher the probability to die in a nursing home instead of a hospital. [34,35] As a consequence, SEP and familial/housing factors could gain even more influence on the place of end-of-life.

The analysis of the three Swiss language regions revealed that death at home was significantly more likely for both men and women in the German speaking than in the French or Italian speaking part. The reason might be cultural differences regarding attitudes towards death and life-prolonging measures, as described for physicians from the three Swiss language areas. [36] We therefore assume that people in the German speaking part more strongly prefer to die at home, especially when the underlying disease is incurable. In a study on main reasons for institutionalization in Switzerland, [37] inability of housekeeping was the most frequent answer, even before medical reasons or need for support.

Strengths and limitations

The strength of our study is the national comprehensiveness and the size of the study population, which minimizes selections bias. We were able to explore a wide variety of socio- demographic characteristics based on information individually linked from the census.

The study has two main limitations: First, we assumed that all deaths not tracked in hospitals or nursing homes occurred at home. Second, we were not able to link all deaths to a census record. This problem was more prevalent in nursing homes (ca. 12%) than in hospitals (ca. 5%). However, linkage success did not substantially vary by region of living, age or sex of the deceased persons. A further limitation was the lack of actual information about income, assets and health insurance coverage of the study population. Our results emphasize the importance of nursing homes as places of death in Switzerland. Our findings might therefore be generalizable foremost to countries with a similar socio-economic setting (e. g., The Netherlands, Norway, Iceland) [34].

Conclusion

Death at home is an unaccomplished wish for a majority of elderly people in Switzerland. Dying in an institution is rather the norm than exception – and this makes it important to scrutinize the reasons why people die where they do. Dying in a hospital appears to be mainly driven by medical reasons. In contrast, living and dying in a nursing home is substantially driven by socio-demographic determinants such as SEP, living alone, housing characteristics and structural (regional) factors. The proportion of deaths occurring in nursing homes may increase in the future [34,35] and as a consequence also the importance of socio-demographic determinants of living conditions at the end-of-life. Individuals with a lower SEP, living alone or having no children, i.e., those with less resources and therefore less freedom of choice are overrepresented in nursing homes. Thus, health policy should aim to empower these groups when having to decide whether to move to a nursing home or to stay in a private home. Since nursing home stays are rather expensive, more public engagement in home care offers may not only meet the request of many concerned persons but also pay off in a macroeconomic view. The interplay between demand and need, between availability of nursing home and hospital beds as well as home care offers, is complex and so are the various push and pull effects exerted by the stakeholders [38].

Acknowledgments

We thank the Swiss Federal Statistical Office for providing mortality and census data and for the support which made the Swiss National Cohort and this study possible. The members of the Swiss National Cohort Study Group are Matthias Egger (Chairman of the Executive Board), Adrian Spoerri and Marcel Zwahlen (all Bern), Milo Puhan (Chairman of the Scientific Board), Matthias Bopp (both Zurich), Nino Künzli (Basel), Fred Paccaud (Lausanne) and Michel Oris (Geneva).

Author Contributions

Analyzed the data: DH MB JB UZ. Contributed reagents/materials/analysis tools: DH MB JB. Contributed to the writing of the manuscript: DH JB MB VK. Conceived and supervised the study and the record linkage and repeatedly edited later versions of the manuscript: MB. Conducted all statistical analyses and wrote the first version of the manuscript: DH. Supervised the statistical analyses and improved the manuscript: JB. Conducted the record linkage and prepared the analysis files: UZ. Contributed important intellectual content and edited the manuscript: VK.

References

1. Clark D (2002) Between hope and acceptance: the medicalisation of dying. BMJ 324: 905–907.
2. Houttekier D, Cohen J, Bilsen J, Deboosere P, Verduyckt P, et al. (2009) Determinants of the Place of Death in the Brussels Metropolitan Region. J Pain Symptom Manage 37: 996–1005. doi:10.1016/j.jpainsymman.2008.05.014.
3. Teno JM, Clarridge BR, Casey V, Welch LC, Wetle T, et al. (2004) Family perspectives on end-of-life care at the last place of care. JAMA J Am Med Assoc 291: 88–93. doi:10.1001/jama.291.1.88.
4. Brogaard T, Neergaard MA, Sokolowski I, Olesen F, Jensen AB (2012) Congruence between preferred and actual place of care and death among Danish cancer patients. Palliat Med 0: 1–10. doi:10.1177/0269216312438468.
5. Foreman LM, Hunt RW, Luke CG, Roder DM (2006) Factors predictive of preferred place of death in the general population of South Australia. Palliat Med 20: 447–453. doi:10.1191/0269216306pm1149oa.
6. Fischer S, Bosshard G, Zellweger U, Faisst K (2004) Der Sterbeort: "Wo sterben die Menschen heute in der Schweiz?" Z Gerontol Geriatr 37: 467–474. doi:10.1007/s00391-004-0216-3.
7. Bowling A (1983) The hospitalisation of death: should more people die at home? J Med Ethics 9: 158–161. doi:10.1136/jme.9.3.158.
8. Townsend J, Frank AO, Fermont D, Dyer S, Karran O, et al. (1990) Terminal cancer care and patients' preference for place of death: a prospective study. BMJ 301: 415–417.

9. Thomas C, Morris SM, Clark D (2004) Place of death: preferences among cancer patients and their carers. Soc Sci Med 58: 2431–2444. doi:10.1016/j.socscimed.2003.09.005.
10. Evans N, Walsh H (2002) The organisation of death and dying in today's society. Nurs Stand 16: 33–38.
11. Rice DP, Fineman N (2004) Economic implications of increased longevity in the United States. Annu Rev Public Health 25: 457–473. doi:10.1146/annurev.publhealth.25.101802.123054.
12. Bickel H (1998) Das letzte Lebensjahr: Eine Repräsentativstudie an Verstorbenen. Wohnsituation, Sterbeort und Nutzung von Versorgungsangeboten. Z Gerontol Geriatr 31: 193–204.
13. Riley GF, Lubitz JD (2010) Long-term trends in Medicare payments in the last year of life. Health Serv Res 45: 565–576. doi:10.1111/j.1475-6773.2010.01082.x.
14. Kelley AS, Ettner SL, Morrison S, Qingling D, Morrison RS, et al. (2011) Determinants of Medical Expenditures in the last 6 Months of Life. Ann Intern Med 154: 235–242. doi:10.1016/j.jpainsymman.2010.10.124.
15. Shugarman LR, Decker SL, Bercovitz A (2009) Demographic and social characteristics and spending at the end of life. J Pain Symptom Manage 38: 15–26. doi:10.1016/j.jpainsymman.2009.04.004.
16. Reich O, Signorell A, Busato A (2013) Place of death and health care utilization for people in the last 6 months of life in Switzerland: a retrospective analysis using administrative data. BMC Health Serv Res 13: 116. doi:10.1186/1472-6963-13-116.
17. Centeno C, Clark D, Lynch T, Racafort J, Praill D, et al. (2007) Facts and indicators on palliative care development in 52 countries of the WHO European region: results of an EAPC task force. Palliat Med 21: 463–471. doi:10.1177/0269216307081942.
18. Gomes B, Calanzani N, Curiale V, Mccrone P, Higginson I (2014) Effectiveness and cost-effectiveness of home palliative care services for adults with advanced illness and their caregivers (Review). Cochrane Database Syst Rev.
19. BfS (2012) Inventar der Datensituation über Palliative Care. Neuenburg: Bundesamt für Statistik BfS.
20. Jaggi A, Junker C, Minder C (2001) Beeinflusst die medizinische Versorgungsstruktur den Anteil Todesfälle im Spital? Sozial- und Präventivmedizin SPM 46: 379–388.
21. Weitzen S, Teno JM, Fennell M, Mor V (2003) Factors associated with site of death: a national study of where people die. Med Care 41: 323–335. doi:10.1097/01.MLR.0000044913.37084.27.
22. Jayaraman J, Joseph K (2013) Determinants of place of death: a population-based retrospective cohort study. BMC Palliat Care 12: 19. doi:10.1186/1472-684X-12-19.
23. Cohen J, Bilsen J, Hooft P, Deboosere P, van der Wal G, et al. (2006) Dying at home or in an institution using death certificates to explore the factors associated with place of death. Health Policy (New York) 78: 319–329. doi:10.1016/j.healthpol.2005.11.003.
24. Faeh D, Bopp M (2010) Educational inequalities in mortality and associated risk factors: German- versus French-speaking Switzerland. BMC Public Health 10: 567. doi:10.1186/1471-2458-10-567.
25. Bopp M, Spoerri A, Zwahlen M, Gutzwiller F, Paccaud F, et al. (2009) Cohort Profile: the Swiss National Cohort-a longitudinal study of 6.8 million people. Int J Epidemiol 38: 379–384. doi:10.1093/ije/dyn042.
26. Medizinische Statistik der Krankenhäuser 2011 - Standardtabellen (2013). Neuenburg: Bundesamt für Statistik BfS.
27. Bopp M, Zellweger U, Faeh D (2011) Routine data sources challenge international diabetes Federation extrapolations of national diabetes prevalence in Switzerland. Diabetes Care 34: 2387–2389. doi:10.2337/dc11-0157.
28. Statistik der sozialmedizinischen Institutionen 2011 – Standardtabellen (2013). Neuenburg: Bundesamt für Statistik BfS.
29. Zellweger U, Bopp M (2010) Record Linkage der Medizinischen Statistik 2000–2006 der Krankenhäuser mit der Swiss National Cohort (SNC). Zurich: Institut für Sozial- und Präventivmedizin der Universität Zürich/Forschung und Dokumentation 32.
30. Zellweger U, Bopp M (2011) Record Linkage der Todesfälle in der Statistik der Sozialmedizinischen Institutionen 2006–2008 mit der Swiss National Cohort. Swiss National Cohort Report Nr. 7. Institut für Sozial- und Präventivmedizin der Universität Zürich/Forschung und Dokumentation 34.
31. Artazcoz L, Rueda S (2007) Social inequalities in health among the elderly: a challenge for public health research. J Epidemiol Community Health 61: 466–467. doi:10.1136/jech.2006.058081.
32. Hosmer DW, Lemeshow S (2000) Applied Logistic Regression, Second Edition. New York: John Wiley & Sons, inc.
33. Klinkenberg M, Visser G, van Groenou MIB, van der Wal G, Deeg DJH, et al. (2005) The last 3 months of life: care, transitions and the place of death of older people. Health Soc Care Community 13: 420–430. doi:10.1111/j.1365-2524.2005.00567.x.
34. Broad JB, Gott M, Kim H, Boyd M, Chen H, et al. (2013) Where do people die? An international comparison of the percentage of deaths occurring in hospital and residential aged care settings in 45 populations, using published and available statistics. Int J Public Health 58: 257–267. doi:10.1007/s00038-012-0394-5.
35. Houttekier D, Cohen J, Surkyn J, Deliens L (2011) Study of recent and future trends in place of death in Belgium using death certificate data: a shift from hospitals to care homes. BMC Public Health 11: 228. doi:10.1186/1471-2458-11-228.
36. Fischer S, Bosshard G, Faisst K, Tschopp A, Fischer J, et al. (2005) Swiss doctors' attitudes towards end-of-life decisions and their determinants. Swiss Med Wkly 135: 370–376.
37. BfS (2011) Eintritt in ein Alters- und Pflegeheim. Neuenburg: Bundesamt für Statistik BfS.
38. BAG (2012) Versorgungsstrukturen für spezialisierte Palliative Care in der Schweiz. Bern: Bundesamt für Gesundheit BAG.

16

Interrelationship of Postoperative Delirium and Cognitive Impairment and Their Impact on the Functional Status in Older Patients Undergoing Orthopaedic Surgery: A Prospective Cohort Study

Chih-Kuang Liang[1,2,3], Chin-Liang Chu[1,3,4], Ming-Yueh Chou[1,3,5], Yu-Te Lin[1,2,3]*, Ti Lu[4], Chien-Jen Hsu[6], Liang-Kung Chen[3,7]*

1 Center for Geriatrics and Gerontology, Kaohsiung Veterans General Hospital, Kaohsiung, Taiwan, **2** Division of Neurology, Department of Medicine, Kaohsiung Veterans General Hospital Kaohsiung, Taiwan, **3** Aging and Health Research Center, National Yang Ming University, Taipei, Taiwan, **4** Department of Psychiatry, Kaohsiung Veterans General Hospital, Kaohsiung, Taiwan, **5** Department of Family Medicine, Kaohsiung Veterans General Hospital, Kaohsiung, Taiwan, **6** Department of Orthopaedics, Kaohsiung Veterans General Hospital, Kaohsiung, Taiwan, **7** Center for Geriatrics and Gerontology, Taipei Veterans General Hospital, Taipei, Taiwan

Abstract

Background: The impact of postoperative delirium on post-discharge functional status of older patients remains unclear, and little is known regarding the interrelationship between cognitive impairment and post-operative delirium. Therefore, the main purpose was to evaluate the post-discharge functional status of patients who experience delirium after undergoing orthopaedic surgery and the interrelationship of postoperative delirium with underlying cognitive impairment.

Method: This prospective cohort study, conducted at a tertiary care medical center from April 2011 to March 2012, enrolled all subjects aged over 60 years who were admitted for orthopaedic surgery. The baseline characteristics (age, gender, BMI, and living arrangement), surgery-related factors (ASA class, admission type, type of surgery, and length of hospital stay), results of geriatric assessment (postoperative delirium, cognition, depressive mood, comorbidity, pain, malnutrition, polypharmacy, ADL, and instrumental [I]ADL) and 1–12-month postoperative ADL and IADL functional status were collected for analysis.

Results: Overall, 9.1% of 232 patients (mean age: 74.7±7.8 years) experienced postoperative delirium, which was significantly associated with IADL decline at only 6 and 12 months postoperatively (RR: 6.22, 95% CI: 1.08–35.70 and RR: 12.54, 95% CI: 1.88–83.71, respectively). Delirium superimposed on cognitive impairment was a significant predictor for poor functional status at 6 and 12 months postoperatively (RR: 12.80, 95% CI: 1.65–99.40 for ADL at the 6th month, and RR: 7.96, 95% CI: 1.35–46.99 at the 12th month; RR: 13.68, 95% CI: 1.94–96.55 for IADL at the 6th month, and RR: 30.61, 95% CI: 2.94–318.54 at the 12th month, respectively).

Conclusion: Postoperative delirium is predictive of IADL decline in older patients undergoing orthopaedic surgery, and delirium superimposed on cognitive impairment is an independent risk factor for deterioration of ADL and IADL functional status. Early identification of cognitive function and to prevent delirium are needed to improve functional status following orthopaedic surgery.

Editor: Stephen D. Ginsberg, Nathan Kline Institute and New York University School of Medicine, United States of America

Funding: This work was supported by grants from the Veteran Affairs Commission of Taiwan. The funders had no role in study design, data collection and analysis, decision to publish, or preparation of the manuscript.

Competing Interests: The authors have declared that no competing interests exist.

* Email: ytlin@vghks.gov.tw (YTL); lkchen2@vghtpe.gov.tw (LKC)

Introduction

Delirium is an acute mental disorder that is characterized by rapid onset and a fluctuating course of consciousness disturbance and inattention, possibly leading to further adverse health consequences in the elderly population [1]. Although delirium is a well-recognized geriatric syndrome, it is often overlooked by clinicians and nurses [2,3]. The incidence of delirium following orthopaedic surgery has been reported to be 4–65%. Considerable variation is seen and is dependent on the type of procedure, with the reported incidence being 35–65% in patients undergoing operative treatment of a hip fracture and 9–15% in patients undergoing elective orthopaedic procedures [4,5]. Risk factors for the development of postoperative delirium in older patients include older age, cognitive impairment, depressed mood, poor baseline physical function, comorbid diseases, type of surgery, and institutionalization before admission [6–10]. Although delirium is a common geriatric syndrome, its etiopathogenesis remains unclear. However, preventive strategies focused on early identification and management of risk factors are believed to be superior to strategies that emphasize treatment of delirium after it occurs [10–13].

Delirium subsequent to surgery is associated with higher rates of in-hospital and long-term mortality [14–20], as well as longer hospital stay, longer intensive care unit stay, and higher chance of discharge to nursing facilities [14–16,21]. Although the adverse impact of postoperative delirium has been clearly identified, the impact of postoperative delirium on long-term functional status remains unclear. Dementia or cognitive impairment has been reported as an independent risk factor for delirium [10], and the overall incidence of new delirium was significantly higher among older patients with dementia than among older patients with no dementia [22]. Moreover, pre-fracture cognitive impairment and post-fracture delirium were also strongly associated with higher mortality rate and risk for institutionalization [23,24], and delirium might be an early indicator for post-discharge cognitive decline [25,26]. Although it can result in long-term cognitive decline, postoperative cognitive decline secondary to delirium does not occur in all patients [10]. To date, little is known regarding the interrelationship between delirium and cognitive impairment and their impact on adverse functional status in older patients. Therefore, the purpose of the present study was to evaluate the impact of postoperative delirium, in the presence of underlying cognitive impairment, on changes in the post-discharge functional status of patients who underwent orthopaedic surgery.

Methods

Study design

This prospective cohort study was conducted in a tertiary care medical center in Southern Taiwan. All subjects aged 60 years and older who were admitted for orthopaedic surgery during the period April 2011 to March 2012 were screened for this study. Patients were excluded for the following reasons: (1) medical conditions that prevented comprehensive geriatric assessment (CGA), or admission or transfer to an intensive care unit before enrollment, (2) inability to complete the comprehensive geriatric assessment (CGA), (3) inability to provide informed consent, (4) limited life expectancy less than 6 months such as in cancer and terminal stage heart failure cases, (5) delirium occurring before enrollment or surgery, and (6) incomplete data. The study protocol was approved by the Institutional Review Board of Kaohsiung Veterans General Hospital and written informed consents were obtained from all participants before the study started. During a one-year period, a total of 232 patients were enrolled with mean age of 74.7±7.8 years (range: 60–93). Among them, 28 (12.1%) patients were admitted to the hospital from the emergency department. The incidence of postoperative delirium was 9.1% (21/232).

Preoperative evaluation

Demographic data and surgery characteristics. Two research nurses interviewed all participants to collect the preoperative demographic data (including age, gender, educational level, living arrangement, and body mass index [BMI]), and data on other characteristics including admission type (emergency or elective surgery), type of surgery (including spinal decompression only, spinal surgery with instrumented fusion, total knee arthroplasty, other elective knee surgery, elective total hip arthroplasty [total hip replacement]/bipolar hemiarthroplasty, revision hip surgery, and open reduction and internal fixation [ORIF]/arthroplasty for hip fracture), ASA (American Society of Anesthesiologists) physical status, and length of hospital stay.

Comprehensive geriatric assessment (CGA). All participants were assessed by trained research nurses using the CGA before preceding the orthopaedic operation, and within the first 24 hours after hospital admission from the outpatient clinics or emergency department. The assessment covered visual and hearing impairments, polypharmacy (defined as currently using >4 prescription drugs for over 2 weeks), depressive symptoms (using the 15-item Chinese Geriatric Depression Scale) [27,28], nutritional status (as determined by the Mini Nutritional Assessment) [29], comorbidity (as evaluated by the Charlson's Comorbidity Index) [30], symptoms of pain (rated on a Visual Analogue Scale) [31], cognitive function (as assessed by the Chinese version of the Mini-Mental State Examination at admission) [32], the Activities of Daily Living (ADL, evaluated by the Barthel Index) [33], and the Lawton-Brody Instrumental ADL (IADL) [34].

Patients were screened for delirium daily by the primary care nurses in the orthopaedic wards after orthopaedic surgery using the Confusion Assessment Method (CAM) [35], and a senior psychiatrist would confirm the diagnosis if the patient was deemed to be confused. The research nurses obtained ADL and IADL scores by conducting telephone interviews of the participating patients or their primary caregivers at 1, 3, 6, and 12 months after hospital discharge.

Statistical analysis

Continuous data are expressed as means ± SD, and categorical data are expressed as percentages. Dichotomous and ordinal variables were compared in those with and without delirium using the Chi-square test or Fisher exact test, and continuous variables were compared using the independent Student *t*-test or Mann-Whitney *U* test when appropriate.

The independent Student *t*-test or Mann-Whitney *U* test were used to compare the ADL or IADL scores between groups based on delirium status at 1, 3, 6, and 12 months. The differences in mean ADL and IADL scores between those with and without delirium at different time points were evaluated using the Analysis of Covariance (ANCOVA) with the inclusion of baseline ADL or IADL scores as covariates. To compare functional changes at 1, 3, 6, and 12 months, ADL or IADL functional decline was defined as lower ADL or IADL score at follow-up than at baseline. Multivariable logistic regression analysis was performed to determine whether delirium was an independent predictor of ADL or IADL decline at follow-up. In this model, age, gender, admission type, type of surgery, hearing impairment, polypharmacy, cognitive impairment, depressive symptoms, BMI, high risk of malnutrition, Charlson's Comorbidity Index (CCI), symptoms of pain, ASA class, and hospital length of stay were entered as explanatory variables.

To evaluate the effect of cognitive problems on long-term functional status (ADL and IADL scores at 1, 3, 6, and 12 months follow-up), four categorical variables representing four groups were defined (no cognitive problem [group A]; cognitive impairment alone indicated by MMSE <24 [group B]; postoperative delirium superimposed on cognitive problems [group C], and delirium only [group D]). ANCOVA was used to compare the mean ADL and IADL scores between these four groups after adjusting for baseline ADL and IADL scores (the covariates). The independent effect of each categorical variable on ADL and IADL outcomes was assessed using multivariable logistic regression

Table 1. Demographic data, functional status, and surgery-related factors in 232 subjects with postoperative delirium or no delirium.

	Total	Postoperative delirium	No delirium	
	N = 232	N = 21	N = 211	
Variables	(% or mean ± SD)	(% or mean ± SD)	(% or mean ± SD)	*p* value
Age	74.7±7.8	81.3±5.2	74.1±7.7	<0.001
Educational level	5.8±4.7	6.4±4.6	5.7±4.7	0.522
Gender (male)	108(46.6%)	17(81.0%)	91(43.1%)	0.001
Admission route				0.149
Emergency room	28(12.1%)	5(23.8%)	23(10.9%)	
Outpatient clinic (elective)	204(87.9%)	16(76.2%)	188(89.1%)	
Living				0.035
Alone	32(13.8%)	1(4.8%)	31(14.7%)	
Institutionalized	10(4.3%)	3(14.3%)	7(3.3%)	
With relatives/friends	190(81.9%)	17(81.0%)	173(82.0%)	
BMI	26.5±4.3	23.7±3.2	26.8±4.2	0.001
Polypharmacy (Yes)	106(45.7%)	13(61.9%)	93(44.1%)	0.118
Psychotic drugs (Yes)	36(15.5%)	4(19.0%)	32(15.2%)	0.751
Visual impairment (Yes)	157(67.7%)	18(85.7%)	139(65.9%)	0.064
Hearing impairment (Yes)	38(16.4%)	8(38.1%)	30(14.2%)	0.010
ADL(BI) before admission	94.1±2.3	85.0±19.9	95.0±1.0	0.034
IADL before admission	5.7±1.4	4.4±1.9	5.8±1.3	0.004
Cognitive impairment at admission (MMSE <24)	91(39.2%)	16(76.2%)	75(35.5%)	<0.001
Presence of depressive symptoms (defined by GDS-15> = 5)	19(8.2%)	1(4.8%)	18(8.5%)	1.000
Risk of malnutrition (screening by MNA)	19(8.2%)	7(33.3%)	12(5.7%)	<0.001
CCI	0.82±1.07	1.71±1.79	0.73±0.93	0.022
Pain VAS score	4.72±1.58	5.14±1.71	4.68±1.56	0.203
ASA				0.124
ASA 1 and 2	225(97.0%)	19(90.5%)	206(97.6%)	
ASA 3	7(3.0%)	2(9.5%)	5(2.4%)	
Length of hospital stay	8.45±4.46	8.42±4.63	8.76±2.221	0.736
Type of surgery				0.090
Elective spine surgery	60(25.9%)	7(11.7%)	53(88.3%)	
Elective knee surgery	100(43.1%)	6(6.0%)	94(94.0%)	
Elective hip arthroplasty	39(17.7%)	1(2.6%)	38(97.4%)	
ORIF/arthroplasty for hip fracture	33(13.4%)	7(21.2%)	26(78.8%)	

BMI: Body Mass Index; ADL: Activities of Daily Living; BI: Barthel Index; IADL: Instrumental Activities of Daily Living; MMSE: Mini-mental State Examination; GDS: Geriatric Depression Scale; MNA: Mini-nutritional Assessment; CCI: Charlson's Comorbidity Index; VAS: Visual Analogue Scale; ASA: American Society of Anesthesiologists physical status; ORIF: open reduction and internal fixation.
Elective Spine Surgery: Spinal decompression only and Spinal surgery with instrumented fusion.
Elective knee surgery: includes total knee replacement (N = 92) and other elective knee surgery (N = 8).
Elective hip arthroplasty: includes total hip replacement, bipolar hemiarthroplasty, and revision hip surgery.

analysis after controlling for age, gender, admission type, type of surgery, hearing impairment, polypharmacy, cognitive impairment, depressive symptoms, BMI, high risk of malnutrition, CCI, symptoms of pain, ASA class, and hospital length of stay and baseline IADL or ADL scores as covariates. For all tests, a P value (two-tailed) less than 0.05 was considered statistically significant. All statistical analyses were performed using IBM SPSS version 21 (SPSS Inc., Chicago, IL).

Results

The effect of delirium on functional status

Demographic characteristics of all 232 patients are summarized in Table 1. Fifty of the 232 patients were lost to follow up and therefore excluded from the evaluation of post-discharge functional status. The demographic characteristics of the excluded patients were similar to those of the enrolled patients except for age (77.0±8.7 years vs 74.1±7.4 years, $p = 0.018$) and BMI (25.2±4.5 vs 26.7±4.1 kg/m^2, $p = 0.015$). The number of patients who underwent spinal decompression only, spinal surgery with

Table 2. Comparing the ADL and IADL scores at baseline and 1, 3, 6, and 12 months of follow-up in groups with delirium.

	Time of follow-up (months)								
	Non-adjusted functional status (mean ± SE)					Adjusted baseline functional status by ANCOVA (mean ± SE)			
Outcomes variables	Baseline	1	3	6	12	1	3	6	12
ADL (BI) scores (mean ± SE)									
Delirium (N = 17)	85.9±4.81#	77.9±5.25#	79.4±5.62#	81.8±5.44#	81.8±5.86#	83.0±2.82#	84.5±2.77#	86.9±3.06#	86.4±3.18#
No delirium (N = 165)	95.6±0.80	93.2±0.93	94.9±0.89	95.2±1.00	95.6±0.99	92.7±0.88	94.4±0.87	94.6±0.96	95.2±1.00
IADL scores (mean ± SE)									
Delirium (N = 17)	4.4±0.40#	3.4±0.45#	3.4±0.47#	3.2±0.53#	2.9±0.53#	4.4±0.28#	4.4±0.28#	4.3±0.33#	4.0±0.33#
No delirium (N = 165)	5.8±0.09	5.3±0.11	5.6±0.11	5.6±0.12	5.7±0.12	5.2±0.09	5.5±0.09	5.5±0.10	5.6±0.10

#p<0.05 for comparing groups by delirium status. ANCOVA: Analysis of Covariance.

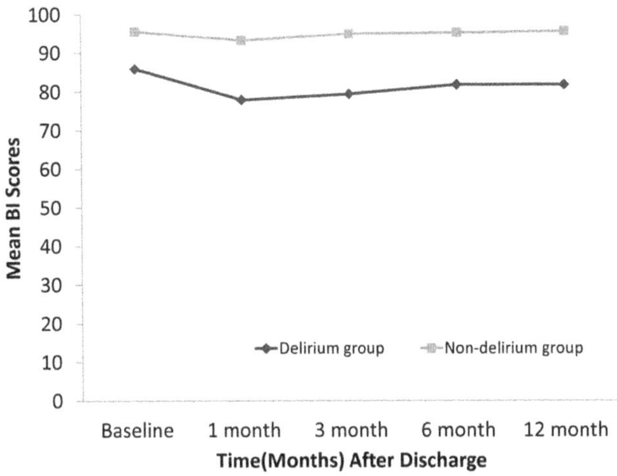

Figure 1. The trend of Barthel Index scores (ADL) (a) and IADL (b) for the delirium and no delirium groups.

instrumented fusion, total knee arthroplasty, other elective knee surgery, elective total hip replacement/bipolar hemiarthroplasty, revision hip surgery, and ORIF/arthroplasty for hip fracture was 7 (3.0%), 53 (22.8%), 92 (39.7%), 8 (3.4%), 31 (13.4%), 8 (3.4%), and 33 (14.2%), respectively. These procedures were grouped into four categories (elective spine surgery, elective knee surgery, elective hip arthroplasty, and ORIF/arthroplasty for hip fracture) for further analysis. Comparing the 50 patients lost to follow up with the 182 included patients, the delirium occurred in a similar proportion of both groups (8.0% [4/50] vs 9.3% [17/182]; data not shown), indicating that delirium did not increase the likelihood of loss to follow up.

At baseline, the 182 enrolled subjects (17 with delirium and 165 without delirium) had an ADL score of 85.9 (standard error [SE] = 4.81) vs 95.6 ([SE] = 0.80) and an IADL score of 4.4 ([SE] = 0.40) vs 5.8 ([SE] = 0.09; Table 2). Figure 1 shows the change in ADL and IADL scores over time after hospitalization for both groups. ADL and IADL scores were significantly different between those who developed post-operative delirium and those who did not. When controlling for baseline ADL, IADL scores remained significantly lower in patients who developed postoperative delirium than in those who did not. Table 3 shows the differences in ADL and IADL decline between the two groups at different follow-up times. Results of univariate logistic regression analysis identified delirium as a predictor of ADL decline at 6 and 12 months (p value: 0.036 vs 0.014), and IADL decline at 3, 6, and 12 months after surgery (p value: 0.033 vs 0.005 vs 0.001). In addition, multivariable logistic regression analysis identified delirium as a predictor of only IADL decline at 6 and 12 months (for IADL at 6 months, adjusted RR: 6.22, 95% CI:1.08–35.70, p value = 0.040; for IADL at 12 months, adjusted RR: 12.54, 95% CI: 1.88–83.71, p value = 0.009).

Impact of combined cognitive problems on functional status

The 182 included patients were divided into four groups based on delirium and cognitive status. The patients in group D (with delirium, but without baseline cognitive impairment) were excluded because of small sample size (N = 4). Baseline ADL and IADL scores were significantly different between patients with no cognitive problems (group A), and those with both baseline cognitive dysfunction and delirium (group C) or with baseline

Table 3. Analysis of the percentage of functional decline and the predicted effect on functional status in groups divided by delirium status using Chi-square test and multivariable logistic regression.

	Percentage of functional decline						Predicted effect on functional decline											
	ADL decline			IADL decline			RR of delirium for ADL decline						RR of delirium for IADL decline					
	Delirium	No delirium		Delirium	No delirium		Unadjusted			Adjusted			Unadjusted			Adjusted		
Follow-up times	N(%)	N(%)	p value	N(%)	N(%)	p value	RR	95% CI	p value	RR	95% CI	p value	RR	95% CI	p value	RR	95% CI	p value
1-month	8/17(47. 1)	46/165(27.9)	0.099	6/13(46.2%)	59/165(35.8)	0.552	2.30	0.84–6.32	0.107	2.45	0.60–9.99	0.210	2.02	0.74–5.52	0.170	1.84	0.47–7.12	0.380
3-month	5/17(29.4)	25/165(15.2)	0.164	6/13(46.2%)	45/165(27.3)	0.045	2.33	0.76–7.20	0.141	1.85	0.36–9.68	0.465	3.00	1.09–8.25	0.033	2.75	0.66–11.47	0.164
6-month	6/15(40.0)	27/160(16.9)	0.040	7/13(53.8)	41/165(24.8)	0.045	3.28	1.08–9.99	0.036	3.68	0.64–21.18	0.144	4.32	1.55–12.08	0.005	6.22	1.08–35.70	0.040
12-month	7/17(41.2)	26/165(15.8)	0.017	8/13(61.5)	39/165(23.6)	0.006	3.74	1.31–10.72	0.014	3.55	0.70–17.91	0.125	5.92	2.06–17.06	0.001	12.54	1.88–83.71	0.009

Covariates after adjusting for ADL: age, gender, admission type, type of surgery, hearing impairment, polypharmacy, MMSE scores, GDS-15 scores, BMI, risk of malnutrition, CCI scores, pain VAS scores, ASA physical status, length of hospital stay, baseline IADL scores.
Covariates after adjusting for IADL: age, gender, admission type, type of surgery, hearing impairment, polypharmacy, MMSE scores, GDS-15 scores, BMI, risk of malnutrition, CCI scores, pain VAS scores, ASA physical status, length of hospital stay, baseline ADL scores.

Table 4. Comparing the ADL and IADL scores at baseline and 1, 3, 6, and 12 months of follow-up in groups divided on the basis of cognitive problems.

	Time of follow-up (months)								
	Non-adjusted functional status (mean ± SE)					Adjusted baseline functional status by ANCOVA (mean ± SE)			
Outcomes variables	Baseline	1	3	6	12	1	3	6	12
ADL (BI) scores (mean ± SE) [a,b]									
Non-cognitive problems (A), N = 109	$97.2\pm0.71^{\$,*}$	$94.2\pm1.10^{*}$	$95.8\pm1.05^{*}$	$96.3\pm1.00^{*}$	$96.8\pm0.89^{*}$	$93.0\pm1.10^{*}$	$94.5\pm1.08^{*}$	$95.0\pm1.19^{*}$	$95.6\pm1.24^{*}$
Cognitive impairment alone (B), N = 56	$92.4\pm1.85^{\$}$	$91.3\pm1.68^{\#}$	$93.2\pm1.62^{\#}$	$92.9\pm2.19^{\#}$	$93.4\pm2.32^{\#}$	$92.6\pm1.53^{\#}$	$94.6\pm1.51^{\#}$	$94.4\pm1.66^{\#}$	$94.8\pm1.72^{\#}$
Delirium superimposed on cognitive impairment (C), N = 13	$87.3\pm5.36^{*}$	$77.7\pm6.01^{*,\#}$	$78.5\pm6.76^{*,\#}$	$79.6\pm6.83^{*,\#}$	$79.2\pm7.42^{*,\#}$	$81.8\pm3.21^{*,\#}$	$82.7\pm3.16^{*,\#}$	$84.2\pm3.47^{*,\#}$	$83.3\pm3.61^{*,\#}$
IADL scores (mean ± SE) [a,b]									
Non-cognitive problems (A), N = 109	$6.1\pm0.09^{*,\$}$	$5.7\pm0.12^{*,\$}$	$5.8\pm0.13^{*,\$}$	$5.9\pm0.14^{*,\$}$	$6.0\pm0.14^{*,\$}$	$5.4\pm0.11^{*}$	$5.5\pm0.11^{*}$	$5.6\pm0.13^{*}$	$5.7\pm0.13^{*}$
Cognitive impairment alone (B), N = 56	$5.3\pm0.20^{\#,\$}$	$4.7\pm0.20^{\#,\$}$	$5.0\pm0.21^{\#,\$}$	$5.0\pm0.22^{\#,\$}$	$5.1\pm0.22^{\#,\$}$	$5.0\pm0.15^{\#}$	$5.4\pm0.15^{\#}$	$5.3\pm0.18^{*}$	$5.4\pm0.18^{\#}$
Delirium superimposed on cognitive impairment (C), N = 13	$4.3\pm0.47^{*,\#}$	$3.3\pm0.49^{*,\#}$	$3.2\pm0.51^{*,\#}$	$3.1\pm0.60^{*,\#}$	$2.7\pm0.58^{*,\#}$	$4.4\pm0.32^{*,\#}$	$4.4\pm0.32^{*,\#}$	$4.2\pm0.38^{*,\#}$	$3.7\pm0.38^{*,\#}$

$^{*}p<0.05$ for comparing C and A; $^{\#}p<0.05$ for comparing C and B; $^{\$}p<0.05$ for comparing A and B.

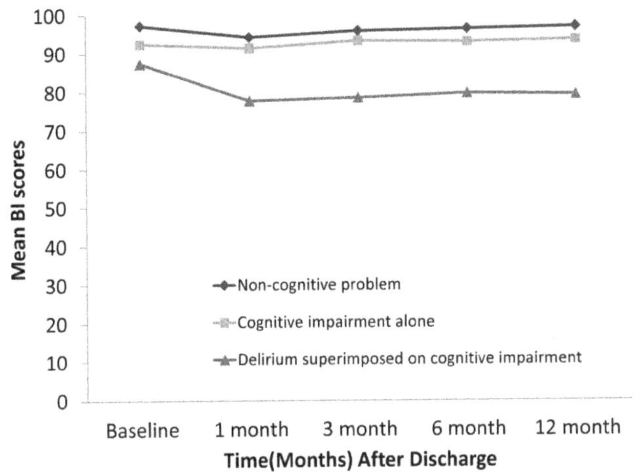

Figure 2. The trend of Barthel Index scores (ADL) (a) and IADL (b) for three groups corresponding to non-cognitive problem, cognitive impairment alone, and delirium superimposed on cognitive impairment.

cognitive dysfunction only (group B; Table 4). In terms of the decline in ADL and IADL scores at 1, 3, 6, and 12 months of follow up, ANCOVA (after adjustment for baseline ADL and IADL values) found significant ADL and IADL decline only in group C (Figure 2). After controlling for confounders (Table 5), multivariable logistic regression still showed the tendency for ADL and IADL to decline in patients in group C at 6 and 12 months (Adjusted RR for ADL at 6 months: 12.80, 95% CI: 1.65–99.40; Adjusted RR for ADL at 12 months: 7.96, 95% CI: 1.35–46.99; Adjusted RR for IADL at 6 months: 13.68, 95% CI: 1.94–96.55; Adjusted RR for IADL at 12 months: 30.61, 95% CI: 2.94–318.54).

Discussion

This prospective study investigated the effects of postoperative delirium on functional status (defined as decline in ADL and IADL scores) in patients who underwent orthopaedic surgery, and examined the interrelationship between underlying cognitive impairment and post-operative delirium. Postoperative delirium was an important predictor for poor IADL but not for poor ADL results. Moreover, delirium superimposed on cognitive problems was a stronger predictor of poor post-discharge functional status than cognitive impairment alone. The risk factors for the development of postoperative delirium identified in this study were in agreement with those identified by previous studies [6–10]. However, the incidence of postoperative delirium was lower in the present study than in previous studies, and the difference might be attributed to the higher percentage of elective surgery patients in our study (elective vs emergency surgery: 87.9% vs 12.1%). Moreover, patients in critical condition and unable to give their informed consent, such as some demented patients, were excluded from our study, thereby reducing the incidence of postoperative delirium.

Postoperative delirium had a strong adverse impact on IADL score after controlling for common geriatric problems, comorbidity, polypharmacy, and surgery-related conditions. A previous study reported that delirium had no significant effect on ADL score 6 months after surgery and attributed the relationship between delirium and mortality to some significant underlying medical problems [36]. An association between postoperative

Table 5. Multivariable logistic regression analysis of the predicted effect on functional status at the 6 and 12-month follow-up in groups divided on the basis of cognitive problems.

	ADL decline								IADL decline							
	at 6 months				at 12 months				at 6 months				at 12 months			
	Unadjusted		Adjusted		Unadjusted		Adjusted		Unadjusted		Adjusted		Unadjusted		Adjusted	
Independent variables	RR	95% CI	RR	95% CI	RR	95% CI	RR	95% CI	RR	95% CI	RR	95% CI	RR	95% CI	RR	95% CI
Cognitive impairment only (B) vs non-cognitive problem (A)	1.44	0.62–3.36	1.50	0.52–4.39	1.04	0.43–2.50	0.99	0.32–3.06	1.54	0.73–3.20	1.95	0.79–4.78	1.5	0.71–3.14	1.88	0.76–4.66
Delirium superimposed on cognitive impairment (C) vs non-cognitive problem (A)	6.75&	1.84–24.78	12.80*	1.65–99.40	6.31&	1.89–21.11	7.96*	1.35–46.99	4.13*	1.27–13.46	13.68&	1.94–96.55	5.98&	1.79–20.03	30.61&	2.94–318.54

*p<0.05, &p<0.01.
Covariates after adjusting for ADL: age, gender, admission type, type of surgery, hearing impairment, polypharmacy, GDS-15 scores, BMI, risk of malnutrition, CCI scores, pain VAS scores, ASA physical status, length of hospital stay, baseline IADL scores.
Covariates after adjusting for IADL: age, gender, admission type, type of surgery, hearing impairment, polypharmacy, GDS-15 scores, BMI, risk of malnutrition, CCI scores, pain VAS scores, ASA physical status, length of hospital stay, baseline ADL scores.

delirium and change in functional status at the time of hospital discharge and/or during follow up has also been shown in past studies [37–39]. However, the focus of most of these studies is short-term functional status. Although Vida et al. reported that delirium had an adverse effect on long-term IADL functional status 18 months after hospitalization, the effect disappeared after controlling for confounders [40]. In contrast to our results showing a relationship of postoperative delirium to IADL functional decline, those of Edelstein et al. demonstrated that decline in basic ADL but not IADL at 1-year follow-up was more likely in hip fracture surgery patients with postoperative delirium [41]. All the patients in the study by Edelstein et al. underwent hip fracture surgery, which has a greater impact on postoperative delirium and functional status than elective orthopaedic surgery. Furthermore, our study placed more emphasis on geriatric problems as confounders, e.g., malnutrition, polypharmacy, mood status, and symptoms of pain, which impact the risk of postoperative delirium as well as postoperative function. To the best of our knowledge, this is the first study to demonstrate the adverse impact of postoperative delirium on post-discharge ADL and IADL functional status after controlling for most geriatric problems considered as potential confounders. The adverse impact of postoperative delirium in this study was more profound on the IADL than ADL score. The baseline ADL scores for patients developing postoperative delirium and not developing postoperative delirium (85.9±4.81 and 95.6±0.80, respectively) indicated only mild impairment. It implied that the adverse effect of postoperative delirium might be reduced in robust elderly patients. Moreover, the predictive effect of delirium on IADL functional status was only noted 6 and 12 months after surgery. Therefore, factors other than delirium might have a greater effect on short-term functional status of elderly patients undergoing orthopaedic surgery.

Although delirium alone is not predictive for ADL decline during follow-up (after adjusting for confounders such as MMSE), delirium superimposed on cognitive impairment was significantly associated with ADL and IADL decline after surgery. In addition, postoperative delirium was more likely to develop in patients with severe cognitive impairment than in patients with moderate cognitive impairment (mean MMSE scores: group A 26.7±1.8 vs group B 19.8±3.8 vs group C 16.0±4.2). Underlying cognitive impairment (MMSE score <24) alone was not associated with postoperative ADL and IADL decline. The effects of severe cognitive impairment and postoperative delirium were highly interactive. Recovery from postoperative functional impairment by elderly patients undergoing orthopaedic surgery was dependent on the cognitive ability to adhere to rehabilitation programs. Givens et al. reported that each additional cognitive or mood disorder was associated with a greater risk of poor functional status [42]. Therefore, the results of this current study not only confirm the need to identify patients at risk for postoperative delirium, but also the highly interactive nature of the effects of baseline cognitive impairment and superimposed delirium on both ADL and IADL decline.

Despite the effort put into it, this study has several limitations. First, 21.6% (50/232) of the study subjects did not complete follow-up interviews. It has been reported that patients who experience delirium are more likely to miss follow-up appointments [43]. Although the incidence of delirium and the demographic data were similar between patients who completed follow-up and those who did not, there may still be a high risk of systematic attrition bias. Followed-up patients may have poorer clinical outcomes, therefore, the impact of delirium on long-term functional status may be underestimated in these patients. Second, the incidence of postoperative delirium was lower in our study than in previously published studies. Though delirium in this study was detected by the CAM and confirmed by a senior psychiatrist, who avoided overestimation, underestimation was still possible because we excluded patients who were admitted or transferred to ICU or unable to give informed consent, e.g., demented patients. Third, although the baseline cognitive function (assessed on admission before orthopaedic surgery) may be influenced by fracture or pain and lead to overestimation of cognitive impairment, it was not a predictor of ADL and IADL decline in our studies. Fourth, use of a wide range of procedures (performed within a single anatomic region) will impact both the risk of delirium as well as postoperative functional status. Because there were few patients undergoing operations, such as spinal decompression only, other elective knee surgery, and revision hip surgery, we treated similar types of surgery as single covariates, grouping them into four categories (elective spine surgery, elective knee surgery, elective hip arthroplasty, and ORIF/arthroplasty for hip fracture). Further work is needed to investigate the link between postoperative delirium and functional status in patients undergoing orthopaedic surgery at single operative site.

In conclusion, this prospective study evaluated the impact of different cognitive factors on ADL and IADL decline in elderly people undergoing orthopaedic surgery, and it was noted that delirium superimposed on cognitive impairment strongly affects both long-term ADL and IADL functional status. Early identification of patients with baseline cognitive impairment and implementation of strategies to prevent delirium may reduce the likelihood of functional decline following orthopaedic surgery in older patients. Further study is needed to confirm this.

Acknowledgments

Our local Institutional Review Board approved the present study protocol. The study was supported by the Veteran Affairs Commission of Taiwan. All authors declare no conflicts of interest.

The authors would like to thank all staff in the Orthopaedic Department for their valuable assistance in collecting the delirium symptom data. We also wish to thank Mr. Zhao-Rong Li, Associate Professor, Department of Business Management, National Kaohsiung Normal University, for his statistical assistance.

Author Contributions

Conceived and designed the experiments: CKL CLC YTL LKC. Performed the experiments: CKL CLC MYC TL CJH. Analyzed the data: CKL CLC LKC. Contributed reagents/materials/analysis tools: CLC MYC TL CJH. Wrote the paper: CKL YTL LKC.

References

1. Inouye SK (2006) Delirium in older persons. N Engl J Med 354: 1157–1165.
2. Élie M, Rousseau F, Cole M, Primeau F, McCusker J, et al. (2000) Prevalence and detection of delirium in elderly emergency department patients. CMAJ 163(8): 977–981.
3. Inouye SK, Foreman MD, Mion LC, Katz KH, Cooney LM Jr (2001) Nurses' recognition of delirium and its symptoms: comparison of nurse and researcher ratings. Arch Intern Med 161(20): 2467–2473.
4. Rudolph JL, Marcantonio ER (2011) Review articles: postoperative delirium: acute change with long-term implications. Anesth Analg 112: 1202–1211.
5. Gustafson Y, Berggren D, Brännström B, Bucht G, Norberg A, et al. (1988) Acute confusional states in elderly patients treated for femoral neck fracture. J Am Geriatr Soc 36: 525–530.
6. Schor JD, Levkoff SE, Lipsitz LA, Reilly CH, Cleary PD, et al. (1992) Risk factors for delirium in hospitalized elderly. JAMA 267: 827–831.

7. Levkoff SE, Evans DA, Liptzin B, Cleary PD, Lipsitz LA, et al. (1992) Delirium. The occurrence and persistence of symptoms among elderly hospitalized patients. Arch Intern Med 152: 334–340.
8. Wu CH, Chang CI, Chen CY (2012) Overview of studies related to geriatric syndrome in Taiwan. J Clin Gerontol Geriatr 3: 14–20.
9. Pompei P, Foreman M, Rudberg MA, Inouye SK, Braund V, et al. (1994) Delirium in hospitalized older persons: outcomes and predictors. J Am Geriatr Soc 42: 809–815.
10. Sanders RD, Pandharipande PP, Davidson AJ, Ma D, Maze M (2011) Anticipating and managing postoperative delirium and cognitive decline in adults. BMJ 343: d4331.
11. Chu CL, Liang CK, Lin YT, Chow PC, Pan CC, et al. (2011) Biomarkers of delirium: Well evidenced or not? J Clin Gerontol Geriatr 2: 100–104.
12. Inouye SK, Bogardus ST Jr, Charpentier PA, Leo-Summers L, Acampora D, et al. (1999) A multicomponent intervention to prevent delirium in hospitalized older patients. N Engl J Med 340: 669–676.
13. Marcantonio ER, Flacker JM, Wright RJ, Resnick NM (2001) Reducing delirium after hip fracture: a randomized trial. J Am Geriatr Soc 49: 516–522.
14. Rudolph JL, Jones RN, Rasmussen LS, Silverstein JH, Inouye SK, et al. (2007) Independent vascular and cognitive risk factors for postoperative delirium. Am J Med 120: 807–813.
15. Norkiene I, Ringaitiene D, Misiuriene I, Samalavicius R, Bubulis R, et al. (2007) Incidence and precipitating factors of delirium after coronary artery bypass grafting. Scand Cardiovasc J 41: 180–185.
16. Marcantonio ER, Flacker JM, Michaels M, Resnick NM (2000) Delirium is independently associated with poor functional recovery after hip fracture. J Am Geriatr Soc 48: 618–624.
17. Robinson TN, Raeburn CD, Tran ZV, Angles EM, Brenner LA, et al. (2009) Postoperative delirium in the elderly: risk factors and outcomes. Ann Surg 249: 173–178.
18. Koster S, Hensens AG, van der Palen J (2009) The long-term cognitive and functional outcomes of postoperative delirium after cardiac surgery. Ann Thorac Surg 87: 1469–1474.
19. Gottesman RF, Grega MA, Bailey MM, Pham LD, Zeger SL, et al. (2010) Delirium after coronary artery bypass graft surgery and late mortality. Ann Neurol 67: 338–344.
20. Lundstrom M, Edlund A, Bucht G, Karlsson S, Gustafson Y (2003) Dementia after delirium in patients with femoral neck fractures. J Am Geriatr Soc 51: 1002–1006.
21. Witlox J, Eurelings LS, de Jonghe JF, Kalisvaart KJ, Eikelenboom P, et al. (2010) Delirium in elderly patients and the risk of postdischarge mortality, institutionalization, and dementia: a meta-analysis. JAMA 304: 443–451.
22. Fick DM, Steis MR, Waller JL, Inouye SK (2013) Delirium superimposed on dementia is associated with prolonged length of stay and poor outcomes in hospitalized older adults. J Hosp Med 8: 500–505.
23. Steiner JF, Kramer AM, Eilertsen TB Kowalsky JC (1997) Development and validation of a clinical prediction rule for prolonged nursing home residence after hip fracture. J Am Geriatr Soc 45: 1510–1514.
24. Holmes J, House A (2000) Psychiatric illness predicts poor outcome after surgery for hip fracture: A prospective cohort study. Psychol Med 30: 921–929.
25. Francis J, Kapoor WN (1992) Prognosis after hospital discharge of older medical patients with delirium. J Am Geriatr Soc 40: 601–606.
26. Koponen H, Stenbäck U, Mattila E, Soininen H, Reinikainen K, et al. (1989) Delirium among elderly persons admitted to a psychiatric hospital: clinical course during the acute stage and one-year follow-up. Acta Psychiatr Scand 79: 579–585.
27. Liao YC, Yeh TL, Ko HC, Luoh CM, Lu HF (1995) Geriatric depression scale (GDS) – a preliminary report of reliability and validity for Chinese version. Changhua Med J 1; 11–17. (in Chinese)
28. Nyunt MS, Fones C, Niti M, Ng TP (2009) Criterion-based validity and reliability of the Geriatric Depression Screening Scale (GDS-15) in a large validation sample of community-living Asian older adults. Aging Ment Health 13: 376–382.
29. Kaiser MJ, Bauer JM, Ramsch C, Uter W, Guigoz Y, et al. (2009) Validation of the Mini Nutritional Assessment Short-Form (MNA-SF): a practical tool for identification of nutritional status. J Nutr Health Aging 13: 782–788.
30. Charlson ME, Pompei P, Ales KL, MacKenzie CR (1987) A new method of classifying prognostic comorbidity in longitudinal studies: development and validation. J Chronic Dis 40: 373–383.
31. Huskisson EC (1974) Measurement of pain. Lancet 2(7889): 1127–1131.
32. Folstein MF, Folstein SE, McHugh PR (1975) Mini-mental status: a practical method for grading the cognitive state of patients for the clinical use. J Psychiatr Res 12: 189–198.
33. Collin C, Wade DT, Davies S, Horne V (1988) "The Barthel ADL Index: a reliability study." Int Disability Study 10: 61–63.
34. Lawton MP, Brody EM (1969) Assessment of older people: Self-maintaining and instrumental activities of daily living. The Gerontologist 9: 179–186.
35. Inouye SK, Van Dyck CH, Alessi CA, Balkin S, Siegal AP, et al. (1990) Clarifying confusion: the confusion assessment method. A new method for detection of delirium. Ann Intern Med 113: 941–948.
36. Francis J, Kapoor WN (1990) Delirium in hospitalized elderly. J Gen Intern Med 5: 65–79.
37. Inouye SK, Rushing JT, Foreman MD, Palmer RM, Pompei P (1998) Does delirium contribute to poor hospital outcomes? A three-site epidemiologic study. J Gen Intern Med 13: 234–242.
38. Marcantonio ER, Flacker JM, Michaels M, Resnick NM (2000) Delirium is independently associated with poor functional recovery after hip fracture. J Am Geriatr Soc 48: 618–624.
39. Quinlan N, Rudolph JL (2011) Postoperative delirium and functional decline after noncardiac surgery. J Am Geriatr Soc 59 Suppl 2: S301–304.
40. Vida S, Galbaud du Fort G, Kakuma R, Arsenault L, Platt RW, et al. (2006) An 18-month prospective cohort study of functional outcome of delirium in elderly patients: activities of daily living. Int Psychogeriatr 18: 681–700.
41. Edelstein DM, Aharonoff GB, Karp A, Capla EL, Zuckerman JD, et al. (2004) Effect of postoperative delirium on outcome after hip fracture. Clin Orthop Relat Res (422): 195–200.
42. Givens JL, Sanft TB, Marcantonio ER (2008) Functional recovery after hip fracture: the combined effects of depressive symptoms, cognitive impairment, and delirium. J Am Geriatr Soc 56: 1075–1079.
43. Rudolph JL, Marcantonio ER, Culley DJ, Silverstein JH, Rasmussen LS, et al. (2008) Delirium is associated with early postoperative cognitive dysfunction. Anaesthesia 63: 941–947.

17

Influence of Municipality-Level Mean Income on Access to Aortic Valve Surgery: A Cross-Sectional Observational Study under Japan's Universal Health-Care Coverage

Seitetsu L. Lee[1], Hideki Hashimoto[2*], Takahide Kohro[7], Hiromasa Horiguchi[6], Daisuke Koide[4], Issei Komuro[1], Kiyohide Fushimi[8], Tsutomu Yamazaki[3], Hideo Yasunaga[5]

1 Department of Cardiovascular Medicine, The University of Tokyo, Tokyo, Japan, **2** Department of Health and Social Behavior, The University of Tokyo, Tokyo, Japan, **3** Clinical Research Support Center, The University of Tokyo, Tokyo, Japan, **4** Department of Clinical Epidemiology and Systems, The University of Tokyo, Tokyo, Japan, **5** Department of Clinical Epidemiology and Health Economics, The University of Tokyo, Tokyo, Japan, **6** Department of Clinical Data Management and Research, Clinical Research Center, National Hospital Organization Headquarters, Tokyo, Japan, **7** Department of Clinical Informatics, Jichi Medical University, Tochigi, Japan, **8** Department of Health Policy and Informatics, Tokyo Medical and Dental University, Tokyo, Japan

Abstract

Background: Universal health-care coverage has attracted the interest of policy makers as a way of achieving health equity. However, previous reports have shown that despite universal coverage, socioeconomic disparity persists in access to high-tech invasive care, such as cardiac treatment. In this study, we aimed to investigate the association between socioeconomic status and care of aortic stenosis in the context of Japan's health-care system, which is mainly publicly funded.

Methods: We chose aortic stenosis in older people as a target because such patients are likely to be affected by socioeconomic disparity. Using a large Japanese claim-based inpatient database, we identified 12,893 isolated aortic stenosis patients aged over 65 years who were hospitalized between July 2010 and March 2012. Municipality socioeconomic status was represented by the mean household income of the patients' residential municipality, categorized into quartiles. The likelihood of undergoing aortic valve surgery and in-hospital mortality was regressed against socioeconomic status level with adjustments for hospital volume, regional number of cardiac surgeons per 1 million population, and patients' clinical status.

Results: We found no significant differences between the highest and lowest quartile groups in surgical indication (odds ratio, 0.84; 95% confidence interval, 0.69–1.03) or in-hospital mortality (1.00; 0.68–1.48). Hospital volume was significantly associated with lower postoperative mortality (odds ratio of the highest volume tertile to the lowest, 0.49; 0.34–0.71).

Conclusions: Under Japan's current universal health-care coverage, municipality socioeconomic status did not appear to have a systematic relationship with either treatment decision for surgical intervention or postoperative survival following aortic valve surgery among older patients. Our results imply that universal health-care coverage with high publicly funded coverage offers equal access to high-tech cardiovascular care.

Editor: Toshiyuki Ojima, Hamamatsu University School of Medicine, Japan

Funding: This study is supported by a Grant-in-Aid for Research on Policy Planning and Evaluation (H22-Policy-031 and, in part, H22-Policy-033) from the Ministry of Health, Labour and Welfare, Japan; by a Grant-in-Aid for Scientific Research B (No. 22390131) from the Ministry of Education, Culture, Sports, Science and Technology, Japan; and by the Funding Program for World-Leading Innovative R&D on Science and Technology (FIRST program) from the Council for Science and Technology Policy, Japan (No. 0301002001001). The funders had no role in study design, data collection and analysis, decision to publish, or preparation of the manuscript.

Competing Interests: The authors have declared that no competing interests exist.

* Email: hidehashimoto-circ@umin.ac.jp

Introduction

Equal access to health care is a major policy concern for achieving health equity in different countries. Universal health coverage (UHC) by means of public funding has been used as a solution. The Medicare program in the United Sates offers near UHC for patients aged 65 years and above. Studies in that country have shown the health benefits and effectiveness in closing the gap across socioeconomic conditions through public health insurance coverage [1,2]. However, investigations in Canada [3,4], Australia [5], and Taiwan [6], where UHC has been in effect for decades, have indicated a persisting access gap to high-quality medical care, such as cardiac interventions, which suggests the need for further action to achieve access equity under UHC.

The "World Health Report 2010" of the World Health Organization [7] proposed that to achieve equal access to health care, UHC needs to strike a balance in the proportion of the population covered, the range of available services, and the proportion of direct costs covered by public funding. The three countries mentioned above provide universal coverage in terms of population and service coverage. However, according to the latest health statistics from the Organisation for Economic Co-operation and Development (OECD) and other data sources, the proportion of health-care spending covered by public funding in those places was lower (Canada, 66.4% in 2010 [8]; Australia, 64.4% in 2010 [8]; Taiwan, 53% in 2005 [9]) than in other OECD countries, such as Japan (81.4%) [8]. Given this background, we hypothesized that high coverage by public funding would make a difference in the level of equal access to high-tech invasive care under a UHC scheme.

To examine this issue, we chose to study surgical treatment for aortic stenosis (AS) among an older population. We did so for several reasons. First, older people are more financially vulnerable owing to limited income sources, and their income gap is greater than that among young people [9]. Second, cardiovascular diseases are the leading cause of death globally. An estimated 17.3 million people died through cardiovascular diseases in 2008, representing 30% of all global deaths, according to a report by the World Health Organization [10]. Moreover, AS is a prevalent cardiac condition among older people, and its impact among cardiovascular diseases has increased owing to the growth of Japan's aged population. A study in the United Kingdom reported that aortic valve surgery has increased remarkably in volume owing to the marked rise in the number of older patients suffering from AS [11]. In Japan, where the total population is 127.1 million (10th largest in the world), people aged 65 and above account for over 23% of that population, and the volume of aortic valve surgery exceeds that of coronary artery bypass graft surgery [12]. Third, treatment for AS mostly has an elective status, which makes the treatment decision more discretionary than with emergency conditions, such as acute coronary syndrome [5]. Thus, if an access gap exists, it is likely that surgical treatment for AS among older people will reveal it. We aimed to investigate whether Japan's health-care strategy is associated with smaller access gap for cardiac intervention in an older population.

Materials and Methods

Data Source and Patient Inclusion

We used a large claim-bill-based database called the Diagnosis Procedure Combination Database [13] to identify patients aged 65 years old and over who were hospitalized for AS between July 2010 and March 2012. The DPC is a Japanese case-mix classification system linked to a per diem inclusive payment scheme for acute-care hospitals under the national health insurance scheme. The database contains administrative claims and discharge data, which are collected with a standardized electronic format nationwide by the Ministry of Health Labour and Welfare for reimbursement purposes. All 82 university teaching hospitals are obliged to adopt the DPC system, but adoption by community hospitals is voluntary. In 2012, the database included all 82 academic hospitals in Japan and about 1,000 voluntarily participating community hospitals, which covered about 50% of acute-care beds in the country.

The data included a unique identifier of hospitals, patients' residential zip code, comorbidity diagnoses on admission coded using the International Classification of Diseases, Tenth Revision (ICD10) codes, surgical procedures coded using the Japanese claims classification (K-code), and clinical data, such as the New York Heart Association (NYHA) functional classification, smoking index, and body mass index. We identified patients with AS (ICD10 code I350) and AS and regurgitation (I352).

Municipality Socioeconomic Status

We used municipality-level socioeconomic status (SES) as a marker of socioeconomic inequality. Following previous studies using a US nationwide representative sample of inpatients [14–19], municipality SES was assessed by mean household income in the municipality in which the patient lived. Mean municipal household income was estimated as the total municipal household income divided by the number of households, which was derived from the "Statistical Observations of Municipalities (*Shi*, *Ku*, *Machi*, and *Mura*) 2012" [20], published by the Statistics Bureau, Ministry of Internal Affairs and Communications, Japan. We investigated 1,894 municipalities; the median population of the municipalities was 30,644 people (interquartile range, 9,847–83,167), and the median number of households in each municipality was 10,993 (interquartile range, 3,614–31,569). We adjusted the estimated mean municipality-level income for regional consumer price calibrators to enable a cross-regional comparison. Finally, the estimated mean income was categorized into quartiles for further analysis. The first, second, third, and fourth quartiles of income (mean household income adjusted for regional price index) were ≤2,799.5, 2,799.6–3,253.2, 3,253.3–3,719.1, and ≥3,719.2 (1,000 yen), respectively.

Study Variables and Outcomes

We obtained data on the patients' demographic and clinical status: age (divided into 65–74 years and ≥75 years old); gender; body mass index (measured on admission, categorized into <18.5, 18.5–29.9, and ≥30 kg/m^2); urgent admission status; pre-hospital dialysis; prior history of stroke; length of stay after surgery; type of surgery (valve repair, aortic valve replacement, replacement of more than two valves, combined surgery with Maze surgery, coronary artery bypass graft, or surgery of the thoracic aorta); and NYHA classification on admission. We defined hospital volume as the number of aortic valve surgery procedures performed during 2011 at each institution and divided the numbers into tertiles (1–35, 36–68, and 69 or more cases/year). We also calculated the number of cardiac surgeons per 1 million population in the municipality.

Statistical Analysis

We conducted descriptive analyses on variables by municipality SES quartiles. *p* values were calculated using the chi-square test for all variables except length of stay after surgery. The *p* value for length of stay after surgery was calculated using the Kruskal-Wallis test. For multivariable analysis, we fitted generalized estimating equation (GEE) models because the data involved observations clustered by hospital. We regressed the surgical indication (likelihood of undergoing aortic valve surgery) on SES with adjustment for age, gender, body mass index, urgent admission status, pre-hospital dialysis, prior history of stroke, NYHA classification on admission, hospital volume, and regional factor (the number of cardiac surgeons per 1 million population). We also regressed in-hospital mortality after surgery on municipality SES with adjustment for the same set of covariates as in the GEE model of surgical indication as well as length of stay after surgery and type of surgery. All statistical analyses were performed using IBM SPSS version 19.0 (IBM SPSS, Armonk, NY, USA).

Ethical concerns

Because of the anonymous nature of the data, the need for informed consent was waived by the Institutional Review Board at The University of Tokyo when the study was approved.

Results

We identified 12,893 older patients with isolated AS who were hospitalized in 393 hospitals between July 2010 and March 2012. Of these patients, 6,784 underwent valve surgery. Table 1 and 2, show the descriptive statistics by municipality SES quartiles. The patients in higher SES quartiles were more likely to be young, thin, smokers, on dialysis, admitted urgently to higher-volume hospitals, and have a diagnosis of lone stenosis (Table 1). The population in the higher SES quartiles was larger. The median population of each SES stratum was 1,812,575 (interquartile range, 1,362,820–5,485,952), 2,631,671 (interquartile range, 1,442,428–5,079,291), 2,855,045 (interquartile range, 2,000,010–7,207,139), and 7,416,336 (interquartile range, 5,581,968–9,058,094), respectively, for the first, second, third, and fourth quartiles of income. Through concerns over low-income patients living in big cities being misclassified as high SES, we also analyzed the database after excluding the five largest cities in Japan (Tokyo, Yokohama, Osaka, Nagoya, and Sapporo), which together account for about 15% of Japan's total population. However, the results of multivariable regression were the same. Surgical treatment was most frequently observed in the lowest municipality SES quartile (56.2%), followed by the highest (52.9%); it was least frequent among the second quartile group (Table 2).

Among surgical patients, as shown in Table 2, the type of combined surgery was not significantly different across municipality SES groups—except for Maze operations, which were most frequent in the highest SES group (8.9%). Aortic valve plasty was most frequently performed in the highest SES group, whereas lone aortic valve replacement was commonest in the lowest SES group. Crude in-hospital mortality was 4.1% in the lowest quartile, 4.3% in the second, 4.4% in the third, and 4.4% in the highest quartile ($p = 0.973$). Age-adjusted in-hospital mortality was 4.1, 4.3, 4.4, and 4.4%, respectively, for the first, second, third, and fourth quartiles of income.

Table 3 shows the results of multivariate logistic regression on surgical indication. The second- and third-lowest municipality SES groups were significantly less likely to undergo surgery than the lowest group. Otherwise, there were no significant disparities across municipality SES groups for surgical indication. Patients with severe NYHA scores, those on dialysis, and those admitted to higher-volume hospitals were more likely to receive surgery, whereas patients aged over 75, admitted urgently, and with low body mass index were less likely to undergo surgery.

Table 4 presents the results on postoperative in-hospital mortality. After adjusting for patient, hospital, and regional factors, municipality SES quartiles exhibited no statistically significant association with mortality. Patients who were older, female, with NYHA class IV, had a stroke history, and were undergoing dialysis had significantly higher mortality, whereas those admitted to high-volume hospitals showed significantly lower in-hospital mortality.

Table 1. Patient and institutional characteristics by municipality-level mean income strata (all patients).

		Municipality-level mean income (lowest to highest)				
n = 12,893		**1st**	**2nd**	**3rd**	**4th**	***p* value**
Patient characteristics						
Number of symptomatic AS patients		3,228	3,183	3,172	3,310	
Age	≥75	70.0%	70.2%	65.9%	66.1%	<0.001
Female		58.3%	60.7%	57.7%	58.5%	0.072
Smoker		31.0%	29.4%	32.5%	35.3%	<0.001
Prior history of stroke		3.0%	2.8%	2.6%	2.3%	0.249
Dialysis		13.0%	12.3%	14.7%	15.0%	0.003
Urgent admission		17.4%	20.4%	22.1%	20.8%	<0.001
Indication for hospitalization	ASR	15.1%	12.9%	11.9%	11.2%	<0.001
	AS	84.9%	87.1%	88.1%	88.8%	
Body mass index	18.5–29.9	85.1%	85.5%	84.4%	84.1%	0.002
	<18.5	10.2%	11.2%	11.7%	12.5%	
	≥30	4.7%	3.2%	3.9%	3.4%	
NYHA class	0–2	40.8%	39.9%	37.5%	39.5%	0.146
	3–4	20.1%	20.0%	20.5%	19.4%	
	data NA	39.1%	40.1%	42.0%	41.1%	
Institutional characteristics						
Hospital volume	1–35	41.8%	39.3%	37.5%	39.8%	<0.001
	36–68	33.5%	32.5%	32.7%	27.3%	
	≥69	24.8%	28.2%	29.9%	33.0%	
Number of patients undergoing surgery		1,814	1,569	1,651	1,750	<.001
(% to total patients)		56.2%	49.3%	52.0%	52.9%	

1st, 2nd, 3rd, and 4th quartiles of income (mean household income adjusted for regional price index): ≤2,799.5, 2,799.6–3,253.2, 3,253.3–3,719.1, ≥3,719.2 (1,000 yen); Hospital volume: the number of aortic valve surgery procedures performed during 2011 at each institution; p values were calculated using the chi-square test.
ASR, aortic stenosis and regurgitation; AS, aortic stenosis, BMI, body mass index; NYHA, New York Heart Association; NA, not available.

Table 2. Process and outcome of surgical patients by municipality-level mean income strata.

		Municipality-level mean income (lowest to highest)				
		1st	**2nd**	**3rd**	**4th**	***p* value**
Combined surgery	CABG	20.4%	22.2%	22.2%	22.4%	0.436
	TAA	1.2%	0.8%	1.0%	1.1%	0.722
	Maze	6.5%	6.9%	6.5%	8.9%	0.018
Type of surgery	Plasty	0.7%	1.0%	2.4%	5.3%	<0.001
	AVR	91.8%	93.7%	89.1%	85.6%	
	DVR	7.6%	5.4%	8.5%	9.1%	
Length of stay after surgery		29 [22–41]	28[22–41]	27[21–39]	26[19–37]	<0.001*
Postoperative in-hospital death		4.10%	4.30%	4.40%	4.40%	0.973

p values were calculated using the chi-square test and *Kruskal-Wallis test.1st, 2nd, 3rd, and 4th quartiles of income (mean household income adjusted for regional price index): ≤2,799.5, 2,799.6–3,253.2, 3,253.3–3,719.1, ≥3,719.2 (1,000 yen); Length of stay is expressed as mean values [interquartile range].
CABG, coronary artery bypass graft; TAA, thoracic aortic aneurysm; AVR, aortic valve replacement; DVR, dual valve replacement.

Discussion

Using a large claim-based database, our analysis did not detect any systematic disparity across municipality SES groups in the outcome of surgical treatment for older AS patients in Japan. However, the second- and third-lowest SES groups were significantly less likely to receive surgery than the lowest group. The trend was not linear but U-shaped. We have no good explanation for this trend.

Patients with AS have not previously been fully investigated with regard to the relationship between their SES and operative outcome. After controlling for the patient's clinical condition and hospital characteristics, a US study using a nationally representative sample [14] reported that municipality household income was linked to unequal postoperative survival following various surgical procedures. That investigation showed municipality-level income to be an independent factor of in-hospital death after aortic valve replacement. By contrast, numerous studies of patients with ischemic heart disease have identified a socioeconomic disparity in access to and clinical outcomes of cardiovascular interventions [3–6,17,21–23]. Unlike these studies', our results did not suggest socioeconomic disparity in surgical indication and subsequent outcome after aortic valve surgery among older AS patients following hospital referral. We conducted a similar analysis with respect to length of stay and cost per day but found no significant differences among the SES groups (data not shown, available from the authors on request). The results of that analysis lend further support to our finding that the indication decision, resource use, and surgical outcome for AS in older people under Japan's UHC coverage do not depend on the local socioeconomic conditions of a patient's residential area.

A possible explanation for our results may relate to the uniqueness of Japan's UHC: the proportion of public funding covering total health expenditure is high [8]. High coverage by public funding is mainly achieved in two ways. One is the reduced copayment for people aged over 75, which has been shown to have a positive health impact among older people [24]. The other is public subsidies to prevent catastrophic payment, whereby out-of-pocket payments that exceed a monthly limit according to annual household income levels are reimbursed [8]. TRICARE is a UHC in the United States with almost full governmental coverage for all active-duty and retired military service personnel as well as their dependents. Previous reports studying the population under TRICARE [25,26] have shown that even in the United States with a wide range of SES, UHC with high publicly funded coverage offered equal access to high-tech care. We suppose that this policy of keeping out-of-pocket payments affordable for a patient's household plays an important role in a patient choosing advanced care, such as cardiovascular interventions. However, there is still a lack of studies examining access to and quality of health care under systems that offer high public coverage. Further investigations are warranted especially in countries with UHC and high publicly funded coverage, such as Germany, Norway, and the Netherlands.

In terms of supply-side control, Japan's UHC is unusual in that its fees are uniform across the nation; this may reduce regional disparity in the allocation of facilities that perform cardiovascular interventions. Using a nationwide registry, Nakamura et al. [27] detailed how Japanese hospitals provide high-quality care for patients with acute myocardial ischemia either during regular hospital hours or after hours regardless of location. Their results support our argument that resources for and the outcome of cardiovascular interventions in Japan do not depend on the local socioeconomic conditions of a patient's residential area. The socioeconomic circumstances under Japan's UHC may enable equal resource use after hospital referral regardless of local SES.

In line with repeated findings in other studies, our analysis confirms the significant impact of hospital volume on the propensity for surgical intervention and in-hospital mortality [28,29]. Since admission to a high-volume hospital was significantly related to higher SES neighborhood, type of surgery, and better surgical outcome, we conducted an additional multivariate analysis that excluded hospital volume: we were concerned that hospital volume may have over-controlled the impact of municipality SES. However, this analysis simply confirmed our former findings. We also checked variance inflation factors for each variable, and all values were less than 2. Hence, we believe that our models were not seriously affected by multicollinearity. We speculate that the observed association between municipality SES and hospital volume may simply reflect the positive effect of treatment in an urban high-volume center.

Policy Implications

Our results suggest that the UHC may have contributed to equal access to and quality of cardiovascular surgery for AS patients in Japan. Small out-of-pocket payments that receive a high level of coverage by public funding may have enabled

Table 3. Multivariate model of GEE for the likelihood of undergoing valve surgery.

		Unadjusted OR	95% CI			Adjusted OR	95% CI		
Municipality-level mean income	4	0.87	0.70	-	1.09	0.84	0.69	-	1.03
	3	0.85	0.69	-	1.03	0.80	0.66	-	0.97
	2	0.76	0.63	-	0.91	0.72	0.60	-	0.86
	1	1				1			
Hospital volume	≥69	3.78	2.96	-	4.82	3.36	2.67	-	4.24
	36–68	3.39	2.81	-	4.08	3.24	2.68	-	3.91
	1–35	1				1			
Number of cardiac surgeons per 1 million population (per one increment)		0.98	0.89	-	1.08	0.97	0.93	-	1.01
Age	≥75	0.62	0.57	-	0.67	0.74	0.67	-	0.81
Female		0.82	0.77	-	0.88	1.02	0.94	-	1.11
Smoker		1.23	1.12	-	1.34	1.13	1.02	-	1.26
NYHA class	Data NA	1.05	0.91	-	1.21	1.17	1.01	-	1.35
	4	0.72	0.56	-	0.91	1.52	1.22	-	1.91
	3	1.38	1.11	-	1.72	1.88	1.54	-	2.29
	2	1.53	1.27	-	1.84	1.63	1.38	-	1.92
	0–1	1				1			
Prior history of stroke		0.95	0.74	-	1.23	1.09	0.85	-	1.39
Dialysis		1.36	1.21	-	1.53	1.38	1.2	-	1.57
Urgent admission		0.30	0.26	-	0.33	0.34	0.29	-	0.38
BMI	≥30	1.02	0.85	-	1.22	0.95	0.78	-	1.16
	<18.5	0.74	0.66	-	0.83	0.78	0.69	-	0.88
	18.5–29.9	1				1			

GEE, generalized estimating equation; Municipality-level mean income represents mean household income adjusted for regional price index. 1st 2nd, 3rd, and 4th quartiles of income: ≤2,799.5, 2,799.6–3,253.2, 3,253.3–3,719.1, ≥ 3,719.2 (1,000 yen); Hospital volume: the number of aortic valve surgery procedures performed during 2011 at each institution.
AS, aortic stenosis; BMI, body mass index; CI, confidence interval; NYHA: New York Heart Association; NA, not available; OR, odds ratio.

Table 4. Multivariate model of GEE for postoperative in-hospital death among surgical patients.

		Unadjusted OR	95% CI		Adjusted OR	95% CI	
Municipality-level mean income	4	1.07	0.76	- 1.49	1.01	0.68	- 1.49
	3	1.07	0.76	- 1.51	1.09	0.73	- 1.64
	2	1.03	0.74	- 1.45	1.15	0.77	- 1.71
	1	1			1		
Hospital volume	≥69	0.58	0.42	- 0.80	0.51	0.35	- 0.73
	36–68	0.66	0.49	- 0.87	0.66	0.47	- 0.92
	1–35	1			1		
Number of cardiac surgeons per one million population (per one increment)		1.05	0.93	- 1.18	1.02	0.89	- 1.17
Age	≥75	1.28	0.99	- 1.67	2.08	1.55	- 2.79
Female		0.88	0.69	- 1.12	1.44	1.02	- 2.03
Smoker		1.14	0.89	- 1.45	1.21	0.89	- 1.63
NYHA class	Data NA	1.99	1.30	- 3.04	1.77	1.11	- 2.81
	4	4.52	2.76	- 7.41	2.76	1.51	- 5.04
	3	1.88	1.16	- 3.03	1.47	0.85	- 2.52
	2	0.81	0.50	- 1.30	0.88	0.53	- 1.47
	0–1	1			1		
Prior history of stroke		1.94	1.11	- 3.37	2.17	1.14	- 4.13
Dialysis		22.06	16.22	- 30.0	23.12	16.34	- 32.7
Urgent admission		2.38	1.78	- 3.18	1.31	0.89	- 1.91
Length of stay after surgery (per one increment)		1.01	1.01	- 1.01	1.00	1.00	- 1.01
BMI	≥30	1.22	0.69	- 2.18	1.28	0.68	- 2.41
	<18.5	2	1.47	- 2.72	1.09	0.76	- 1.56
	18.5–29.9	1			1		
Combined surgery	CABG	1.53	1.18	- 1.98	1.26	0.93	- 1.70
	TAA	2.8	1.31	- 6.00	2.58	1.04	- 6.42
	Maze	1.18	0.75	- 1.86	1.01	0.60	- 1.71
Type of surgery	DVR	0.91	0.51	- 1.62	0.81	0.42	- 1.55
	AVR	0.43	0.26	- 0.69	0.43	0.24	- 0.79
	Plasty	1			1		

GEE, generalized estimating equation; Income represents mean household income adjusted for regional price index. 1st, 2nd, 3rd, and 4th quartiles of income: ≤2,799.5, 2,799.6–3,253.2, 3,253.3–3,719.1, ≥3,719.2 (1,000 yen);
Hospital volume: the number of aortic valve surgery procedures performed during 2011 at each institution;
OR, odds ratio; CI, confidence interval; AS, aortic stenosis; BMI, body mass index; NYHA, New York Heart Association; CABG, coronary artery bypass graft; TAA, thoracic aortic aneurysm; AVR, aortic valve replacement; DVR, dual valve replacement; NA, not available.

patients to undergo medically appropriate treatment regardless of their SES. Full reimbursement under the UHC and uniform fees across the nation may also reduce regional disparities in facilities that perform cardiovascular interventions. The socioeconomic circumstances achieved under Japan's UHC may have enabled equal resource use after hospital referral regardless of municipality SES. Recently, there has been discussion about the weakened financial sustainability of Japan's health-care system and the possible change to a more austere policy in the near future. We suggest that further monitoring will be necessary to examine how such policy changes could impact the relationship between SES and the outcome with high-tech cardiovascular care.

Strengths and Limitations of This Study

The key strength of our study is that we covered 98.6% of the patients who underwent isolated aortic valve surgery in 2011; we based this figure on the annual report of the Japanese Association for Thoracic Surgery [12]. However, several limitations should be acknowledged. First, we could not obtain information about individual SES, and the aggregated income data we used may have ignored regional income disparity; this could have led to an underestimation of the socioeconomic gradient of a surgical indication and outcome. Further, we established a regional composite SES index based on a previous study [30], which included unemployment rate, dwelling area per household, proportion of households receiving public assistance, percentage of persons with higher education, per capita income, percentage of owned houses, and percentage of aged single households. However, the tendency and results using the regional composite SES index were the same as those when we employed the municipality-level mean income. A review article [31] about SES and health in the Japanese population concluded that income and SES exhibited a significant relationship, and so we adopted municipality-level mean income as a proxy for municipality SES.

Second, the claims data we used in this analysis suffered from a lack of detailed clinical information and possible miscoding of diagnoses, which may have caused our null findings. Third, our model for surgical indication failed to exhibit good model fitness, which indicates that factors influencing the surgical indication may have been incorrectly specified in our model. However, our results are in accordance with a 7-year longitudinal nationwide report from the United States [32]; it showed that differences between ethnic groups in undergoing cardiovascular procedures narrowed markedly once a serious illness developed and there was adequate insurance coverage. Fourth, 30-day mortality would be more robust to confounding by length of stay for assessing postoperative mortality. However, we were unable to use 30-day mortality in our model owing to data limitations (median value of postoperative length of stay in surgical patients, 21 days; interquartile range, 16–30). Instead, we used length of stay after surgery as a covariate of the model. Finally, through lack of proper data, we were unable to consider the effects of SES on waiting time for elective surgery, timing of hospital referral, and mid-term outcome of patients: the DPC database included in-patient data only. Future investigation using a population based on registry data is warranted. Whether the mid-term outcome differs across socioeconomic groups requires further investigation.

Conclusions

Under the current Japanese health-care system, municipality SES did not appear to influence systematically either the treatment decision for surgical intervention or postoperative survival following aortic valve surgery. Our results imply that a UHC with high coverage by public funding allows equal access to high-tech care. According to the three-dimensional model of UHC, policy makers should carefully design their systems if they aim to achieve equity in health-care access within a population in light of underlying socioeconomic disparities.

Author Contributions

Conceived and designed the experiments: SLL H. Hashimoto HY. Analyzed the data: SLL H. Hashimoto HY. Contributed reagents/ materials/analysis tools: HY H. Horiguchi KF. Wrote the paper: SLL H. Hashimoto TK. Intellectual input and critical review/comments: DK IK TY HY.

References

1. Ayanian JZ, Weissman JS, Schneider EC, Ginsburg JA, Zaslavsky AM (2000) Unmet health needs of uninsured adults in the United States. JAMA 284: 2061–2069.
2. McWilliams JM, Meara E, Zaslavsky AM, Ayanian JZ (2009) Differences in control of cardiovascular disease and diabetes by race, ethnicity, and education: U.S. trends from 1999 to 2006 and effects of medicare coverage. Ann Intern Med 150: 505–515.
3. Pilote L, Joseph L, Belisle P, Penrod J (2003) Universal health insurance coverage does not eliminate inequities in access to cardiac procedures after acute myocardial infarction. Am Heart J 146: 1030–1037.
4. Pilote L, Tu JV, Humphries K, Behouli H, Belisle P, et al. (2007) Socioeconomic status, access to health care, and outcomes after acute myocardial infarction in Canada's universal health care system. Med Care 45: 638–646.
5. Korda RJ, Clements MS, Kelman CW (2009) Universal health care no guarantee of equity: comparison of socioeconomic inequalities in the receipt of coronary procedures in patients with acute myocardial infarction and angina. BMC Public Health 9: 460.
6. Wang JY, Wang CY, Juang SY, Huang KY, Chou P, et al. (2014) Low socioeconomic status increases short-term mortality of acute myocardial infarction despite universal health coverage. Int J Cardiol 172: 82–87.
7. World Health Organization (2010) World health report 2010, Health systems financing: the path to universal coverage Available: http://www.who.int/whr/2010/en/ Accessed 2014 May 27
8. Ikegami N, Yoo BK, Hashimoto H, Matsumoto M, Ogata H, et al. (2011) Japanese universal health coverage: evolution, achievements, and challenges. Lancet 378: 1106–1115.
9. Murata C, Yamada T, Chen CC, Ojima T, Hirai H, et al. (2010) Barriers to health care among the elderly in Japan. Int J Environ Res Public Health 7: 1330–1341.
10. World Health Organization (2013) Cardiovascular diseases Fact sheet No 317 Available: http://www.who.int/mediacentre/factsheets/fs317/en/
11. Dunning J, Gao H, Chambers J, Moat N, Murphy G, et al. (2011) Aortic valve surgery: marked increases in volume and significant decreases in mechanical valve use–an analysis of 41,227 patients over 5 years from the Society for Cardiothoracic Surgery in Great Britain and Ireland National database. J Thorac Cardiovasc Surg 142: 776–782 e773.
12. Amano J, Kuwano H, Yokomise H (2013) Thoracic and cardiovascular surgery in Japan during 2011: Annual report by The Japanese Association for Thoracic Surgery. Gen Thorac Cardiovasc Surg 61: 578–607.
13. Matsuda S IK, Kuwabara K, Fujimori K, Fushimi K, Hashimoto H (2009) Development and use of the Japanese case-mix system. Eurohealth 14: 25–29.
14. Bennett KM, Scarborough JE, Pappas TN, Kepler TB (2010) Patient socioeconomic status is an independent predictor of operative mortality. Ann Surg 252: 552–557; discussion 557–558.
15. Kelz RR, Gimotty PA, Polsky D, Norman S, Fraker D, et al. (2004) Morbidity and mortality of colorectal carcinoma surgery differs by insurance status. Cancer 101: 2187–2194.
16. Yeates K, Wiebe N, Gill J, Sima C, Schaubel D, et al. (2009) Similar outcomes among black and white renal allograft recipients. J Am Soc Nephrol 20: 172–179.
17. Alter DA, Naylor CD, Austin P, Tu JV (1999) Effects of socioeconomic status on access to invasive cardiac procedures and on mortality after acute myocardial infarction. N Engl J Med 341: 1359–1367.
18. Casale SN, Auster CJ, Wolf F, Pei Y, Devereux RB (2007) Ethnicity and socioeconomic status influence use of primary angioplasty in patients presenting with acute myocardial infarction. Am Heart J 154: 989–993.
19. van Walraven C, Wong J, Forster AJ (2013) Influence of neighborhood household income on early death or urgent hospital readmission. J Hosp Med 8: 261–266.

20. The Statistics Bureau, Ministry of Internal Affairs ans Communications, Japan (2012) Social Observations of Shi, Ku, Machi, Mura Available: http://www.stat.go.jp/english/data/sougou/index.htm and http://www.stat.go.jp/data/ssds/index.htm
21. Chaix B, Rosvall M, Merlo J (2007) Neighborhood socioeconomic deprivation and residential instability: effects on incidence of ischemic heart disease and survival after myocardial infarction. Epidemiology 18: 104–111.
22. Morrison C, Woodward M, Leslie W, Tunstall-Pedoe H (1997) Effect of socioeconomic group on incidence of, management of, and survival after myocardial infarction and coronary death: analysis of community coronary event register. BMJ 314: 541–546.
23. Winkleby M, Sundquist K, Cubbin C (2007) Inequities in CHD incidence and case fatality by neighborhood deprivation. Am J Prev Med 32: 97–106.
24. Nishi A, McWilliams JM, Noguchi H, Hashimoto H, Tamiya N, et al. (2012) Health benefits of reduced patient cost sharing in Japan. Bull World Health Organ 90: 426–435A.
25. Ambrosio A, Brigger MT (2014) Surgery for Otitis Media in a Universal Health Care Model: Socioeconomic Status and Race/Ethnicity Effects. Otolaryngol Head Neck Surg 151: 137–141.
26. Walker A, Hatch Q, Drake T, Nelson DW, Fitzpatrick E, et al. (2014) Predictors of appendiceal perforation in an equal access system. J Surg Res 190: 87–92.
27. Nakamura M, Yamagishi M, Ueno T, Hara K, Ishiwata S, et al. (2013) Current treatment of ST elevation acute myocardial infarction in Japan: door-to-balloon time and total ischemic time from the J-AMI registry. Cardiovasc Interv Ther 28: 30–36.
28. Committee for Scientific A, Kazui T, Osada H, Fujita H (2007) An attempt to analyze the relation between hospital surgical volume and clinical outcome. Gen Thorac Cardiovasc Surg 55: 483–492.
29. Sakata R, Kuwano H, Yokomise H (2012) Hospital volume and outcomes of cardiothoracic surgery in Japan: 2005–2009 national survey. Gen Thorac Cardiovasc Surg 60: 625–638.
30. Fukuda Y, Nakamura K, Takano T (2007) Higher mortality in areas of lower socioeconomic position measured by a single index of deprivation in Japan. Public Health 121: 163–173.
31. Kagamimori S, Gaina A, Nasermoaddeli A (2009) Socioeconomic status and health in the Japanese population. Soc Sci Med 68: 2152–2160.
32. Daumit GL, Hermann JA, Coresh J, Powe NR (1999) Use of cardiovascular procedures among black persons and white persons: a 7-year nationwide study in patients with renal disease. Ann Intern Med 130: 173–182.

18

Missed Opportunities for Early Access to Care of HIV-Infected Infants in Burkina Faso

Malik Coulibaly[1]*, Nicolas Meda[1,2], Caroline Yonaba[3], Sylvie Ouedraogo[4], Malika Congo[5], Mamoudou Barry[6], Elisabeth Thio[1], Issa Siribié[1], Fla Koueta[4], Diarra Ye[4], Ludovic Kam[3], Stéphane Blanche[7], Phillipe Van De Perre[8], Valériane Leroy[9], for the MONOD Study Group ANRS 12206¶

1 Projet MONOD ANRS 12206, Centre de Recherche Internationale pour la Santé, Site ANRS Burkina, Université de Ouagadougou, Ouagadougou, Burkina Faso, **2** Centre Muraz, Bobo Dioulasso, Burkina Faso, **3** Service de Pédiatrie, CHU Yalgado Ouédraogo, Ouagadougou, Burkina Faso, **4** Service de Pédiatrie Médicale, CHU Charles de Gaulle, Ouagadougou, Burkina Faso, **5** Laboratoire de Bactériologie - Virologie CHU Yalgado Ouédraogo, Ouagadougou, Burkina Faso, **6** Service de laboratoire, CHU Charles de Gaulle, Ouagadougou, Burkina Faso, **7** Groupe hospitalier Necker- Enfants malades, Paris, France, **8** Inserm U1058, Université Montpellier 1, Montpellier, France, **9** Inserm, U897, Institut de Santé Publique, Epidémiologie et Développement (ISPED), Université de Bordeaux, Bordeaux, France

Abstract

Objective: The World Health Organization (WHO) has recommended a universal antiretroviral therapy (ART) for all HIV-infected children before the age of two since 2010, but this implies an early identification of these infants. We described the Prevention of Mother-to-Child HIV Transmission (PMTCT) cascade, the staffing and the quality of infrastructures in pediatric HIV care facilities, in Ouagadougou, Burkina Faso.

Methods: We conducted a cross-sectional survey in 2011 in all health care facilities involved in PMTCT and pediatric HIV care in Ouagadougou. We assessed them according to their coverage in pediatric HIV care and WHO standards, through a desk review of medical registers and a semi-structured questionnaire administered to health-care workers (HCW).

Results: In 2011, there was no offer of care in primary health care facilities for HIV-infected children in Ouagadougou. Six district hospitals and two university hospitals provided pediatric HIV care. Among the 67 592 pregnant women attending antenatal clinics in 2011, 85.9% were tested for HIV. The prevalence of HIV was 1.8% (95% Confidence Interval: 1.7%–1.9%). Among the 1 064 HIV-infected pregnant women attending antenatal clinics, 41.4% received a mother-to-child HIV transmission prevention intervention. Among the HIV-exposed infants, 313 (29.4%) had an early infant HIV test, and 306 (97.8%) of these infants tested received their result within a four-month period. Among the 40 children initially tested HIV-infected, 33 (82.5%) were referred to a health care facility, 3 (9.0%) were false positive, and 27 (90.0%) were initiated on ART. Although health care facilities were adequately supplied with HIV drugs, they were hindered by operational challenges such as shortage of infrastructures, laboratory reagents, and trained HCW.

Conclusions: The PMTCT cascade revealed bottle necks in PMTCT intervention and HIV early infant diagnosis. The staffing in HIV care and quality of health care infrastructures were also insufficient in 2011 in Ouagadougou.

Editor: Julian W. Tang, Alberta Provincial Laboratory for Public Health/University of Alberta, Canada

Funding: The study was supported in part by the MONOD ANRS 12206 project granted by the European and Developing Countries Clinical Trial Partnership (EDCTP), the CRP-santé in Luxembourg and the French ANRS-Inserm. Dr. Malik Coulibaly is a fellow PhD candidate of the Doctoral School of Society, Politics and Public Health, Bordeaux, France funded by the MONOD consortium. The content of this publication is solely the responsibility of the authors and does not necessarily represent the official views of any of the institutions mentioned above. The funders had no role in study design, data collection and analysis, decision to publish, or preparation of the manuscript.

Competing Interests: The authors have declared that no competing interests exist.

* Email: coulmalik@yahoo.fr

¶ Membership of the MONOD Study Group ANRS 12206 is provided in Appendix S1.

Introduction

Despite the efficacy of Prevention of Mother-To-Child- HIV Transmission (PMTCT), Human Immunodeficiency Virus (HIV) pediatric infection still occurs in Africa because of the lack of operational access to this intervention. Without any intervention, mortality of HIV infected children can reach up to 35% before the first birthday and up to 52% before the second birthday [1,2], and the untreated survivors would need substantial care [3]. However early antiretroviral treatment routinely started before 12 weeks of age significantly increases infant survival by 76%, reduces morbidity and enhances immunological benefits [4,5,6,7]. The 2010 World Health Organization (WHO) revised guidelines recommend early antiretroviral treatment in all HIV infected children less than two years of age, regardless of their immune status [8]. These guidelines also recommend a routine Early Infant Diagnosis (EID) from six-weeks of age of all HIV-exposed children. EID requires sophisticated technology before 18 months of age because of the persistence of maternal antibodies in infants [9]. In addition, the uptake at each step in the EID cascade highlights that even with the highest reported level of uptake, nearly half of HIV-infected infants may not successfully complete the cumulative cascade [10]. In sub-Saharan Africa, HIV-exposed infants continue to suffer from insufficient access to EID and antiretroviral therapy. In 2010, a survey was conducted in Burkina Faso, Ghana and Côte d'Ivoire, to identify the major challenges regarding HIV prophylaxis for children in West Africa [11]. The results of this survey indicated that only a small proportion of HIV-exposed newborns received antiretroviral prophylaxis. Scaling-up management of early pediatric HIV infection remains challenging in West African countries in 2011. But there is a need to increase the PMTCT coverage and to trace the children born in the setting of the PMTCT programs [12]. It is crucial to identify the barriers at the national level. Burkina Faso is a West-African developing country where HIV prevalence was about 1.0% in 2010 [13]. HIV EID in children born to HIV-infected mothers is organized in cascade from the district health care facilities, towards district hospital laboratories, to the university hospital laboratories. There are few data on the full PMTCT cascade coverage and postnatal services in regard to infants born to HIV-infected mothers. Problems are related to resource management, and lack of assessment of sites.

We described the access to pediatric HIV diagnosis and care in Ouagadougou, the capital of Burkina Faso. We also assessed the health care facilities regarding the conformance of staff and infrastructures with WHO standards for the care of HIV infected infants in Ouagadougou in 2010–2011.

Methods

Access to HIV care for infants in Burkina Faso

Burkina Faso is administratively divided into 13 regions, 45 provinces and 351 rural and urban municipalities. In 2011, the public health system was organized around four types of hospitals: district, confessional, regional, and university hospitals. Besides the public health facilities, Burkina Faso had also a large number of private health care facilities and traditional healers [14].

The "big" Ouagadougou equated the Center region with a population of 2 136 582 inhabitants in 2011, of whom 39.7% were children less than 15 years of age [14]. The Center region was the most populous and urbanized of the 13 administrative regions of Burkina Faso, with a land area of 2 869 square kilometers [15]. We identified in this region two university hospitals, five district hospitals, one confessional hospital, eight hospitals without surgical units, and 81 primary health care facilities [16]. According to the 2010 health and demographic survey, the HIV prevalence in Ouagadougou was estimated at 2.1% (95% CI: 1.5–2.7) in 2010 [13].

PMTCT services are integrated in the national health system. All pregnant women who come for antenatal care in a health care facility are expected to be counseled for HIV testing. In case of consent, HIV screening is performed on-site using rapid HIV antibody tests, with a simultaneous HIV result delivery. The pregnant women who attend antenatal consultation with a documented positive result are also tested for the sake control, unless that they are already treated with antiretroviral drugs. In any case, there were included in the PMTCT cascade.

In Burkina Faso, the option A of PMTCT was still recommended in 2011 and HIV-infected pregnant women were eligible to antiretroviral treatment on the basis of CD4 count. Pregnant women with more than 350 cells/mm^3 CD4 count were prescribed zidovudine at 28 weeks gestation in antepartum. In intrapartum, at onset of labor, a single dose of nevirapine and the first dose of zidovudine/lamivudine were given. In postpartum, a daily zidovudine/lamivudine was given for seven days. Whenever the pregnant women's CD4 count was inferior or equal to 350 cells/mm^3 a triple antiretroviral therapy was started as soon as diagnosed, and continued for life. Infants received a daily nevirapine dose from birth up to one week after the complete cessation of breastfeeding. When mothers were not breastfeeding or were on antiretroviral drugs, infants were given *a* daily nevirapine dose up to six weeks of age. Infant breastfeeding was the most recommended feeding option.

After delivery, HIV-infected mothers and their children were advised to go to the nearest health care facility for a postnatal visit and an EID preformed since six weeks of age. This EID was based on a first deoxyribonucleic acid polymerase chain reaction (DNA PCR) test on a Dried Blood Spot (DBS) and was scheduled once a month. The DBS were sent for processing by the corresponding district hospital to one of the three laboratories in Ouagadougou region (the university hospital Yalgado Ouédraogo, the university hospital Charles de Gaulle, and the Saint Camille hospital). All HIV tests results were sent back to the health care facilities via the corresponding district hospitals. In case of a first positive DBS result, a second DNA PCR test is performed on a blood sample to confirm HIV infection [17].

Context and study design

The study was conducted in the implementation phase of the MONOD ANRS 12206 clinical trial (ClinicalTrial.gov registry n°NCT01127204), which was approved by the national ethics committee and the Burkina Faso Ministry of Health. The study was conducted in the capital of the country (Ouagadougou). Health professionals who were interviewed and parents of children who were enrolled for treatment provided a clear written consent. The ethics committee approved the consent procedure. The informed consent was waived for the use of aggregate register data.

The ANRS 12206 MONOD trial is a randomized controlled trial whose aim is to assess a simplified once daily antiretroviral treatment in virologically suppressed HIV infected children initially treated with a triple therapy containing lopinavir/ritonavir before the age of two (Appendix S1).

We undertook a cross-sectional survey from January 2011 to January 2012, to evaluate the performance of PMTCT cascade, and the conformance of infrastructures and staff in health care facilities with pediatric HIV services in Ouagadougou.

Study site and population

We included all the health care facilities providing PMTCT services, infant HIV diagnosis and antiretroviral treatments in Ouagadougou. We first used their 2011 aggregate data to document the PMTCT cascade. Then, in each health care facility, we interviewed all the heads of the various services: health districts, health care facilities, PMTCT services, laboratories, pharmacies, pediatric services, statistics and epidemiology surveillance division, and human resource services.

Data collection

We used 2010 and 2011 Ministry of Health statistical yearbook, as the reference figures [14,16]. We designed a semi-structured questionnaire with three sections according to the staff targeted: pediatric, laboratory and pharmacy services. Two medical epidemiologists, one midwife and one sociologist carried out the desk review and interviewed the selected health professionals. The questionnaire reviewed variables related to PMTCT statistics (cascade of HIV care from antenatal services to EID of HIV-exposed children at six weeks of age and antiretroviral treatment care for HIV-infected children), infrastructures, laboratory reagents, essential drug management and health professionals staffing (doctors, nurses, pharmacists, and laboratory technicians). The staff interviews helped to check registers and identify difficulties faced in providing early HIV infant diagnosis and treatment, and possible solutions.

In 2011, there were 103 health care facilities providing PMTCT services in Ouagadougou and we collected data from all of them. In each health care facility, there was a statistics manager who was in charge of collecting data monthly in a register provided by the Ministry of Health. Pregnant women received for antenatal consultation were recorded in a register that was later used by the statistics manager. A report was then sent to the district head of statistics and epidemiology surveillance division, who compiled the different health care facility reports with Excel software. In our study, we monthly recorded data in term of aggregate number of the different variables related to the PMTCT cascade, from the health care facility registers as well as the district registers, for comparison. In case of discrepancies, we monitored the data recording process to correct the errors. Finally, we were able to document individual data for the HIV-infected children diagnosed and transferred to HIV pediatric care for antiretroviral treatment in the MONOD trial.

For drug management, we checked the registers where the drug management was recorded to determine the availability of drugs and stock-outs. We checked the availability of antiretroviral drugs needed for the national guideline treatment: zidovudine or stavudine or abacavir, lamivudine or emtricitabine, nevirapine or efavirenz, and lopinavir/ritonavir. For opportunistic infection treatment and prophylaxis, we checked the availability of the following drugs: cotrimoxazole, nistatine, miconazole, amphotericine B, ciprofloxacine, ceftriaxone, acyclovir, and anti-tuberculosis drugs.

Finally, we checked the laboratory reagent management and availability with the responsible of laboratories in the corresponding registers.

To document the PMTCT cascade, we used the Ministry of Health method to estimate the expected number of pregnancies, based on the expected number of births multiplied by 1.10 [14]. The expected number of births is equal to the number of women of childbearing age multiplied by the corrected fertility rate of the Center region, equal to 0.1247. The logic of multiplying the expected number of births by 1.10 to obtain the number of expected pregnancies comes from a study of Sedgh et al. who found that 10% of pregnancies end in abortions in Western Africa [18].

Essential infrastructure requirement for health care centers

In 2008, WHO published an operational manual for HIV high prevalence resource constraint settings, to assess health care facilities serving HIV infected people [19].

The WHO defines health care facility's space, design, power supply, water, hygiene and sanitation, and equipment requirements to be able to deliver quality HIV prevention, care and treatment services. We assessed health care facilities using the following WHO criteria: space, privacy and confidentiality, infection control (tuberculosis infection and HIV infection), safe water supply and hygiene (sanitation, hand washing and other hygiene practices, waste management, latrine/toilet, and cleaning), communications, power, and fire safety. The standards require using color-coded waste containers and fire extinguishers. Space requirement is at least 9 m^2 for consultation room, 2.25 m^2 for counseling room, 9 m^2 for laboratory specimen analysis room, and 9 m^2 for pharmacy room [19].

We checked the space available in pediatric consultation ward, laboratory, and pharmacy rooms. This criteria was classified as conform if the available space was superior or equal to that required by the WHO standards. We also checked other qualitative criteria such as the availability of power supply, infection control and the respect of privacy and confidentiality by health professionals. The conformance was good if all the criteria were met. For laboratory tests, we assessed the capacity for performing the required tests in hospitals, without neither shortages of laboratory reagents nor failure of medical devices.

Finally, the conformance was good if antiretroviral drugs and drugs for opportunistic infection treatment and prophylaxis were available to treat HIV infected children with a regimen recommended by the national guidelines.

Statistical analysis

The prevalence of HIV infected pregnant women was calculated by dividing the number of HIV infected pregnant women by the total number of pregnant women screened for HIV infection. The 95% confidence intervals were determined according to the following formula: $(P - Z_{1-\frac{\alpha}{2}}\sqrt{\frac{P(1-P)}{n}} + \frac{1}{2n}, P + Z_{1-\frac{\alpha}{2}}\sqrt{\frac{P(1-P)}{n}} + \frac{1}{2n})$ [20] where p = prevalence, n = sample size. We described the coverage of pediatric HIV services and the flow from HIV-exposed children to access to ART, of HIV-infected children. The cascade of care was compiled on Microsoft Excel software using proportions. All the proportions of the PMTCT cascade were calculated by dividing the total number of favorable cases by the number of eligible cases with their 95% confidence intervals according to the formula previously mentioned.

Results

From the 103 health care facilities providing PMTCT services in Ouagadougou in 2011, 127 health professionals were interviewed: 7 (5.5%) pediatricians, 5 (3.9%) general practitioners, 10 (7.9%) pharmacists, 5 (3.9%) nurse-epidemiologists, 75 (59.1%) nurses, 7 (5.5%) midwives, 9 (7.1%) pharmacist assistants, 5 (3.9%) laboratory technicians, 2 (1.6%) biologists, and 2 (1.6%) human resource managers.

Staffing in pediatric HIV health services

In 2010, there was no HIV treatment for HIV-infected children in primary health care facilities in Ouagadougou. All pediatric HIV care was provided by the six district hospitals, and two university hospitals. In these hospitals, a total of 225 health professionals were directly involved in pediatric HIV infection care, and among them 40% worked in the two university hospitals (Table 1). Overall, 10.7% were pediatricians, 4.4% general practitioners, 19.1% nurses, 5.8% counselors, 8.9% pharmacists, and 29.8% laboratory technicians. Six of the eight hospitals had at least one pediatrician.

In 2010, the total population of children less than 15 years old in the whole region was estimated at 811 115 [16]. With an HIV prevalence of 0.26% in children less than 15 years old [11], we estimated the number of HIV infected children less than 15 to be about 2 109 (811 115×0.26%) in Ouagadougou. With 24 pediatricians in this area (10.7% of the overall staff dedicated to pediatric HIV care), one pediatrician was responsible for 33 797 (811 115/24) children less than 15 years age of whom 88 (2 109/24) were HIV infected.

Table 1. Staff involved in HIV pediatric care per health district or university hospitals, and qualification, in Ouagadougou, in 2010.

	Pediatricians	General practitioners	Pharmacists	Laboratory technicians	Psychologist/ counselors	Nurses	Others	Total
District hospitals	8	9	6	38	6	30	36	133
Mean per hospital	1.6	1.8	1.2	7.6	1.2	6	7.2	26.6
University hospital	16	1	14	29	7	13	12	92
Mean per hospital	8	0.5	7	14.5	3.5	6.5	6	46

Others: pharmacy assistants and laboratory assistants.

When evaluating the conformance of health staff requirements of the WHO standards in the health district hospitals [19], the staff is overall insufficient: general practitioners are less than 1/10 000, and pharmacists are less than 1/20 000 in all the five health districts of Ouagadougou. We had more than 1/4000 nurses in four health districts. Overall, both physician and pharmacist staff were scarce.

PMTCT cascade

In 2011, out of the 76 935 expected pregnancies in the Center region, 67 592 attended at least one antenatal consultation (87.8%). Among the pregnant women attending antenatal consultation, 58 036 accepted to be HIV-tested (85.9%) and the HIV prevalence was 1.8% (95% CI: 1.7%–1.9%). Furthermore, 441 out of the 1 064 HIV-infected pregnant women (41.4%) benefitted from a PMTCT intervention (option A). Then, only 313 (29.4%) HIV-exposed infants (0–18 months) had an HIV virologic test on a DBS, and 306 (97.8%) among these infants tested received their results, usually within a month, but sometimes within a four-month period. Still among the infants tested, 40 children were initially identified as HIV-infected, and 33 (82.5%) out the infants tested, were referred to the MONOD study sites before the age of two for an HIV test confirmation using a deoxyribonucleic acid polymerase chain reaction (DNA PCR). With three children identified as false positive (9%) and 30 (91%) confirmed to be HIV-infected, the HIV prevalence was estimated to be 9.6% (95% CI: 6.3%–12.9%). Finally, 27 children (90.0%) were enrolled in the MONOD ANRS 12206 trial and treated with a triple lopinavir/ritonavir based therapy (Table 2). Their median age at diagnosis was 13 months [IQR: 7–19].

Seven children (17.5%) were not referred for HIV care. One of them died before his laboratory result was released. The six remaining did not come back for their laboratory results and we were not able to contact them because of missing telephone numbers or addresses in the health care facility registers.

Among the six (18.2%) children who were referred to MONOD clinical sites, but were not enrolled in the trial to start an antiretroviral therapy, two died before being able to initiate treatment because of their advanced stage of HIV disease. One was lost to-follow-up after his father refusal to consent for treatment, and three were finally controlled as HIV-negative and not eligible for antiretroviral treatment.

Infrastructures

The conformance of infrastructures was globally gauged "not conform" because of two criteria: safe waste management and fire safety. Indeed, none of the health care facilities had either segregate color-coded waste containers or fire extinguishers.

Essential laboratory tests and apparatus

The availability of essential laboratory tests was checked in health care facilities (Table 3). The lack of some of the laboratory tests was associated to either a failure/lack of the corresponding laboratory apparatus or a reagent shortage. The table 4 displays the reasons for the laboratory non conformance. In addition, lack of apparatus maintenance has been underlined in all the health care facilities.

Essential drugs

The availability of essential antiretroviral drugs was quite good in 2010, and the conformance was judged to be good in spite of few shortages which did not affect the treatment of HIV-infected patient according to national guidelines. A shortage of seven days

Table 2. The PMTCT cascade until HIV pediatric care in Ouagadougou, 2011.

Designation	Number	Percentage (%)	Confidence Interval 95%
Pregnant women expected	76 935	100%	-
Pregnant women attending antenatal consultation	67 592	87.8 (100%)	[87.6–88.0]
Pregnant women having been counseled for HIV testing	60 156	89.0	[88.8–89.2]
Pregnant women having been HIV-tested	58 036	85.9 (100%) (96.5% of the counseled women)	[85.6–86.1]
HIV-infected pregnant women	1 064	1.8 (100%)	[1.7–1.9]
Pregnant women exposed to PMTCT intervention	441	41.4	[38.4–44.4]
HIV-exposed infants having been HIV-tested using DBS	313	29.4 (100%)	[26.6–32.2]
DBS tests results returned	306	97.8	[96.0–99.6]
Infants identified as HIV-infected on the first DBS test (100%)	40	12.8	[8.9–16.6]
HIV-infected infants referred to pediatric care	33	82.5	[71.9–95.5]
Infants confirmed as HIV-infected on the second test (DNA PCR on blood sample)	30	9.6 (100%)	[6.3–12.9]
HIV-infected infants initiated on antiretroviral therapy	27	90.0	[79.2–100.0]

100% is the reference number.
DNA PCR = deoxyribonucleic acid polymerase chain reaction.
DBS = dried blood spot.

was observed for lopinavir/ritonavir, lamivudine and abacavir in Charles de Gaulle university hospital in 2010. In addition, Bogodogo district hospital noticed a shortage of 30 days for the combination lamivudine + nevirapine + stavudine (triomune junior). The drugs for opportunistic infections were available and conform to WHO standards, but they were not free of charge for HIV-infected patients in 2010, except anti-tuberculosis drugs and cotrimoxazole.

Discussion

This cross-sectional survey assessed for the first time the staff, the infrastructures and the PMTCT cascade from prenatal PMTCT up to pediatric HIV care, in all health care facilities providing pediatric HIV care services in Ouagadougou. We documented that only 40% of HIV-infected women received a PMTCT intervention and less than a third of HIV-exposed children were tested during the postnatal period. Moreover, it provides a description of the health care system in this country, useful to understand some of the weaknesses of the system when it comes to the issue of EID in all HIV exposed children, and their access to antiretroviral therapy.

There are several drawbacks in our observations. Firstly, the incompleteness of the data collected may be the source of information bias in this study. Our study method was partially based on desk review, where we checked the statistics in the available registers. Unfortunately, we could not get all the information related to our objectives. For instance, it had not been possible to routinely determine the duration of laboratory reagent shortage. Secondly, we were not able to really link one-to-one the PMTCT with the postnatal data, and we assumed that each HIV-pregnant woman was supposed to give one alive pregnancy outcome, without taking into account multiple pregnancy outcomes or stillbirth. Furthermore, some of the infants tested in 2011, had their mothers attend their first antenatal consultation in the preceding years, and some of the pregnant women tracked in 2011 will give birth in 2012 as well, resulting in a kind of compensation allowing the PMTCT and EID coverage estimates. Consequently, we feel that these figures were accurate enough to understand the overall patient flow throughout the health care system services. Thirdly, the conformance of health care services was determined with respect to the WHO standards, ideally suitable for district hospitals [19]. These standards might not be suitable when applied to university hospitals, where a higher standard of care is expected. Lastly, in terms of representativeness, our results showed a similar proportion of antenatal consultations among pregnant women in Ouagadougou, compared to the rest of the country (88%) [14]. As a matter of fact, Ouagadougou had a greater number of private health facilities compared to the rest of the country [14], and their statistics were

Table 3. Conformance of Ouagadougou hospitals according to WHO standards, in 2010.

WHO criteria of conformance	District hospital	University hospital
	N=6	N=2
	# conform/N	# conform/N
Infrastructure		
Room space >9 m^2	6/6	2/2
Power (electricity) available	6/6	2/2
Tap water available	6/6	2/2
Tuberculosis infection control (ventilated waiting rooms, cough control, good patient flow)	6/6	2/2
HIV infection control (injection safety, appropriate use and disposal of sharps, personal protective equipment for staff, post exposure prophylaxis available)	6/6	2/2
Waste management (3 color-containers available)	0/6	0/2
Privacy of patient's test protected	6/6	2/2
Communication (land line available)	6/6	2/2
Fire extinguisher available	0/6	0/2
Conclusion	**Not conform**	**Not conform**
Laboratory test available		
Rapid HIV antibody test	4/6	2/2
DBS	6/6	2/2
CD4 count	1/6	1/2
Hemoglobin determination	5/6	2/2
Serum alanin aminotransferase	4/6	2/2
Serum creatinin & blood urea nitrogen	4/6	2/2
Bilirubin determination	4/6	2/2
Lactic acid	5/6	2/2
Blood sugar	4/6	2/2
Tuberculosis diagnostics	6/6	2/2
Pregnancy test	6/6	2/2
Urine dipstick for sugar and protein	6/6	2/2
Conclusion	**Not conform**	**Not conform**
Drugs available		
Antiretroviral drugs	6/6	2/2
Opportunistic infection drugs	6/6	2/2
Conclusion	**Conform**	**Conform**
Staff		
One general practitioner for 10 000	0/6	Not applicable*
One pharmacist for 20 000	0/6	Not applicable*
One nurse for 4 000	4/6	Not applicable*
Conclusion	**Not conform**	**Not applicable**

*The university hospitals are located in the center region, but patients are referred from the whole country.

not included in our figures. As a result, the number of antenatal consultations was lower than that was really carried out in Ouagadougou. However, in our study, we considered all pregnant women who were on PMTCT antiretroviral protocol with the hypothesis that their children would be referred to the public system if they were found to be HIV-infected.

Our study helped to identify major challenges facing EID and antiretroviral treatment access for children in Burkina Faso. A survey conducted in Burkina Faso, Ghana and Côte d'Ivoire, from January 2010 to February 2011 had already reported the lack of access to child PMTCT prophylaxis [11]. Our results confirm that in the urban setting of Ouagadougou. The level of missed opportunities was so high that it was difficult to cover sufficiently with PMTCT intervention, the mother-infant couple, estimated at 59%, as well as to offer EID to all HIV-exposed children, reaching 71%. We also conclude that these missed opportunities should be greater at the national level considering the fact that the health

Table 4. Reasons for Ouagadougou laboratory non conformance in 2010.

	District hospitals N=6		University hospitals N=2	
Laboratory tests non available	**Lack or apparatus failure**	**Reagent shortage**	**Lack or apparatus failure**	**Reagent shortage**
Rapid HIV antibody test	Non applicable	2	Non applicable	0
CD4 count	5	5	1	0
Hemoglobin determination	1	0	0	0
Serum alanin aminotransferase	1	1	0	0
Serum creatinin & blood urea nitrogen	1	1	0	0
Bilirubin determination	1	1	0	0
Lactic acid	1	0	0	0
Blood sugar	1	1	0	0

care system would be more complex and thus weaker at the rural level in comparison to the urban one.

Some factors could explain these missed opportunities and could be separately addressed. Firstly, the low awareness of HIV prevention and care services in the community could explain the non-attendance of EID services or the rejection of these services by families. In Burkina Faso, only 20.1% of the population attended the secondary school in 2008/2009 [21] and therefore we think that substantial efforts should be developed to make them aware of the benefit of PMTCT services. In addition, men should also be targeted in education, because they are likely to be reluctant to carrying out HIV screening, and they can greatly support their wives in using PMTCT services [22,23].

Secondly, we highlighted the lack of adequate quantitative and qualitative health care workers (HCW) to cover the needs. At the six-week postnatal visit for instance, due to the fact that nurses were not all trained to perform DBS, the DBS could only be performed one day in a month. Mothers who would like have their infant HIV-tested could only return on this unique day, leading to a high attrition rate because of the inadequate offer of this simple service.

Thirdly, the inaccessibility to EID services is also related to the health system organization, as the current DBS sample circuit and transportation is too complicated and should be simplified. Indeed, the need to go through each district hospital while the final laboratory test is performed in each university laboratory hospital should be considered. It would be more efficient to perform the DBS directly in the health care facilities, to limit the lost to follow-up rate. In the neighboring country of Côte d'Ivoire, we had a similar problem of low coverage rate of EID, favored by the civil war, with only 24% of the HIV exposed children early diagnosed in 2010 [24]. In comparison, a study carried out in 2008, showed that DNA polymerase chain reaction testing in routine was 35.2% for children hospitalized in Malawi, but their age was not specified [25].

Similarly, the low PMTCT intervention coverage is related to problems in the health service organization. When a pregnant woman attends antenatal consultation in a health care facility, she is counseled and screened for HIV with a rapid HIV antibody test. In case of HIV infection, she is referred to the referent district hospital in order to carry out the other tests such as CD4 count, before visiting a doctor who would prescribe an option A antiretroviral treatment, mainly based on nevirapine. Then, she is later sent back in the former health care facility, to pursue her antenatal follow-up. Although not documented, we assume that some pregnant women could not reach the district hospitals, thus increasing the number of lost to follow-up. This could explain why a lot of pregnant women attend antenatal consultation but do not benefit from PMTCT intervention, when they are HIV-infected.

Fourthly, there are also laboratory related challenges, with the need to offer routine services while the HIV-prevalence is still low, leading to frequent laboratory reagent shortages. Thairu et al. also confirmed our results about maintenance and reagent stock management, in their study in Burkina Faso and Zimbabwe [26]. A frequently-cited barrier to expansion of EID programs is the cost of the required laboratory assays.

Thus, substantial sequential barriers explain the low PMTCT and EID complete cascade coverage, and the lack of personnel and infrastructure requirements. A review reported that even with the highest reported levels of uptake, nearly half of HIV-infected infants may not complete the cascade successfully [10].

Additionally, we raise the overall problem of the EID strategy performances. In settings with low HIV prevalence or well performing PMTCT program, vertical transmission rates may be as low as 2% at six weeks and the positive predictive value of a single test will be approximately 50%, meaning that only half of infants who are tested positive are truly infected [27,28]. For this reason, a confirmatory test is essential, especially in the context of a low HIV prevalence country such as Burkina Faso. Indeed, in our study, the high rate of false positive DBS (9%) highly affects the positive predictive value of the national HIV screening strategy. Acknowledging this, the test confirmation is a priority and laboratories should implement reliable quality control system and constantly work on maintaining high quality standards of EID.

Antiretroviral access for HIV-infected children looked good in our study when compared to the estimates of the Ethiopian study, where only 8.4% of positive babies had access to antiretroviral treatment [29]. But, it is important to point out the contribution of the Monod trial implementation in our results, which set up a network whose aim was to improve the coverage of pediatric antiretroviral therapy beyond the EID.

A shortage of some antiretroviral drugs was observed in two health care facilities for several days, as a result of delays in reporting. In effect, antiretroviral drugs are provided by the Ministry of Health division for HIV/AIDS (Comité Ministériel de Lutte contre le Sida), and they required periodic reports, before delivery. Hence, a delay in providing a report will ultimately end in a delay in drug supply.

Moreover, while all antiretroviral drugs were free of charge in Burkina Faso in 2010, the opportunistic infection drugs are charged to families. It has already been reported that having to pay for HIV treatment and laboratory tests, increases the risk of lost to follow-up [30].

When analyzing the conformance of health centers with respect to the PMTCT cascade, we can point out that the infrastructure requirements are almost met, and that the absence of fire extinguishers and segregate color-codes waste containers, did not affect antenatal consultation rate which is quite good in a developing country setting such as this. However, the non conformance to laboratory test requirements explained why we observed an attrition of the cascade at the number of children tested for HIV infection. The conformance of pharmacies was found to be good and consequently two-third of HIV infected children were treated. The missed opportunity for treatment was related to communication and pregnant women HIV testing circuit problem.

Globally, the causes of non conformance at the district and university hospitals are almost similar because they are public centers (except Saint Camille hospital), run by the Ministry of Health. The causes could be a lack of resources, or a mismanagement of the available resources.

The problem could be alleviated by improving the communication process between the peripheral health services and the national procurement system. The community awareness should also be improved and contextualized to the socio-cultural needs of the region.

Moreover, training in a large scale on DBS practicing and in HIV care among HCW would be useful and promote task shifting activities [31,32,33]. Finally, characteristics of the health care facilities could be determinant in improving the pediatric HIV care in Africa as reported in the HEART project [34]: characteristics associated with favorable children enrolment in care are nutritional support, linkages with associations of people living with HIV, access to EID and integration of PMTCT services. Applying the South African strategies to improve antiretroviral treatment in the province of KwaZulu-Natal could be beneficial. In addition to training all the staff in contact with mothers and children, they carried out campaigns aimed at increasing HIV testing during immunization and clinics, routinely testing of HIV in children with tuberculosis and malnutrition, and systematically testing for HIV, all children admitted at hospital [35]. However, in Burkina Faso, as the HIV prevalence is lower than that of South Africa, it would be more efficient to start the systematic HIV diagnosis by screening first the children with rapid HIV antibody tests. Expanding these characteristics to improve pediatric HIV treatment in Burkina Faso, warrants further evaluation for improving the scaling up of pediatric HIV care. Finally, as it was reported in South Africa, it is possible to improve the identification of HIV-infected children and ensure a prompt start on ART when needed with relatively simple measures, limited staffing and budgets [35].

Despite an overall good access to prenatal services in Ouagadougou in 2011, there are still many missed opportunities for both the prevention of mother-to-child transmission and the early access to diagnosis and antiretroviral therapy for HIV-infected children before two years of life. The government should look forward to improving the awareness and education among the population, training health care workers for HIV diagnosis and care, facilitating the access to EID and making health care facilities more attractive to families. In addition, the DBS circuit should be simplified to avoid lost to follow-up. Early access to EID and to antiretroviral therapy will require political willingness and leadership to address these health system barriers in Burkina Faso.

Acknowledgments

We acknowledge the Head of Ministry of Health division for AIDS (Comité Ministériel de Lutte contre le Sida), in Burkina Faso, Dr Marie-Joseph Sanou, the regional Director of Health, Dr Amédée Prosper Djiguemdé and all heads of health care facilities in Ouagadougou and their staff for their contribution to data collection. We are grateful to the French GIP ESTHER for its assistance to HIV infected children in Burkina Faso. We would like to give special thanks to Pr Louis Rachid Salmi for his helpful suggestion on using WHO standards.

Author Contributions

Conceived and designed the experiments: M. Coulibaly NM VL PV SB DY LK CY SO MB IS ET M. Congo. Performed the experiments: M. Coulibaly IS ET. Analyzed the data: M. Coulibaly IS VL. Contributed reagents/materials/analysis tools: CY M. Congo MB NM VL PV. Wrote the paper: M. Coulibaly VL SB PV NM FK. Edit the manuscript: VL SB PV ET MB LK CY SO IS DY FK M. Congo.

References

1. Newell ML, Brahmbhatt H, Ghys PD (2004) Child mortality and HIV infection in Africa: a review. AIDS 18 Suppl 2: S27–34.
2. Newell ML, Coovadia H, Cortina-Borja M, Rollins N, Gaillard P, et al. (2004) Mortality of infected and uninfected infants born to HIV-infected mothers in Africa: a pooled analysis. Lancet 364: 1236–1243.
3. Desmonde S, Coffie P, Aka E, Amani-Bosse C, Messou E, et al. (2011) Severe morbidity and mortality in untreated HIV-infected children in a paediatric care programme in Abidjan, Cote d'Ivoire, 2004–2009. BMC Infect Dis 11: 182.
4. Goetghebuer T, Le Chenadec J, Haelterman E, Galli L, Dollfus C, et al. (2012) Short- and long-term immunological and virological outcome in HIV-infected infants according to the age at antiretroviral treatment initiation. Clin Infect Dis 54: 878–881.
5. Prendergast AJ, Penazzato M, Cotton M, Musoke P, Mulenga V, et al. (2012) Treatment of young children with HIV infection: using evidence to inform policymakers. PLoS Med 9: e1001273.
6. Prendergast A, Mphatswe W, Tudor-Williams G, Rakgotho M, Pillay V, et al. (2008) Early virological suppression with three-class antiretroviral therapy in HIV-infected African infants. AIDS 22: 1333–1343.
7. Violari A, Cotton MF, Gibb DM, Babiker AG, Steyn J, et al. (2008) Early antiretroviral therapy and mortality among HIV-infected infants. N Engl J Med 359: 2233–2244.
8. WHO (2010) Antiretroviral therapy for HIV infection in infants and children: Towards universal access. Recommendations for a public health approach. 2010 revision.
9. Nielsen K, Bryson YJ (2000) Diagnosis of HIV infection in children. Pediatr Clin North Am 47: 39–63.
10. Ciaranello AL, Park JE, Ramirez-Avila L, Freedberg KA, Walensky RP, et al. (2011) Early infant HIV-1 diagnosis programs in resource-limited settings: opportunities for improved outcomes and more cost-effective interventions. BMC Med 9: 59.
11. Tchidjou HK, Maria Martino A, Goli LP, Diop Ly M, Zekeng L, et al. (2012) Paediatric HIV infection in Western Africa: the long way to the standard of care. J Trop Pediatr 58: 451–456.
12. Ndondoki C, Brou H, Timite-Konan M, Oga M, Amani-Bosse C, et al. (2013) Universal HIV screening at postnatal points of care: which public health approach for early infant diagnosis in Cote d'Ivoire? PLoS One 8: e67996.

13. Ministère de l'Economie et des Finances Burkina Faso (2011) Enquête Démographique et de Santé et à indicateurs Multiples (EDSBF-MICS IV) 2010. Ouagadougou, Burkina Faso. 50 p. Available: www.measuredhs.com/pubs/pdf/PR9/PR9.pdf. Accessed 2012 September 12.
14. Ministère de la Santé Burkina Faso (2012) Annuaire statistique 2011. Ouagadougou, Burkina Faso. 244 p. Available: http://www.sante.gov.bf/phocadownload/Annuaire_statistique_2011.pdf. Accessed 2013 May 27.
15. Institut National de la Statistique et de la Démographie Burkina Faso (2011) La région du centre en chiffres. Ouagadougou, Burkina Faso. 7 p. Available: http://www.insd.bf/n/contenu/statistiques_regions/regions_en_chiffres_en_2011/reg_chif_c_2011.pdf. Accessed 2014 August 4.
16. Ministère de la Santé Burkina Faso (2011) Annaire statistique 2010. Ouagadougou, Burkina Faso. 204p. Availaible: http://www.sante.gov.bf/phocadownload/Publications_statistiques/Annuaire/annuaire_statistique_sante_2010.pdf. Accessed: 2014 October 5.
17. Ministère de la Santé Comité Ministériel de Lutte contre le SIDA Burkina Faso (2008) Normes et protocoles de prise en charge médicale des personnes vivant avec le VIH au Burkina Faso. Ouagadougou.
18. Sedgh G, Henshaw S, Singh S, Ahman E, Shah IH (2007) Induced abortion: estimated rates and trends worldwide. Lancet 370: 1338–1345.
19. WHO (2008) Operations Manual for Delivery of HIV Prevention, Care and Treatment at Primary Health Centres in High-Prevalence, Resource-Constrained Settings. Geneva, Switzerland. 392 p.
20. Forthofer RN, Lee ES, Hernandez M (2007) Biostatistics: A guide to Design, Analysis, and Discovery: Elsevier. 502 p.
21. Institut National de la Statistique et de la Démographie Burkina Faso (2013) Tableau 05.34: Evolution du taux brut de scolarisation de l'ensemble du secondaire (en %). Ouagadougou, Burkina Faso. Available: http://www.insd.bf/n/contenu/tableaux/T0534.htm. Accessed 2013 May 27.
22. Desgrees-Du-Lou A, Brou H, Djohan G, Becquet R, Ekouevi DK, et al. (2009) Beneficial effects of offering prenatal HIV counselling and testing on developing a HIV preventive attitude among couples. Abidjan, 2002–2005. AIDS Behav 13: 348–355.
23. Brou H, Djohan G, Becquet R, Allou G, Ekouevi DK, et al. (2008) Sexual prevention of HIV within the couple after prenatal HIV-testing in West Africa. AIDS Care 20: 413–418.
24. Folquet-Amonissani M, Dainguy M. E, Amani-Bossé C, Elian-Kouakou J, Méa-Assandé V, et al. Early infant diagnosis and access to pediatric HIV care: barriers and challenges in Abidjan, Ivory Coast in 2011; 2012; Washington DC, USA.
25. Van Rompaey S, Kimfuta J, Kimbondo P, Monn C, Buve A (2011) Operational assessment of access to ART in rural Africa: the example of Kisantu in Democratic Republic of the Congo. AIDS Care 23: 686–693.
26. Thairu L, Katzenstein D, Israelski D (2011) Operational challenges in delivering CD4 diagnostics in sub-Saharan Africa. AIDS Care 23: 814–821.
27. WHO (2010) WHO recommendations on the diagnosis of HIV infection in infants and children. Geneva, Switzerland. 64 p.
28. WHO (2014) March 2014 supplement to the 2013 consolidated guidelines on the use of antiretroviral drugs for treating and preventing HIV infection recommendations for a public health approch. Geneva, Swetzerland. 128 p.
29. Nigatu T, Woldegebriel Y (2011) Analysis of the prevention of mother-to-child transmission (PMTCT) service utilization in Ethiopia: 2006–2010. Reprod Health 8: 6.
30. Leroy V, Malateste K, Rabie H, Lumbiganon P, Ayaya S, et al. (2013) Outcomes of antiretroviral therapy in children in Asia and Africa: a comparative analysis of the IeDEA pediatric multiregional collaboration. J Acquir Immune Defic Syndr 62: 208–219.
31. Zachariah R, Ford N, Philips M, Lynch S, Massaquoi M, et al. (2009) Task shifting in HIV/AIDS: opportunities, challenges and proposed actions for sub-Saharan Africa. Trans R Soc Trop Med Hyg 103: 549–558.
32. Creek T, Tanuri A, Smith M, Seipone K, Smit M, et al. (2008) Early diagnosis of human immunodeficiency virus in infants using polymerase chain reaction on dried blood spots in Botswana's national program for prevention of mother-to-child transmission. Pediatr Infect Dis J 27: 22–26.
33. Oga MA, Ndondoki C, Brou H, Salmon A, Bosse-Amani C, et al. (2011) Attitudes and practices of health care workers toward routine HIV testing of infants in Cote d'Ivoire: the PEDI-TEST ANRS 12165 Project. J Acquir Immune Defic Syndr 57 Suppl 1: S16–21.
34. Adjorlolo-Johnson G, Wahl Uheling A, Ramachandran S, Strasser S, Kouakou J, et al. (2013) Scaling up pediatric HIV care and treatment in Africa: clinical site characteristics associated with favorable service utilization. J Acquir Immune Defic Syndr 62: e7–e13.
35. Bland RM, Ndirangu J, Newell ML (2013) Maximising opportunities for increased antiretroviral treatment in children in an existing HIV programme in rural South Africa. BMJ 346: f550.

19

High Utility of Contact Investigation for Latent and Active Tuberculosis Case Detection among the Contacts: A Retrospective Cohort Study in Tbilisi, Georgia, 2010–2011

Tsira Chakhaia[1]*, Matthew J. Magee[2,3], Russell R. Kempker[4], Medea Gegia[1], Leila Goginashvili[5], Ucha Nanava[5], Henry M. Blumberg[3,4]

1 University Research Co., LLC. Branch in Georgia, USAID Georgia TB Prevention Project, Tbilisi, Georgia, **2** Division of Epidemiology and Biostatistics, School of Public Health, Georgia State University, Atlanta, Georgia, United States of America, **3** Departments of Epidemiology and Global Health, Rollins School of Public Health, Emory University, Atlanta, Georgia, United States of America, **4** Division of Infectious Diseases, Department of Medicine, School of Medicine, Emory University, Atlanta, Georgia, United States of America, **5** National Center for Tuberculosis and Lung Disease, Tbilisi, Georgia

Abstract

Setting: The study was conducted at the National Center for Tuberculosis and Lung Diseases (NCTBLD) in Tbilisi, Georgia.

Objective: To assess the utility of contact investigation for tuberculosis (TB) case detection. We also assessed the prevalence and risk factors for active TB disease and latent TB infection (LTBI) among contacts of active pulmonary TB cases.

Design: A retrospective cohort study was conducted among the contacts of active pulmonary TB cases registered in 2010–2011 at the NCTBLD in Tbilisi, Georgia. Contacts of active TB patients were investigated according to an "invitation model": they were referred to the NCTBLD by the index case; were queried about clinical symptoms suggestive of active TB disease; tuberculin skin testing and chest radiographs were performed. Demographic, laboratory, and clinical data of TB patients and their contacts were abstracted from existing records up to February 2013.

Results: 869 contacts of 396 index cases were enrolled in the study; a median of 2 contacts were referred per index case. Among the 869 contacts, 47 (5.4%) were found to have or developed active TB disease: 30 (63.8%) were diagnosed with TB during the baseline period (co-prevalent cases) and 17 (36.2%) developed active TB disease during the follow-up period (mean follow up of 21 months) (incident TB cases). The incidence rate of active TB disease among contacts was 1126.0 per 100 000 person years (95% CI 655.7–1802.0 per 100,000 person-years). Among the 402 contacts who had a tuberculin skin test (TST) performed, 52.7% (95% CI 47.7–57.7%) had LTBI.

Conclusions: A high prevalence of LTBI and active TB disease was found among the contacts of TB cases in Tbilisi, Georgia. Our findings demonstrated that an "invitation" model of contact investigation was an effective method of case detection. Therefore, contact investigation should be scaled up in Georgia.

Editor: Giovanni Delogu, The Catholic University of the Sacred Heart, Rome, Italy

Funding: This work was supported by the National Institutes of Health (NIH) (http://nih.gov/) Fogarty International Center (D43TW007124), NIH NIAID (K23AI103044), the Atlanta Clinical and Translational Science Institute (NIH/NCATS UL1TR000454), and the Emory Global Health Institute. The funders had no role in study design, data collection and analysis, decision to publish, or preparation of the manuscript.

Competing Interests: T. Chakhaia and M. Gegia are employed by University Research Co., LLC. There are no patents, products in development or marketed products to declare.

* Email: tschakhaia@gmail.com

Introduction

Investigating the contacts of patients with tuberculosis (TB) is a priority public health measure employed in high-income countries to detect new TB cases and identify those close contacts who would benefit from latent tuberculosis infection (LTBI) treatment to prevent progression to active TB disease [1]. The U.S. Centers for Disease Control and Prevention (CDC) has indicated that contact investigation has played an important role in decreasing the incidence of TB in the U.S. [2]. In contrast, TB contact

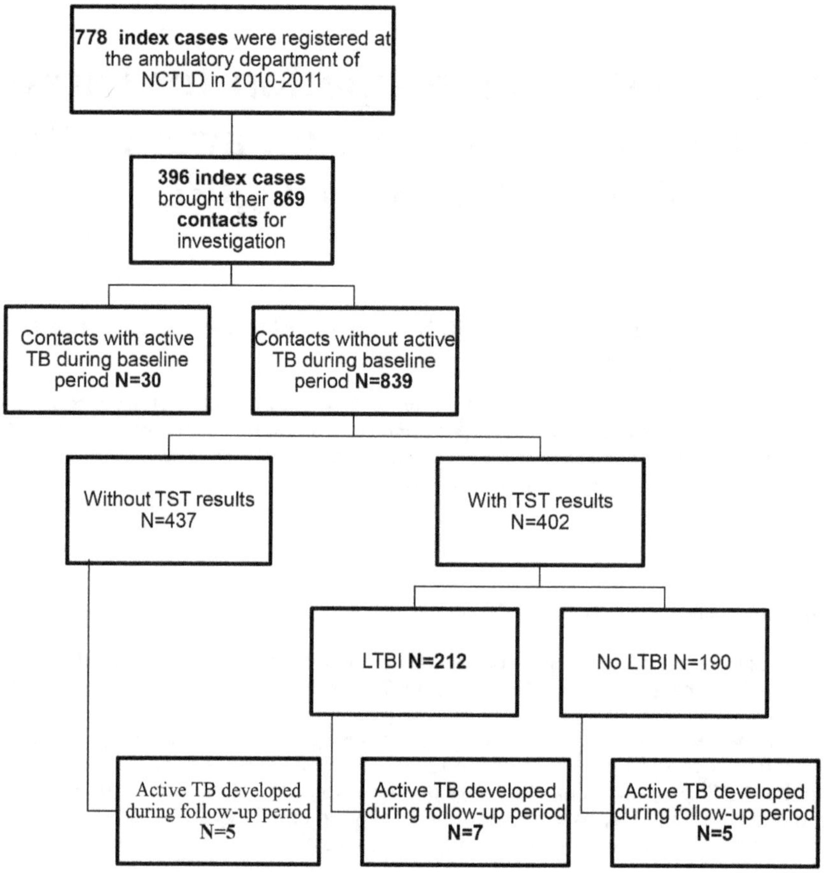

Figure 1. Contact investigation study flow, Tbilisi, Georgia, 2010–2011.

investigation has typically been a low public health priority in most high TB incidence low- and middle-income countries (LMIC) [3,4]. In recent years, there has been increasing interest in contact investigation in resource-limited countries. The World Health Organization (WHO) currently recommends contact investigation in two high-risk populations including children <5 years of age and HIV-infected persons, or when the index case has any of the following characteristics: sputum smear positive [SS (+)] pulmonary TB, multidrug-resistant TB (MDR-TB) or extensively drug-resistant TB (XDR-TB), HIV-infection, or is a child <5 years of age [5,6]. However, WHO indicates that contact investigations may not necessarily be indicated because of competing demands on time and resources and it is frequently not carried out in most LMIC [5,6].

The country of Georgia has a high burden of TB including MDR-TB disease [7,8]. In 2012, the incidence rate of TB in Georgia was 116 per 100,000 persons and approximately 9.2% of new cases and nearly a third of retreatment cases had MDR-TB [9]. In 2010–2011, an "invitation" model of contact investigation was implemented: only contacts who presented to health care facilities in conjunction with an index TB case (cases of new or recurrent pulmonary TB in persons from households (HH) or other settings in which others may have been exposed) were investigated [10]. Per National TB Program (NTP) guidelines, contacts did not come in for study follow-up visits nor were visited by health care workers. Currently, most contacts investigated are referred to a health care facility by the TB index case.

In Georgia and most LMICs in the Caucuses region, limited data exists regarding the prevalence of LTBI and the impact of performing contact investigations for TB case finding among HH and close contacts of patients with TB. Previously published epidemiologic investigations of LTBI in Georgia have been conducted only among healthcare workers and internally displaced persons (IDP) [11,12]. To our knowledge, no data exists regarding the rates of TB among the contacts of active TB patients. Therefore, the overall purpose of our study was to assess the utility of contact investigation for TB case finding. The primary objectives were to 1) determine the prevalence of active TB disease and LTBI at baseline and 2) determine the incidence of active TB disease among contacts of pulmonary TB cases during the follow-up period. A secondary objective of the study was to identify risk factors associated with LTBI and active TB disease among contacts.

Materials and Methods

Study design and Setting

A retrospective cohort study was conducted at the ambulatory department of the National Center for Tuberculosis and Lung Diseases (NCTBLD) in Tbilisi, Georgia. Study data for TB patients and their contacts were abstracted from NCTBLD medical records and NTP database from January 2010 through February 2013. Given the retrospective nature of the study, informed consent was not obtained; however, we only used routinely collected programmatic data and all personal identifiers were removed prior to statistical analyses. The Institutional

Review Boards of the NCTBLD of Georgia and Emory University reviewed and approved the study protocol.

Participants

Index cases were defined as cases of new or recurrent pulmonary TB in persons from HH or other setting in which others may have been exposed, as defined by the WHO [5]. Eligible index cases for the study included all patients with pulmonary TB who registered in the ambulatory department of the NCTBLD from January 1, 2010 to December 31, 2011 and who referred contacts to a health care facility for investigation. Index cases with acid-fast bacilli (AFB) SS (+) specimens were instructed by physicians to refer their HH contacts to the NCTBLD. In addition, sputum smear negative [SS (−)] index cases who voluntary referred their contacts to the NCTBLD were also included in this investigation. Contacts were defined as any persons who were exposed to an index case, according to WHO criteria [5]. Eligible contacts for this study included any contacts referred to the NCTBLD by an enrolled index patient including HH (defined as person who shared the same enclosed living space for one or more nights or for frequent or extended periods during the day with the index case during the 3 months before commencement of the current treatment episode [5]) and other non-HH, close contacts (defined as a person who is not in the household but shared an enclosed space, such as a social gathering place, workplace or facility, for extended periods during the day with the index case during the 3 months before commencement of the current treatment episode [5]). All enrolled contacts were investigated during the baseline period – less than 2 months after the index patient TB treatment start date [13].

Table 1. Socio-demographic and clinical characteristics of index tuberculosis (TB) cases, Tbilisi, Georgia, 2010–2011.

TB Patients' characteristics		TB patients who referred contacts to a health care facility for investigation (index cases)	TB patients who did not referred contacts to a health care facility for investigation	Total	OR (95%CI)
		N = 396 (%)	N = 382 (%)	N = 778	
All TB patients					
Gender	Male	248 (62.6)	241 (63.1)	489 (62.9)	0.98 (0.73–1.31)
	Female	148 (37.4)	141 (36.9)	289 (37.1)	1
Age (years)	0–4	0 (0.0)	0 (0.0)	0 (0.0)	N/A
	5–14	3 (0.8)	7 (1.8)	10 (1.3)	1
	15–24	66 (17.8)	81 (21.2)	147 (19.5)	1.90 (0.47–7.64)
	25–34	122 (32.9)	96 (25.1)	218 (29.0)	2.97 (0.75–11.77)
	35–44	76 (20.5)	87 (22.8)	163 (21.6)	2.04 (0.51–8.16)
	45–54	59 (15.9)	62 (16.2)	121 (16.1)	2.22 (0.55–8.99)
	55–64	29 (7.8)	29 (7.6)	58 (7.7)	2.33 (0.55–9.92)
	> = 65	16 (4.3)	20 (5.2)	36 (4.8)	1.87 (0.42–8.40)
	missing	25	0	25	
Case definition	New	281 (78.7)	290 (76.9)	571 (77.8)	1.11 (0.78–1.57)
	Previously treated	76 (21.3)	87 (23.1)	163 (22.2)	1
	Missing	39	5	44	
AFB smear	SS (+)	276 (89.9)	146 (39.1)	422 (62.1)	13.84 (9.05–21.16)
	SS (−)	31 (10.1)	227 (60.9)	258 (37.9)	1
	Missing	89	9	98	
AFB Culture	Positive	303 (95.9)	224 (66.7)	527 (80.8)	11.65 (6.40–21.23)
	Negative	13 (4.1)	112 (33.3)	125 (19.2)	1
	Missing	80	46	126	
MDR TB status	MDR TB	97 (27.6)	55 (14.4)	152 (20.7)	2.26 (1.56–3.27)
	Non MDR TB	255 (72.4)	327 (85.6)	582 (79.3)	1
	Missing	44	0	44	
Adult index cases[1]					
Work status	Unemployed	281 (87.8)	302 (83.9)	583 (85.7)	1.38 (0.89–2.14)
	Employed	39 (12.2)	58 (16.1)	97 (14.3)	1
	Missing	41	8	49	
History of incarceration	Yes	37 (11.4)	39 (11.3)	76 (11.3)	1.01 (0.63–1.63)
	No	288 (88.6)	306 (88.7)	594 (88.7)	1
	Missing	36	23	59	

[1]index cases>17 years of age.

Abbreviations: AFB–Acid-fast bacilli; SS–sputum smear; MDR–Multidrug-resistant

Table 2. Age and gender distribution of the contacts of the index cases with tuberculosis (TB) disease, Tbilisi, Georgia, 2010–2011.

Contacts' Characteristics		Contact of TB patient n = 869	
		n	%
Gender	Male	373	42.9
	Female	496	57.1
Age (years)	0–4	131	15.1
	5–14	198	22.8
	15–24	148	17.0
	25–34	112	12.9
	35–44	93	10.7
	45–54	90	10.4
	55–64	57	6.6
	>=65	40	4.6

Contacts were evaluated for clinical symptoms; chest radiography (CXR) and tuberculin skin tests (TSTs) were performed. Nurses at the NCTBLD performed a TST on contact who agreed to be tested using the Mantoux method and the TST was read 48–72 hours after administration [14]. Clinicians used clinical symptoms, the TST result, and chest radiograph findings to identify contacts who were suspected of having active TB disease. All persons suspected of having TB had sputum collected for AFB sputum smear microscopy and culture. All TB screening tests were performed as standard practice within the framework of the NTP and thus there was no charge for the contact. According to the WHO recommendations and per Georgia NTP standards, children aged <5 years who were contacts of drug-susceptible TB index cases and were not diagnosed with active TB disease were offered a 6-month course of isoniazid preventive treatment (IPT) [5].

Within the framework of our retrospective study, prospective follow-up study visits of the contacts were not performed. The data for all contacts during the follow-up period was abstracted from the NTP active TB database. If a contact was registered in the National TB Program as a TB case, this contact was classified as an active TB case. Contacts were classified as TB free at the end of the study period if they were not registered as an active TB case in the NTP database.

Definitions

The primary study outcomes included the presence of secondary active TB cases and LTBI among contacts. A secondary TB case was defined as active pulmonary or extrapulmonary TB disease among a contact confirmed by a positive AFB culture for *M. tuberculosis* or a clinical diagnosis of TB by a NCTBLD clinician (based on compatible symptoms and radiographic findings). Secondary cases were classified as either co-prevalent or incident TB cases. Co-prevalent TB cases were defined by the presence of active TB disease among contacts during the baseline period. Incident TB cases were defined as the development of active TB disease during the follow-up period among those contacts without active TB disease at baseline. The follow-up period was defined≥2 months after the index patient started therapy for TB up to 2 years or until the end of the study period (February 2013) [13]. For contacts who developed active TB disease, the follow-up period ended on their TB treatment initiation date. Incident TB cases among contacts were confirmed through reviewing the Georgia NTP TB database (NTP surveillance covers nearly all active TB cases in Georgia). A contact with LTBI was defined as any contact person with a positive TST who did not have active TB disease during baseline investigation [5]. An induration of five or more millimeters was defined as a positive TST [14,15].

Additional data abstracted from the medical record or the Georgian NTP surveillance database included socio-demographic and clinical characteristics of both index cases and contacts. Clinical characteristics included AFB smear status, TB treatment status (newly diagnosed case vs. retreatment TB case) and the presence or absence of MDR TB (defined as resistance to at least isoniazid and rifampin) [16]. All sputum specimens were processed at the Georgian National TB Reference Laboratory in Tbilisi, Georgia according to WHO recommendations [17,18]. Index

Table 3. Active TB disease among contacts, Tbilisi, Georgia, 2010–2011.

Months following initiation of TB treatment in index case	Total number of contacts followed, N	Active TB among contacts, N (%)	Person-Years	Rate of active TB disease per 100 000 person years (95%CI)	Rate Ratio (95%CI)
0–2	869	30 (63.8)	N/A	N/A	N/A
3–6	839	6 (12.8)	419.0	1432.0 (525.5–3117.0)	18.40 (2.22–152.80)
7–12	833	3 (6.4)	832.42	360.4 (74.3–1053.0)	4.63 (4.81–44.51)
13–18	830	7 (14.9)	1216.42	575.5 (231.4–1186.0)	7.39 (0.90–60.09)
19–24	623	1 (2.1)	1284.92	77.8 (1.9–433.6)	1

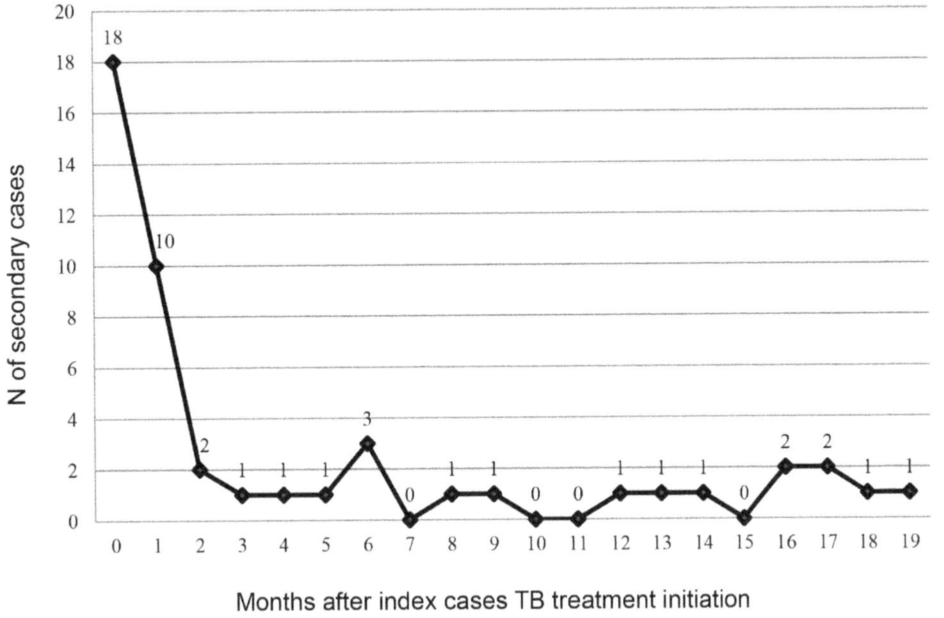

Figure 2. Timing of diagnosis of co-prevalent and incident TB cases among the contacts of index cases, Tbilisi, Georgia, 2010–2011 (n = 47).

patients with higher AFB smear grade were defined as those patients with AFB smear≥2+.

Statistical methods

Data management and statistical analyses were conducted using SPSS v.19.0 (IBM, USA) and OpenEpi v.2.3.1 (Open source). Separate analyses were performed among co-prevalent TB, incident TB, and LTBI cases. The prevalence of active TB disease among contacts during the baseline period was calculated by dividing the number of co-prevalent TB cases by the number of all contacts in the study. The incidence rate of active TB disease among contacts was calculated by dividing the number of incident TB cases by the total number of person-years of follow-up among all contacts at risk of active TB (i.e., excluding co-prevalent TB cases). The prevalence of LTBI among the contacts during the baseline period was calculated by dividing the number of contacts with LTBI by the total number of contacts who did not have active TB disease and had TST performed during the baseline period. We performed univariate analyses to determine factors associated with active TB disease and LTBI among the contacts. To compare rates of incident active TB among the contacts stratified by index patients' and their contacts characteristics, we used exact methods to calculate unadjusted rate ratios (RR) and 95% confidence intervals (CI) [19]. To assess the factors associated with overall active TB disease as well as with prevalent LTBI among the contacts, Mantel-Haenszel chi-square analysis was used to estimate odds ratios (OR) and 95% CI for all active TB cases and LTBI comparisons. A two-sided p-value <0.05 was considered statistically significant.

Results

Between January 2010 and December 2011, 778 active pulmonary TB cases were registered at the ambulatory department of the Georgian NCTBLD (Figure 1). Compared to TB patients who did not refer their contacts to a health care facility for investigation (i.e. those who would be eligible as index patients), enrolled index patients were more likely to be AFB SS (+), culture positive, and have MDR TB (Table 1). A total of 396 (50.9%) index TB cases brought in 869 contacts for investigation; a median of 2 (IQR = 2) contacts were referred per index case. The median age of index cases was 34 years (IQR = 20) and 62.6% were male. Most adult index patients were unemployed (87.8%) and 11.4% had a history of incarceration. The large majority of index cases had culture-confirmed TB (95.9%) and positive AFB sputum smear microscopy (89.9%). Two index cases were AFB smear and culture negative. The prevalence of MDR TB among index cases was 27.6% (Table 1). The median age of contacts was 22 years (IQR = 33) including 131 (15.1%) who were <5 years of age (Table 2).

Active TB disease

Among 869 contacts, 47 (referred by 44 index patients) [5.4% (95% CI 4.0–7.1%)] were found to have active TB at baseline or developed active TB disease during follow-up period. This included 33 cases of pulmonary TB and 14 cases of extrapulmonary TB. Among the 47 contacts with active TB disease, 30 (63.8%)–15 bacteriologically confirmed TB cases and 15 clinically diagnosed TB cases – were found to have active TB during the baseline period (co-prevalent cases) and 17 (36.2%)–8 bacteriologically confirmed TB cases and 9 clinically diagnosed TB cases – developed active TB during the follow-up period (incident TB cases) (Table 3, Figure 1, 2).

During the follow up period 17 of 869 contacts developed active TB for an overall rate of incident active TB of 1126.0 per 100,000 person years (95% CI 655.7–1802.0). During the follow-up period (mean follow up of 21 months), the rate of developing active TB disease among contacts who did not have TB at baseline was highest 3–6 months after their baseline investigation with a rate of 1432.0 per 100,000 person-years. The rate of developing active TB during this 3–6 month period was significantly higher than during the 19–24 months follow-up period (RR = 18.40, 95% CI 2.22–152.80) (Table 3). Among 129 contacts <5 years old who did not have active TB during the baseline period, 4 developed active TB during follow-up period for a rate of 1806.0 per 100,000 person-years. We did not detect any significant predictors of those at increased risk for developing incident TB disease among contacts (Table 4). Out of 17 contacts with incident TB, 7 contacts had LTBI, 5 contacts did not have LTBI and 5 contacts did not perform TST during baseline investigation (Figure 1). We did not detect any significant difference at increased risk for developing incident TB disease between the contacts with or without LTBI.

There was an increased risk of co-prevalent and incident active TB disease among the contacts of previously treated index patients (OR 2.15; 95% CI 1.10–4.19) compared to the contacts of newly diagnosed index TB cases. There was a trend towards increased risk of prevalent and incident active TB disease among contacts aged 15–24 years compared to other age groups (RR 2.41; 95% CI 0.92–6.27) but the difference was not statistically significant (Table 5). The co-prevalence of active TB during the baseline period was 3.5% (30/869) and was lower among young children (1.5% in those <5 years old) compared to children and adults (3.8% in those ≥5 years old) (data not shown).

Latent TB infection

Among those contacts without active TB during the baseline period, 402 (47.9%) of 839 contacts agreed to have a TST performed and 437 (52.1%) declined to have a TST performed. The prevalence of LTBI among this group that had a TST

Table 4. Active incident TB among contacts by age, gender and their index cases' characteristics, Tbilisi, Georgia, 2010–2011.

Socio-demographic and clinical characteristics		N of active incident TB	Rate of active incident TB per 100 000 person years (95%CI)	Rate Ratio (95%CI)
Contacts' Characteristics				
All Contacts		17	1126.0 (655.7–1802.0)	
Gender	Male	7	1070.0 (430.1–2204.0)	1
	Female	10	1169.0 (560.4–2149.0)	1.09 (0.42–2.87)
Age (years)	0–4	4	1806.0 (492.1–4624.0)	6.28 (0.70–56.15)
	5–14	1	287.7 (7.3–1603.0)	1
	15–24	6	2317.0 (850.1–5042.0)	8.05 (0.97–66.87)
	25–34	4	2041.0 (556.0–5225.0)	7.09 (0.79–63.46)
	>=35	2	411.5 (4983.0–1486.0)	1.43 (0.13–5.77)
LTBI	Yes	7	1842 (740.8–3796)	1.23 (0.39–3.87)
	No	5	1502 (487.7–3505)	1
Index cases' characteristics				
All Index cases				
Gender	Male	10	1095.0 (525.0–2013.0)	1
	Female	7	1173.0 (471.7–2417.0)	1.07 (0.41–2.82)
Age (years)	0–34	11	1533.0 (765.1–2742.0)	2.71 (0.86–8.50)
	≥35	4	566.0 (154.2–1449.0)	1
	Missing	2		
Case Definition	Previously treated	4	1499.0 (408.3–3837.0)	1.54 (0.49–4.83)
	New	11	974.4 (486.4–1743.0)	1
	Missing	2		
AFB smear	≥SS(2+)	7	1190.0 (478.6–2453.0)	1.74 (0.51–5.94)
	<SS(2+)	4	684.6 (186.5–1753.0)	1
	Missing	6		
MDR TB Status	MDR TB	1	289.7 (7.3–1614.0)	1
	non MDR TB	14	1369.0 (748.4–2297.0)	4.73 (0.62–35.93)
	Missing	2		
Adult index cases[1]				
Work status	Unemployed	13	1182.0 (629.3–2021.0)	1.05 (0.24–4.63)
	Employed	2	1131.0 (137.0–4086.0)	1
	Missing	2		
History of incarceration	No	13	1137.0 (605.6–1945.0)	1
	Yes	2	1333.0 (161.5–4817.0)	1.17 (0.26–5.18)
	Missing	2		

[1]index cases>17 years of age.

Abbreviations: AFB – Acid-fast bacilli; SS – sputum smear; MDR – Multidrug-resistant.

Table 5. Active Co-prevalent and incident TB among contacts by age, gender and their index cases' characteristics, Tbilisi, Georgia, 2010–2011.

Socio-demographic and clinical characteristics		Contact Status			OR (95%CI)
		Active TB disease N=47 (%)	No TB disease N=822 (%)	Total N=869 (%)	
Contacts' Characteristics					
All contacts					
Gender	Male	18 (38.3)	355 (43.2)	373 (42.9)	0.82 (0.45–1.49)
	Female	29 (61.7)	467 (56.8)	496 (57.1)	1
Age (years)	0–4	6 (12.8)	125 (15.2)	131 (15.1)	1.31 (0.43–3.99)
	5–14	7 (14.9)	191 (23.2)	198 (22.8)	1
	15–24	12 (25.5)	136 (16.5)	148 (17.0)	2.41 (0.92–6.27)
	25–34	7 (14.9)	105 (12.8)	112 (12.9)	1.82 (0.62–5.33)
	≥35	15 (31.9)	265 (32.3)	280 (32.2)	1.54 (0.62–3.86)
Index cases' characteristics					
All Index cases					
Gender	Male	29 (61.7)	496 (60.3)	525 (60.4)	1.06 (0.58–1.94)
	Female	18 (38.3)	326 (39.7)	344 (39.6)	1
Age (years)	0–34	26 (59.1)	388 (49.8)	414 (50.3)	1.46 (0.79–2.70)
	≥35	18 (40.9)	391 (50.2)	409 (49.7)	1
	Missing			46	
Case Definition	Previously treated	14 (33.3)	144 (18.9)	158 (19.6)	2.15 (1.10–4.19)
	New	28 (66.7)	619 (81.1)	647 (80.4)	1
	Missing			64	
AFB smear	≥SS (2+)	18 (56.3)	329 (51.2)	347 (51.5)	1.22 (0.59–2.50)
	<SS(2+)	14 (43.8)	313 (48.8)	327 (48.5)	1
	Missing			195	
MDR TB Status	MDR TB	13 (31.0)	192 (25.6)	205 (25.9)	1.30 (0.66–2.55)
	non MDR TB	29 (69.0)	557 (74.4)	586 (74.1)	1
	Missing			78	
Adult index cases[1]					
Work status	Unemployed	33 (89.2)	603 (86.4)	636 (86.5)	1.30 (0.45–3.75)
	Employed	4 (10.8)	95 (13.6)	99 (13.5)	1
	Missing			68	
History of incarceration	No	35 (89.7)	623 (88.1)	658 (88.2)	1.18 (0.41–3.40)
	Yes	4 (10.3)	84 (11.9)	88 (11.8)	1
	Missing			57	

[1]index cases>17 years of age.
Abbreviations: AFB – Acid-fast bacilli; SS – sputum smear; MDR – Multidrug-resistant.

performed was 52.7% (95% CI 47.7–57.7%) (212 out of 402 had LTBI) (Figure 1). We did not detect any characteristics of index patients or contacts that were statistically significantly associated with risk of LTBI. IPT was taken by 14 (16.9%) of 83 children aged <5 years old who were the contacts of drug-susceptible TB index cases. None of the contacts receiving IPT developed active TB disease, while one child who did not receive IPT developed active TB disease during the follow-up period.

Discussion

There is increasing interest in the utility of contact investigation in LMIC where contact investigation has traditionally not been part of TB control efforts [20]. In 2010–2011 an "invitation" model of contact investigation (where index patients are asked to invite their contacts to be investigated at a health care facility), was implemented within the NTP of Georgia. Our study demonstrated that an "invitation" model of contact investigation, which is a type of passive contact investigation, was an efficient method. We found a high prevalence of active TB cases (3.5%) among contacts of index patients during the baseline period. The invitation model of contact investigation requires few resources, can be easily implemented into ongoing TB control activities and may significantly increase TB case finding in other LMIC's, which do not currently include contact investigations in their national TB program strategy.

We found the invitation model of contact investigation to be an efficient mechanism to implement TB contact investigations without significantly increasing costs. Nonetheless, previous studies have noted active TB contact investigations to have higher yields. A study performed in rural Malawi reported a higher yield of TB cases that were identified among the HH contacts of SS (+) pulmonary TB cases by using active case finding; TB prevalence by passive case finding among HH contacts was 191 per 100,000 and TB prevalence with active case finding was 1735.0 per 100,000 [21]. Another study from Lima, Peru, concluded that inclusion of active case finding importantly increased the identification of TB cases [22]. Significant more resources are required for active contact tracing which has been a barrier to implementation of contact investigation in many LMIC.

As noted, we found a high prevalence (3.5%) of active TB cases among contacts of index patients (30 TB cases among 869 contacts) during the baseline period. Another 17 contacts developed active TB disease during the follow-up period. TB incidence was similar in contacts with or without LTBI. Random error could account for the non-significance in rate ratios that was observed in our study. Because the sample size of our study population was relatively modest, random error is a possible explanation. Overall, we found a high proportion (5.4%) of active TB cases among contacts of index patients. We also found an increased risk of developing active TB disease among the contacts of previously treated index patients which may be due to very prolonged exposure to an infectious index case. Most of the TB cases among contacts (64%) were co-prevalent TB cases, indicating that active TB disease was identified among contacts during the contact investigation at baseline.

Our study also had important findings regarding LTBI. We observed that LTBI was highly prevalent among contacts of index patients; more than half of the contacts without active TB disease who agreed to undergo TST had prevalent LTBI. The prevalence of LTBI among the general population in Georgia is poorly defined so it is not clear how the prevalence of LTBI in contacts compares to the general population although we hypothesize that it is likely significantly higher among contacts. Despite WHO recommendations that all contacts of non-MDR TB cases who are <5 years of age should receive IPT [5,23], relatively few children in our study received such treatment for LTBI (15%). The low level of LTBI treatment among young children who were contacts suggests that health care workers in Georgia may benefit from additional training regarding the benefits of IPT and changes should be made to implement current policy and WHO based recommendations on use of IPT in young children. Our findings that IPT was infrequently used for those children <5 years old, who were the contacts of drug-susceptible index cases is also consistent with the knowledge, attitudes, and practices survey conducted among healthcare workers in Georgia. According to this study, many health care workers in Georgia had incomplete knowledge about LTBI [24].

Our findings are the first data reported from Georgia on the utility of contact investigation. The finding of a high prevalence of active TB disease and LTBI among contacts of index TB cases provides data on the utility of contact investigation and in our setting this was done with limited resources using an "invitation" model. A systematic review and meta-analysis of active TB and LTBI among close contacts of index cases with pulmonary TB in LMIC showed that 4.5% of all household contacts had active TB disease at the time of investigation and 51.4% had LTBI [25]. In most reports, incident TB cases among contacts occurred within the first year (particularly within the first 6 months) after detection of the index case [26].

Our study is subject to several limitations. First, because the study included only contacts of index TB cases that received care from NCTBLD in Tbilisi, the cohort may not be representative of the entire country of Georgia. Moreover, contact investigations conducted at the time of the study were passive ("invitation") and required index patients to refer their contacts to the NCTBLD for evaluation. Consequently, the contacts evaluated in our study may not be generalizable to all TB contacts. However, given the substantial resources needed to conduct investigations on all TB contacts, our "invitation" approach may be a very cost effective way to evaluate contacts and detect new TB cases. Second, because we did not perform genotyping of *M. tuberculosis* strains, we were not able to compare transmission patterns and were unable to definitively determine if transmission occurred from the contacts' index patient or from another source. Future studies that use strain identification of *M. tuberculosis* with genotyping methods among index patients and their contacts are needed to confirm our findings. Third, all TB contacts were not systematically screened for active TB during the follow-up period which could have resulted in an underestimation of the incidence of TB among contacts. Similarly, if contacts developed TB but did not seek care at the NCTBLD the case would not have been identified.

Conclusion

The burden of active TB disease and LTBI was high among the contacts of active TB cases in this study carried out in Tbilisi, Georgia. We demonstrated that an "invitation" model of contact investigation was an efficient method to expand TB case finding among contacts of index TB cases in a recourse-limited setting. Our results suggest that in LMIC such as Georgia, aggressive and timely contact investigation may efficiently enhance TB case finding among recent contacts. Public health interventions are needed to scale up contact investigations and more aggressively identify contacts of index TB cases.

Author Contributions

Conceived and designed the experiments: TC MJM RRK MG LG UN HMB. Performed the experiments: TC MJM RRK MG LG UN HMB. Analyzed the data: TC MJM RRK MG LG UN HMB. Contributed reagents/materials/analysis tools: TC MJM RRK MG LG UN HMB. Wrote the paper: TC MJM RRK MG LG UN HMB.

References

1. National Tuberculosis Controllers Association, Centers for Disease Control and Prevention. (2005) Guidelines for the investigation of contacts of persons with infectious tuberculosis. Recommendations from the National Tuberculosis Controllers Association and CDC. MMWR Recomm Rep 54: 1–47.
2. Taylor Z, Nolan CM, Blumberg HM (2005) Controlling tuberculosis in the United States. Recommendations from the American Thoracic Society, CDC, and the Infectious Diseases Society of America. MMWR Recomm Rep 54: 1–81.
3. Dye C, Floyd K (2006) Tuberculosis. In: Jamison DT, Breman JG, Measham AR, Alleyne G, Claeson M et al., editors. Disease Control Priorities in Developing Countries. 2nd ed. Washington (DC).
4. Arnadottir T (2009) Tuberculosis and Public Health. Policy and Principles in Tuberculosis Control: Paris, France: International Union Against Tuberculosis and Lung Diseases.
5. World Health Organization. (2012). Recommendations for Investigating Contacts of Persons with Infectious Tuberculosis in Low- and Middle-Income Countries. Geneva.

6. Tuberculosis Coalition for Technical Assistance. (2009) International Standards for Tuberculosis Care (ISTC), second edition: Tuberculosis Coalition for Technical Assistance, The Hague.
7. Mdivani N, Zangaladze E, Volkova N, Kourbatova E, Jibuti T, et al. (2008) High prevalence of multidrug-resistant tuberculosis in Georgia. Int J Infect Dis 12: 635–644.
8. Lomtadze N, Aspindzelashvili R, Janjgava M, Mirtskhulava V, Wright A, et al. (2009) Prevalence and risk factors for multidrug-resistant tuberculosis in the Republic of Georgia: a population-based study. Int J Tuberc Lung Dis 13: 68–73.
9. World Health Organization. (2013) Global tuberculosis report 2013 (in IRIS). Geneva: World Health Organization. xi, 289 p. p.
10. Fair E, Miller C (2013) What to Monitor and Evaluate in TB Contact Investigation: Tanzania Experience and Lessons Learned. 44th Union World Conference on Lung Health. Paris, France.
11. Whitaker JA, Mirtskhulava V, Kipiani M, Harris DA, Tabagari N, et al. (2013) Prevalence and incidence of latent tuberculosis infection in georgian healthcare workers. PLoS One 8: e58202.
12. Weinstock DM, Hahn O, Wittkamp M, Sepkowitz KA, Khechinashvili G, et al. (2001) Risk for tuberculosis infection among internally displaced persons in the Republic of Georgia. Int J Tuberc Lung Dis 5: 164–169.
13. Hill PC, Ota MO (2010) Tuberculosis case-contact research in endemic tropical settings: design, conduct, and relevance to other infectious diseases. Lancet Infect Dis 10: 723–732.
14. American Thoracic Society., Centers for Disease Control and Prevention. (2000) Targeted tuberculin testing and treatment of latent tuberculosis infection. MMWR Recomm Rep 49: 1–51.
15. Centers for Disease Control and Prevention. (2013) Latent Tuberculosis Infection: A Guide for Primary Health Care Providers.
16. World Health Organization. (2013) definitions and reporting framework for tuberculosis - 2013 revision. Euro Surveill 18: 20455.
17. Drobniewski FA, Hoffner S, Rusch-Gerdes S, Skenders G, Thomsen V, et al. (2006) Recommended standards for modern tuberculosis laboratory services in Europe. Eur Respir J 28: 903–909.
18. Gegia M, Cohen T, Kalandadze I, Vashakidze L, Furin J (2012) Outcomes among tuberculosis patients with isoniazid resistance in Georgia, 2007–2009. Int J Tuberc Lung Dis 16: 812–816.
19. Martin DO, Austin H (1996) Exact estimates for a rate ratio. Epidemiology 7: 29–33.
20. Fox GJ, Barry SE, Britton WJ, Marks GB (2013) Contact investigation for tuberculosis: a systematic review and meta-analysis. Eur Respir J 41: 140–156.
21. Zachariah R, Spielmann MP, Harries AD, Gomani P, Graham SM, et al. (2003) Passive versus active tuberculosis case finding and isoniazid preventive therapy among household contacts in a rural district of Malawi. Int J Tuberc Lung Dis 7(11): 1033–1039.
22. Becerra MC, Pachao-Torreblanca IF, Bayona J, Celi R, Shin SS, et al. (2005) Expanding tuberculosis case detection by screening household contacts. Public Health Reports 120: 271–277.
23. Rieder HL (2003) Contacts of tuberculosis patients in high-incidence countries. Int J Tuberc Lung Dis 7: S333–336.
24. Mirtskhulava V WJ, Kipiani M, Harris D, Blumberg HM. Latent tuberculosis infection and tuberculosis infection control knowledge, attitudes, and practices survey of health care workers in the country of Georgia; 2012; Kuala-Lumpur, Malaysia. International Union against Tuberculosis and Lung Diseases (The Union). pp. S237.
25. Morrison J, Pai M, Hopewell PC (2008) Tuberculosis and latent tuberculosis infection in close contacts of people with pulmonary tuberculosis in low-income and middle-income countries: a systematic review and meta-analysis. Lancet Infect Dis 8: 359–368.
26. Ling DL, Liaw YP, Lee CY, Lo HY, Yang HL, et al. (2011) Contact investigation for tuberculosis in Taiwan contacts aged under 20 years in 2005. Int J Tuberc Lung Dis 15: 50–55.

20

Taurolidine Lock Is Superior to Heparin Lock in the Prevention of Catheter Related Bloodstream Infections and Occlusions

Evelyn D. Olthof[1], Michelle W. Versleijen[2], Getty Huisman-de Waal[1,3], Ton Feuth[4], Wietske Kievit[4], Geert J. A. Wanten[1]*

1 Intestinal Failure Unit, Department of Gastroenterology and Hepatology, Radboud University Medical Center, Nijmegen, The Netherlands, **2** Department of Nuclear Medicine, Netherlands Cancer Institute - Antoni van Leeuwenhoek, Amsterdam, The Netherlands, **3** Scientific Institute for Quality of Healthcare, Radboud University Medical Center, Nijmegen, The Netherlands, **4** Department of Health Evidence, Radboud University Medical Center, Nijmegen, The Netherlands

Abstract

Background and Aims: Patients on home parenteral nutrition (HPN) are at risk for catheter-related complications; mainly infections and occlusions. We have previously shown in HPN patients presenting with catheter sepsis that catheter locking with taurolidine dramatically reduced re-infections when compared with heparin. Our HPN population therefore switched from heparin to taurolidine in 2008. The aim of the present study was to compare long-term effects of this catheter lock strategy on the occurrence of catheter-related bloodstream infections and occlusions in HPN patients.

Methods: Data of catheter-related complications were retrospectively collected from 212 patients who received HPN between January 2000 and November 2011, comprising 545 and 200 catheters during catheter lock therapy with heparin and taurolidine, respectively. We evaluated catheter-related bloodstream infection and occlusion incidence rates using Poisson-normal regression analysis. Incidence rate ratios were calculated by dividing incidence rates of heparin by those of taurolidine, adjusting for underlying disease, use of anticoagulants or immune suppressives, frequency of HPN/fluid administration, composition of infusion fluids, and duration of HPN/fluid use before catheter creation.

Results: Bloodstream infection incidence rates were 1.1/year for heparin and 0.2/year for taurolidine locked catheters. Occlusion incidence rates were 0.2/year for heparin and 0.1/year for taurolidine locked catheters. Adjusted incidence ratios of heparin compared to taurolidine were 5.9 (95% confidence interval, 3.9–8.7) for bloodstream infections and 1.9 (95% confidence interval, 1.1–3.1) for occlusions.

Conclusions: Given that no other procedural changes than the catheter lock strategy were implemented during the observation period, these data strongly suggest that taurolidine decreases catheter-related bloodstream infections and occlusions in HPN patients compared with heparin.

Editor: Daniel Schneditz, Medical University of Graz, Austria

Funding: This study was supported by a research grant from: Geistlich Pharma (Wolhusen Switzerland). The funders had no role in study design, data collection and analysis, decision to publish, or preparation of the manuscript.

Competing Interests: The authors of this manuscript have the following competing interests: GJAW has performed research and given presentations that were supported by fees from Geistlich and grants from Geistlich Pharma, Fresenius Kabi and Baxter. EDO, MWJV, GJHW, TF and WK declare no conflict of interest.

* Email: Geert.Wanten@radboudumc.nl

Introduction

Catheter-related bloodstream infections (CRBSIs) remain the major, potentially life-threatening, complication of home parenteral nutrition (HPN) therapy. As such, CRBSIs pose a massive burden on the patients'quality of life and hospital resources due to the frequent need for hospital admission, surgical and medical interventions and, eventually, the need for intestinal transplantation when venous access becomes irreversibly compromised [1].

Patient-, therapy- and device-related risk factors for CRBSIs have been characterized previously in detail [2]. The nature of the underlying disease leading to intestinal failure may increase the risk of CRBSI [3]. Also factors that are related to the composition of the parenteral nutrition formulation, such as caloric content and the presence of a lipid emulsion play a role [4], as well as the frequency and duration of the use of the venous access device [5]. The presence of a venous access device that bypasses the natural host barriers by directly connecting the external environment to the patients' central bloodstream, has been identified as an independent risk factor for the occurrence of CRBSIs [6]. The magnitude of the risk also depends on catheter material [5], site of catheter insertion [7], and catheter coating [8]. Finally, the agent that is used to lock the central venous catheter (CVC) after infusion of the parenteral nutrition is increasingly being recognized as pivotal in the prevention of CRBSIs [9].

Several lock solutions, some of which include (combinations of) anticoagulants, fibrinolytic agents, antiseptics and antibiotics, have been introduced, but failed because of side effects, microbial resistance issues or lack in effectiveness [10]. Taurolidine, a microbiocidal agent, has a broad spectrum activity against bacteria and fungi [11]. The suggested microbiocidal activity of taurolidine involves a chemical interaction with the microbial cell wall resulting in irreparable injury [12]. Taurolidine has shown to reduce the risk for CRBSIs in several patient groups who depend on a reliable central venous access device [9,13–19]. A recent meta-analysis confirms these beneficial effects, but also emphasizes low power and methodological flaws of the currently available studies [20].

A randomized trial in our own tertiary HPN referral center comparing the catheter lock strategy using 2% taurolidine (Taurosept) and low dose (150 U/mL) heparin on the recurrence of CRBSIs was preliminary terminated due to the dramatic decrease in CRBSIs in taurolidine locked catheters that became apparent because of the open label character of this study [9]. Although the sample size of this formal randomized trial was very low (heparin: n = 14), taurolidine (n = 16), we considered the results evident enough to switch from low dose heparin to 2% taurolidine catheter locking in all of our HPN patients in the fall of 2008. In the present study, we provide further evidence that taurolidine may be more effective in preventing catheter-related complications in HPN patients compared to heparin, using a comprehensive dataset of long-term catheter locking, covering the period from 2000 to late 2008 (using low-dose heparin) and the period from 2008 to 2011 (using taurolidine). The study comprises 212 patients, 745 central venous catheters and more than 200,000 catheter days, and provides by far the most robust dataset in this field so far. Importantly, none of our HPN practice procedures or materials, other than the catheter lock strategy, changed during the complete observation period.

Patients and Methods

Ethics

The research ethics committee of the Radboud University Nijmegen Medical Centre (CMO Regio Arnhem-Nijmegen) approved this retrospective study under the protocol number (CMO: 2014/167). This ethics committee confirmed that individual written informed consent was not needed. Data was collected, anonymized and de-identified by the treating physician (GW). Subsequently data were entered in a database and statistical analysis was performed.

Patients

We enrolled all consecutive patients on long-term (>3 months and >1/week used for HPN/fluid administration) HPN or fluids using a central venous catheter (Hickman or Port-A-Cath (PAC, implantable port)) at the Radboud University Medical Centre, Nijmegen, the Netherlands, between January 1st, 2000 and November 1st, 2011 (n = 212). Medical records of all patients were reviewed. Patients were categorized into one of five underlying disease groups, based on the indication for fluid/HPN treatment: motility disorder, short bowel with stoma, short bowel without stoma, impaired intestinal absorption (mainly due to radiation enteritis), or other. Data on time and site of catheter insertion were checked in operation reports.

Cleaning protocol of catheter

Only single lumen catheters were placed. During the observation period of this study, none of our cleaning protocol procedures changed. In general, patients are trained in procedures including catheter handling and HPN/fluid administration during an inpatient training period of 1 to 2 weeks in our hospital.

Independent of the access type, the patient's or care-givers's hands are washed and subsequently disinfected with chlorhexidine in ethanol prior to HPN/fluid administration or cleaning of the exit site or skin. Cleaning protocols for Hickman catheter and PAC in our hospital are described in more detail in the following text.

For Hickman catheters, the catheter exit site is covered direct after catheter insertion with a Tegaderm pad (3M Health Care, Neuss, Germany) which is replaced every 96 hours. The exit site is disinfected by circular movements from the exit site to the outer circumference. Every circle is disinfected with a new sterile swap. The first 10 centimeters of the catheter is disinfected with a sterile swap and chlorhexidine in ethanol. After drying, the exit site is covered with a new Tegaderm pad. After 3 weeks, the catheter cuff has grown in the surrounding tissues and sutures for line fixation are removed. From then on, the exit site is no longer covered with a Tegaderm pad and is cleaned daily by washing with water and soap and drying with a clean towel.

For PACs, after placement the wound is covered with sterile compresses. Before HPN/fluid administration, the skin overlying the subcutaneous port is cleaned with chlorhexidine by the described circular movement method above. After HPN administration, the puncture-site is covered with a sterile compress for a few minutes, until (minor) bleeding ends.

Catheter lock solution

Central venous catheters were locked after every administration of HPN or fluids. After a successful open label randomized controlled trial [9], all HPN patients with a Hickman or PAC switched from low dose (150 U/mL) heparin to 2% taurolidine (Taurosept) in 2008. Of every individual patient the date of switching from heparin to taurolidine was used for data analysis.

In case a catheter was locked with heparin and subsequently with taurolidine, only the period before starting taurolidine was analyzed, since catheter related complications after start of taurolidine could possibly be a consequence of a carry-over effect of locking with heparin, since a biofilm that originated from the heparin period might lead to a CRBSI in the taurolidine period. In that case, the total number of catheter days was calculated from insertion of the catheter to the starting date of the catheter lock solution taurolidine (Figure 1).

Catheter related bloodstream infections and occlusions

CRBSIs were defined by the presence of symptoms (fever, chills) associated with positive blood cultures (blood drawn from peripheral vein and/or from venous access device) in the absence of other evident infectious foci that likely could explain the bloodstream infection. Episodes with fever and/or chills without positive blood cultures were only considered a bloodstream infection in case blood samples were drawn under antibiotic treatment (possibly leading to negative blood cultures) and in case patients were showing signs of sepsis [5]. The date of the CRBSI was the date of the first positive blood culture. A CRBSI was considered polymicrobial when different pathogens were found in the peripheral and/or venous access blood culture. All pathogens, were classified as Gram positive or Gram negative bacteria or yeast.

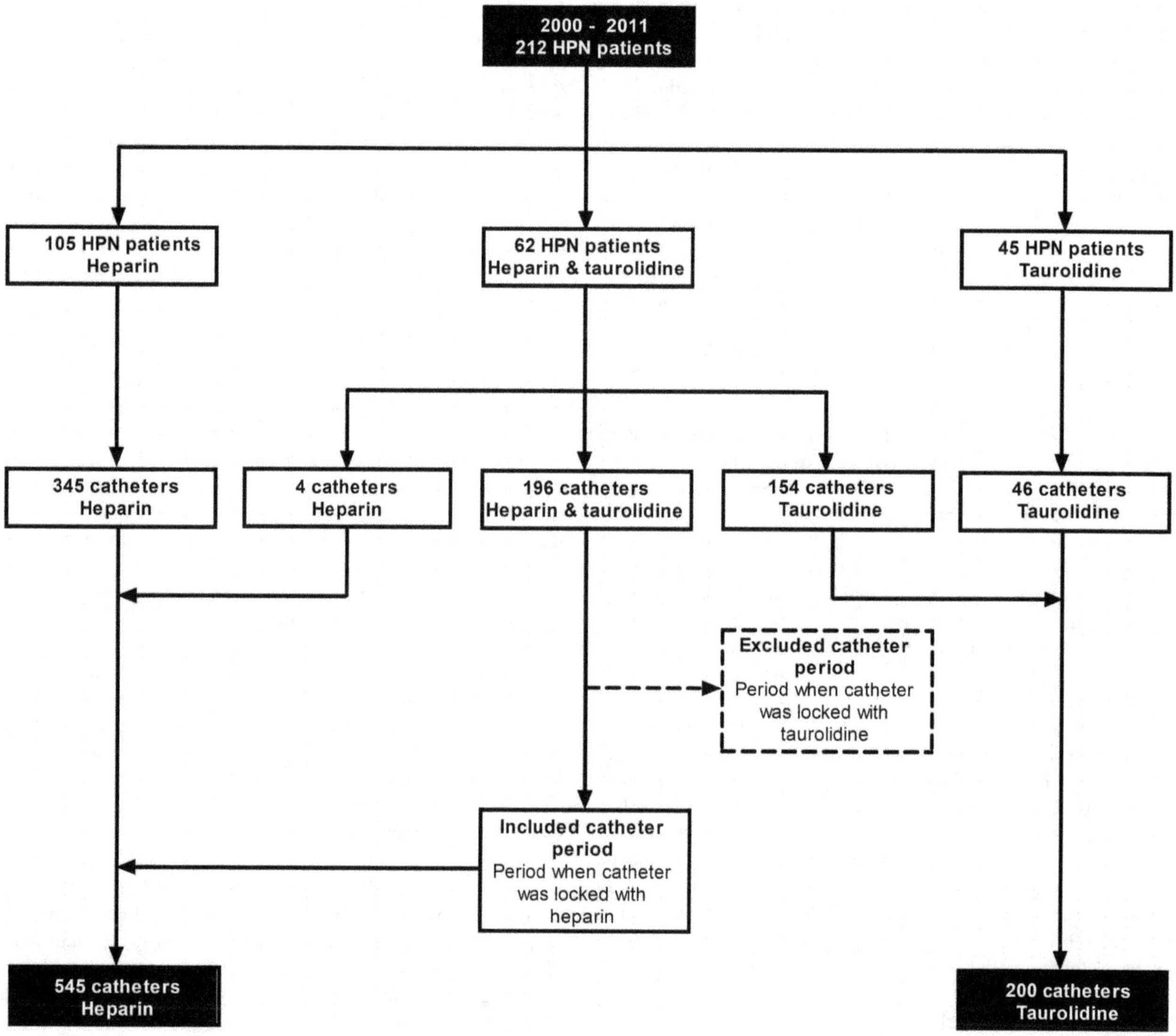

Figure 1. Flowchart of numbers of patients and catheters.

Catheter occlusions were defined by an obstruction of the central venous catheter, described in the medical record, or a vascular occlusion of more than 50% of a vein near the insertion side of the central venous catheter, described in report of a duplex scan. The date of occlusion was the date of the first time that this occlusion was described.

Treatment

Data on the use of anticoagulants and immune suppressive medication, and the type of HPN/fluid formulation and the frequency of HPN/fluid administrations per week was obtained from pharmacy prescriptions. Catheters were described as catheters which were exposed to only fluids, only HPN or a combination of both.

Hospital admission

We evaluated hospital admission data in the pre (2006–2007) and post (2009–2011) taurolidine eras. The transition year 2008 included hospital admissions with taurolidine and heparin locked catheters. No detailed hospital admission data were available of the period before 2006. All hospital admissions for in-hospital training of aseptic catheter techniques were excluded from analysis, since these admissions were not due to complications. Hospital admission were presented as the days that the patients were admitted to our ward in one year divided by the total number of catheter days in that year.

Adverse events

Adverse events resulting in discontinuation of the use of taurolidine were reported. If possible, patients switched first to another taurolidine-containing lock in the form of taurolidine-citrate (Taurolock) and in case of repeated adverse effects switched to saline.

Statistical analysis

Characteristics of patients, vascular accesses and CRBSIs were presented as number (n) with percentage (%), or mean with 95% confidence interval (CI), or median with 25th and 75th percentile. Chi-square test for categorical data and Mann Whitney U test for continuous data were used to compare the heparin and taurolidine group in Table 1 and 2. Statistical significance was accepted if the probability of a type I error did not exceed 5%. We analyzed incidence rates and incidence rate ratios (i.e., the complication incidence rate that occurred with catheters locked with heparin divided by those locked with taurolidine) of CRBSIs and occlusions using random effects model with Poisson distributions for counts. Random effects for patients were incorporated in the modeling process to account for repeated vascular access periods within a patient. Possible confounders in the relation between catheter lock solution and complication rate were identified and reported, based on biological and clinical rationales [5], or a change of 10% or more on unadjusted complication rate ratios by a covariate. Adjusted complication incidence rate ratios for heparin over taurolidine were calculated with respect to these confounders. The NLMIXED procedure of SAS System for Windows version 9.2 was used (SAS Institute Inc, Cary, NC). Statistical significance was accepted if the probability of a type I error did not exceed 5%. To provide information about statistical significance, we reported 95% CI where appropriate. In case data were missing from medical records these were considered to be completely at random and were excluded from analyses.

Results

Study population

212 HPN patients were included in the study: 62 patients had multiple catheters that were initially locked with heparin and later catheters that were locked with taurolidine, 105 patients had catheters that were exclusively locked with heparin, and 45 patients had their catheters exclusively locked with taurolidine (Figure 1). Most patients were male (n (%): 102 (61%) and 74 (69%) in heparin and taurolidine group, respectively). Patients started HPN at a mean (95% CI) age of 48 years (18–78 years) in the heparin group and 49 years (22–77 years) in the taurolidine group. The major indications for HPN (n (%)) use were motility disorder and short bowel syndrome with or without a stoma; 46 (28%), 32 (19%) and 69 (41%) patients in the heparin group, and 40 (37%), 28 (26%) and 34 (32%) patients in the taurolidine group, respectively. Less common indication of HPN was impaired intestinal absorption; 9 (5%) and 4 (4%) patients in the heparin and taurolidine group, respectively. All remaining patients were classified as other HPN indication (n (%)); 11 (7%) patients with heparin locked catheters and 1 (1%) patient with taurolidine locked catheters. The majority of patients (n (%)) was trained at our tertiary referral centre in aseptic catheter handling and parenteral nutrition administration; this concerned 143 (86%) patients for the heparin and 83 (78%) patients for the taurolidine group.

Vascular accesses

The characteristics of a total of 745 central venous catheters, of which 545 were locked with heparin and 200 with taurolidine were included (Figure 1) and analyzed (Table 1). In both groups Hickman catheters (about 70%) were used more frequently than PACs (about 30%). Around 75% of the catheters were inserted in the jugular or subclavian veins; in the heparin group the subclavian vein (62%) was the most common insertion place, while in the taurolidine group the jugular vein (52%) was mostly used. Catheter survival (days: median (25th–75th percentile)) was longer in the taurolidine group (209 days (65–611 days)) compared to the heparin group (120 days (43–310 days)). The total number of catheter days was 147,842 for the 545 heparin locked catheters and 71,112 for the 200 taurolidine locked catheters. Patients with catheters in the taurolidine group were more experienced in the administration of HPN/fluids (probably a consequence of having had heparin locked catheters before), since the median (25th–75th percentile) duration from the start of HPN/fluid use to the creation of the venous access was longer; 214 days (34–765 days) for the heparin group and 564 days (103–1489 days) for the taurolidine group. Most catheters were used more than 5 days a week (75% and 71%, in the heparin and taurolidine group, respectively). HPN only was administered in 53% and 59%, in the heparin and taurolidine group, respectively, whilst a combination of HPN and fluids was administered in 32% and 31%, respectively. A minority, 6% of heparin and 8% of taurolidine catheters, was used for fluid administration only. Half of the catheters (53% and 55% in heparin and taurolidine group, respectively) were inserted in patients who used anticoagulants, and less than a quarter (15% and 21% in heparin and taurolidine group, respectively) of the catheters were inserted in patients who used immune suppressive medication.

Bloodstream infections and occlusion incidence rates

CRBSIs were 464 and 43 times detected in heparin and taurolidine locked catheters, respectively. Table 2 presents the characteristics of these CRBSIs. Forty-four percent of CRBSIs had both a positive blood culture of peripheral and venous access origin. The majority of CRBSIs (74 and 65% in heparin and taurolidine group, respectively) was based on a single type of pathogen. The most common microbial species that caused these CRBSIs were Gram-positive bacteria, followed by Gram-negative bacteria and fungi.

Table 3 shows the unadjusted incidence rates and the adjusted (for confounders) incidence rate ratios of heparin over taurolidine. Bloodstream infection incidence rates (per access year (95% CI)) were 1.1 per access year (0.9–1.3 per access year) in the heparin group and 0.2 per access year (0.1–0.2 per access year) in the taurolidine group. The bloodstream infection incidence ratio, of heparin compared to taurolidine incidence rates, adjusted for confounders (underlying disease, anticoagulant use, immune suppressive use, HPN/fluid frequency per week, composition of infusional fluid, place of catheter insertion and HPN/fluid use before creation catheter), was 5.9 (95% CI, 3.9–8.7).

Catheter related vascular occlusions were 137 and 34 times detected in heparin and taurolidine locked central venous catheters, respectively. As presented in Table 3, occlusion rates (per access year (95% CI)) were slightly lower in the taurolidine group (0.1 per access year (0.1–0.2 per access year)) compared to the heparin group (0.2 per access year (0.2–0.3 per access year)). The occlusion incidence ratio, of heparin compared to taurolidine incidence rates, adjusted for confounders (underlying disease, anticoagulant use, immune suppressive use, HPN/fluid frequency per week, composition of infusional fluid, place of catheter insertion and HPN/fluid use before creation catheter), was 1.9 (95% CI, 1.1–3.1).

Hospital admissions

From 2006 towards the end of 2011 the number of HPN-related admission days at our 15-bed clinical ward remained stable at a mean (± SD) of 1173±159 days per year, while the HPN population increased from 61 to 133 patients, hence the number of catheter days increased from 21,619 to 45,960. Therefore, the ratio of hospital admission days per catheter day decreased by 60% from 0.055 in two pre-taurolidine years to 0.022 in 2011 (Figure 2).

Table 1. Vascular access characteristics.

	Heparin (n = 545)	Taurolidine (n = 200)	p-value
Duration of HPN/fluid use before creation catheter (days: median (25th–75th percentile))	214 (34–765)	564 (103–1489)	0.000*
Unknown (n (%))	7 (1)	0 (0)	
Type of vascular access (n (%))			0.536
Hickman	368 (68)	140 (70)	
Port à cath	177 (32)	60 (30)	
Place of catheter insertion (n (%))			0.000*
Subclavian vein	337 (62)	57 (29)	
Jugular vein	63 (12)	105 (52)	
Femoral vein	33 (6)	19 (9)	
Inferior caval vein	13 (2)	6 (3)	
Unknown	99 (18)	13 (7)	
Catheter survival (days)			0.000*
Median (25th–75th percentile)	120 (43–310)	209 (65–611)	
Total number of catheter days of all catheters	147,842	71,112	
Number of catheters still in place (n (%))			0.000*
Yes	1 (0)	80 (40)	
No	544 (100)	120 (60)	
Composition of infusional fluid (n (%))			0.380
HPN alone	290 (53)	118 (59)	
Fluid alone	30 (6)	16 (8)	
HPN & fluid	178 (32)	61 (31)	
Unknown	47 (9)	5 (2)	
HPN/fluid administration frequency, per week (n (%))			0.529
1	3 (1)	1 (1)	
2	5 (1)	4 (2)	
3	32 (6)	14 (7)	
4	34 (6)	18 (9)	
5	50 (9)	21 (11)	
6	44 (8)	11 (5)	
7	319 (58)	111 (55)	
Unknown	58 (11)	20 (10)	
Immune suppressive use (n (%))			0.121
Yes	83 (15)	41 (21)	
No	437 (80)	154 (77)	
Unknown	25 (5)	5 (2)	
Anticoagulant use (n (%))			0.932
Yes	288 (53)	111 (55)	
No	220 (40)	83 (42)	
Unknown	37 (7)	6 (3)	

Variables are shown per vascular access. Patients may have had multiple vascular accesses, total number of patients assessed is 212 (Figure 1). Characteristics were presented as number of events (n) with percentage (%) or median with 25th and 75th percentile. A p-value lower than 0.05 was considered statistically significant.

Adverse events

Since the switch from heparin to taurolidine 8 of the 107 patients reported adverse events possibly related to use of taurolidine, and did not continue using pure taurolidine as a result. One patient experienced an anaphylactic-like reaction (vomiting, shortness of breath and urticaria) within minutes after the first administration and switched to saline for catheter locking. Five patients, who experienced a burning sensation, PAC occlusion, dizziness, nausea or pain and paresthesia, switched first to taurolidine-citrate, but experienced similar adverse reactions and switched thereafter successfully to saline. Two patients who experienced palpitations or discomfort over the chest switched successfully to taurolidine-citrate.

Table 2. Characteristics of catheter related bloodstream infections.

	Heparin	Taurolidine	p-value
Origin positive blood cultures (n (%))			0.000*
Peripheral	34 (7)	15 (35)	
Catheter	217 (47)	9 (21)	
Both	206 (44)	19 (44)	
Unknown	6 (1)	0 (0)	
Type of bloodstream infection (n (%))			0.147
Monomicrobial	345 (74)	28 (65)	
Polymicrobial	113 (24)	15 (35)	
Unknown	6 (2)	0 (0)	
Type of pathogens in peripheral blood culture (n (%))**			0.093
Gram positive bacteria	164 (57)	24 (55)	
Gram negative bacteria	94 (32)	11 (25)	
Yeast	26 (9)	9 (20)	
Unknown	6 (2)	0 (0)	
Type of pathogens in catheter blood culture (n (%))**			0.332
Gram positive bacteria	313 (55)	24 (57)	
Gram negative bacteria	209 (37)	12 (29)	
Yeast	43 (7)	6 (14)	
Unknown	6 (1)	0 (0)	

Characteristics were presented as number of events (n) with percentage (%). *A p-value lower than 0.05 was considered statistically significant. **More pathogens than CRBSI, because of polymicrobial infections and differences in positive blood cultures between blood cultures of peripheral and venous access origin.

Discussion

The availability and maintenance of an adequate and reliable venous access remains the foremost worry in long-term HPN care, with catheter related complications, mainly infections and occlusions, causing the majority of problems. This study presents by far the most robust data set so far to demonstrate that the use of taurolidine as catheter lock versus low-dose heparin decreases catheter related complications. During an observation period spanning over 200,000 catheter days, we found an impressive six times higher chance of developing CRBSI in heparin compared to taurolidine locked catheters. Also, a two times higher risk for developing catheter occlusions in heparin locked compared to taurolidine locked catheters was observed. Interestingly, we saw that this decrease in catheter complications was accompanied by a steep decrease in strain on healthcare resources in the form of diminished hospital admissions. Importantly, none of our other HPN-related procedures or techniques changed during this period suggesting that the type of catheter lock was instrumental in these observations.

The observed effectiveness of taurolidine to prevent CRBSI found in our study is in agreement with previous research in various patient populations [9,21–25]. A meta-analysis including six studies covering 86,000 catheter days found a slightly lower

Table 3. Catheter related bloodstream infection and occlusion incidence rates and incidence rate ratios in heparin and taurolidine locked catheters.

	Incidence rate per access year (95% CI)	Adjusted incidence rate ratio (95% CI)*
Catheter related bloodstream infection		
Heparin	1.1 (0.9–1.3)	
Taurolidine	0.2 (0.1–0.2)	
Heparin/taurolidine ratio		**5.9 (3.9–8.7)**
Catheter related occlusion		
Heparin	0.2 (0.2–0.3)	
Taurolidine	0.1 (0.1–0.2)	
Heparin/taurolidine ratio		**1.9 (1.1–3.1)**

Data were analyzed using random effects model with Poisson distributions for counts. *Adjusted values are corrected for: underlying disease, anticoagulant use, immune suppressive use, HPN/fluid frequency per week, composition of infusional fluid, and duration of HPN/fluid use before creation catheter. Random effects for patients were incorporated to account for repeated vascular access periods within a patient.

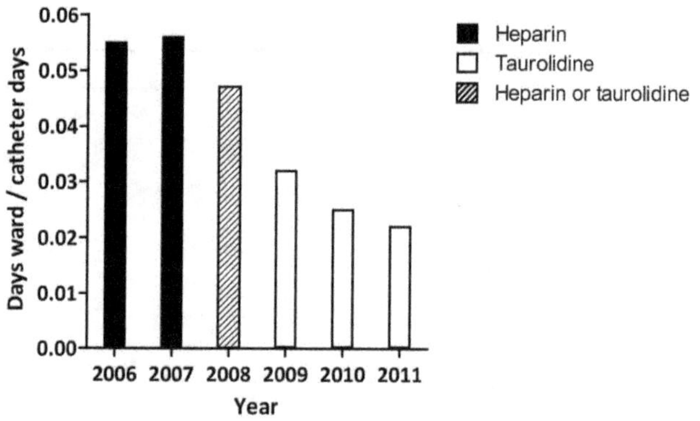

Figure 2. Hospital admissions in period 2006 until 2011. Catheters were locked with heparin (2006–2007) and taurolidine (2009–2011). In 2008 admissions of both lock strategies were included. Data are presented as the days that the patients were admitted to our ward divided by the total number of catheter days.

than our study, but still an impressive three times (confidence interval: 1.8–4.8) higher risk for the development of CRBSI in CVCs locked with heparin compared to taurolidine. Due to small sample sizes as well as methodological deficiencies of the included studies in the meta-analysis these results should be interpreted with caution [20]. Also because these studies contain different heterogeneous patient populations with distinct risk profiles for the development of CRBSIs, and because the effects of diverse taurolidine containing lock solutions, which differ in taurolidine concentration and the presence of other agents such as citrate and/or heparin, were pooled. Concerning the latter, minor differences between extremely diluted pure taurolidine and taurolidine-citrate(-heparin) solutions in the inhibition of growth of yeast, Gram negative and Gram positive bacteria *in vitro* have been found. The clinical relevance of these minor differences between different taurolidine solutions remains however unclear in the absence of clinical comparative studies [26].

Although taurolidine has shown to be able to decrease thrombus weight, but is not as effective as heparin in this respect [27], we observed a lowered incidence of catheter related occlusions with its use. Previous studies described a relationship between the number of CRBSI and occlusions, possibly due to infection-induced activation of the coagulation system [28]. In the same vein, the decrease in catheter related occlusions in our study may be the result of diminished vascular damage because of the lower infection rate [28]. In contrast, the earlier mentioned meta-analysis (with its described limitations) found no significant difference between taurolidine and heparin-treated CVCs in incidence of catheter occlusions [20].

The sharp decrease in catheter related complications that we observed after switching from catheter locking with heparin to taurolidine had a highly significant impact on the clinical burden that HPN care imposes on our clinical ward, as proven by the sharp decrease in number of days that HPN patients spent within the hospital. Keeping in mind that in Europe in general the cost of each case of catheter infection lies between 4,000 to 13,000 Euros [29], and the costs in the Netherlands for one year taurolidine locking (1,800 Euro per year) are about 300 Euros more than for heparin locking (1,500 Euro per year), taurolidine seems from a financial point of view promising. Still, a formal cost-effectiveness analysis is necessary to confirm that taurolidine is cost-effective.

In our study, approximately 7 percent of all patients who locked their catheter with taurolidine experienced (mostly mild) side effects, that urged us to stop the use of (any) taurolidine or switch to a different taurolidine formulation. This switch mostly resulted in similar side effects after which the patient used saline as a catheter lock. Only one probable anaphylactic reaction was observed and we did not dare to rechallenge this patient with the same or another taurolidine preparation. Although theoretically anaphylaxis seems unlikely due to the metabolization of taurolidine into taurine and carbon dioxide, other constituents such as polyvinylpyrrolidone (PVP-17), that is used as a stabilisator/emulgator, might cause these problems, as described in a case study [30]. Side effects have been described before for taurolidine with citrate in a paediatric patient population with haematological malignancies. Twenty percent of the paediatric patients had side effects ranging from discomfort in chest and neck, perioral dysaesthesia, abnormal taste sensations to nausea, and half of these patients using the lock solution taurolidine with citrate was urged to stop with these lock solution because of the side effects they experienced [22].

The statistical significant differences between the taurolidine and heparin locked catheters in HPN/fluid use before the creation of the catheter and the vascular acces *in situ* duration (Table 1) are a direct consequence of the fact that 62 of the 212 patients first locked their catheters with heparin and subsequently locked with taurolidine (Figure 1). The number of catheters that are still *in situ* are significantly higher in the taurolidine group (Table 1), primarily because the HPN population switched to taurolidine and none of the catheters were locked with heparin at the end of this study.

The place of catheter insertion is significantly different between the two groups. However, the place of insertion is dependent of different factors. The choice of venous access depends on the estimated length of parenteral nutrition dependency, the condition of the veins and the personal preference of the patient, with respect to esthetics (visibility of access device) and need for (self-)puncturing. Patients who have had more complications, may have less options left for venous access. A comparison between the place of insertion between catheters locked with taurolidine and heparin is therefore difficult. A recent systematic review did find similar risks for catheter-related complications in subclavian and internal jugular central venous catheters [31].

A significant difference was found in the origin of positive blood cultures between heparin and taurolidine locked catheters (Table 2). We could not explain these differences. When we compare the type of pathogens that caused the CRBSI in the heparin and the taurolidine locked catheters (Table 2), it is interestingly to observe that in taurolidine locked catheters a higher percentage of the CRBSIs is caused by yeasts. This might theoretically be a consequence of the fact that yeast are less sensitive to taurolidine, since *in vitro* studies showed that higher taurolidine concentrations are necessary to eliminate yeasts compared to bacteria [11].

The results of the statistical analysis in Table 1 and 2 should be interpreted with care, since the variables were not corrected for overrepresentation of patients who had multiple vascular accesses. To control for overrepresentation of certain patients, we used a specific statistical model that accounts for repeated measurements in the Poisson analysis, presented in Table 3. Variables of Table 1 and 2 were added as a covariate in the Poisson analysis, based on biological and clinical rationales, or based on the fact that the covariate changed the unadjusted complication rate ratios with 10% or more.

The retrospective nature of this study obviously has its pro's and con's. This study setting enabled us to collect and analyze a substantial number of patients (212), catheters (745) and catheter days (>200,000) from a single center, which makes this by far the most extensive study in this field so far, with only a limited amount of missing data. The downside remains that this study setting hampers the drawing of any conclusions on causal relations.

A limitation of the study is that the diagnoses was based on the presence of symptoms (fever, chills) in association with positive blood cultures and in the absence of other evident infectious foci that likely could explain such an infection. Because of the retrospective nature of the study, it was not possible to use the differential-time-to positivity criteria for diagnoses of CRBSI.

We chose to include all venous accesses of a single patient instead of only the first, since most long-term HPN patients are likely to have more than one catheter over, making our approach more representative for clinical practice. Since none of our other HPN-related procedures or techniques changed during this period, except for the locking strategy, we don't think that bias was introduced by the fact that the cohorts of heparin and taurolidine catheters had not the same observation period.

An important remaining question is whether taurolidine should be used in all HPN patients or only in those who have a high risk for developing CRBSIs, also in light of the fact that it remains unclear from our study design whether the difference in infection rates between both strategies is caused by promotion of infections by heparin and/or prevention of this problem by taurolidine. We hope to shed light on this issue in a multicenter randomized controlled trial that is currently ongoing and which investigates the effectiveness of taurolidine versus saline in preventing CRBSI (ClinicalTrials.gov number, NCT01826526).

Despite the limitations of the study, we suggest that the long-term use of the lock solution taurolidine is more effective in preventing catheter related bloodstream infections and occlusions in HPN patients with CVCs than heparin.

Acknowledgments

We kindly thank Marcia Tummers for her assistance during statistical analysis.

Author Contributions

Conceived and designed the experiments: EDO MWJV GJAW. Performed the experiments: EDO MWJV GJHW. Analyzed the data: EDO TF WK. Contributed reagents/materials/analysis tools: GJAW. Wrote the paper: EDO MWJV GJHW TF WK GJAW.

References

1. Wanten G, Calder PC, Forbes A (2011) Managing adult patients who need home parenteral nutrition. BMJ 342: d1447.
2. Dreesen M, Foulon V, Spriet I, Goossens GA, Hiele M, et al. (2013) Epidemiology of catheter-related infections in adult patients receiving home parenteral nutrition: a systematic review. Clin Nutr 32: 16–26.
3. O'Keefe SJ, Burnes JU, Thompson RL (1994) Recurrent sepsis in home parenteral nutrition patients: an analysis of risk factors. JPEN J Parenter Enteral Nutr 18: 256–263.
4. Wanten GJA, Calder PC (2007) Immune modulation by parenteral lipid emulsions. Am J Clin Nutr 85: 1171–1184.
5. Versleijen MW, Huisman-de Waal GJ, Kock MC, Elferink AJ, van Rossum LG, et al. (2009) Arteriovenous fistulae as an alternative to central venous catheters for delivery of long-term home parenteral nutrition. Gastroenterology 136: 1577–1584.
6. Tokars JI, Cookson ST, McArthur MA, Boyer CL, McGeer AJ, et al. (1999) Prospective evaluation of risk factors for bloodstream infection in patients receiving home infusion therapy. Ann Intern Med 131: 340–347.
7. Bozzetti F, Mariani L, Bertinet DB, Chiavenna G, Crose N, et al. (2002) Central venous catheter complications in 447 patients on home parenteral nutrition: an analysis of over 100.000 catheter days. Clin Nutr 21: 475–485.
8. Lai NM, Chaiyakunapruk N, Lai NA, O'Riordan E, Pau WS, et al. (2013) Catheter impregnation, coating or bonding for reducing central venous catheter-related infections in adults. Cochrane Database Syst Rev 6: CD007878.
9. Bisseling TM, Willems MC, Versleijen MW, Hendriks JC, Vissers RK, et al. (2010) Taurolidine lock is highly effective in preventing catheter-related bloodstream infections in patients on home parenteral nutrition: a heparin-controlled prospective trial. Clin Nutr 29: 464–468.
10. Pittiruti M, Hamilton H, Biffi R, MacFie J, Pertkiewicz M (2009) ESPEN Guidelines on Parenteral Nutrition: central venous catheters (access, care, diagnosis and therapy of complications). Clin Nutr 28: 365–377.
11. Nösner K, Focht J (1994) In-vitro-Wirksamkeit von Taurolidin und 9 Antibiotika gegen klinische Isolate aus chirurgischem Einsendegut sowie gegen Pilze. Chirurgische Gastroenterologie 10: 80–89.
12. Caruso F, Darnowski JW, Opazo C, Goldberg A, Kishore N, et al. (2010) Taurolidine antiadhesive properties on interaction with E. coli; its transformation in biological environment and interaction with bacteria cell wall. PLoS One 5: e8927.
13. Al-Amin AH, Sarveswaran J, Wood JM, Burke DA, Donnellan CF (2013) Efficacy of taurolidine on the prevention of catheter-related bloodstream infections in patients on home parenteral nutrition. J Vasc Access 14: 379–382.
14. Chu HP, Brind J, Tomar R, Hill S (2012) Significant reduction in central venous catheter related bloodstream infections in children on home parenteral nutrition after starting treatment with taurolidine line lock. J Pediatr Gastroenterol Nutr.
15. Jurewitsch B, Jeejeebhoy KN (2005) Taurolidine lock: the key to prevention of recurrent catheter-related bloodstream infections. Clin Nutr 24: 462–465.
16. Jurewitsch B, Lee T, Park J, Jeejeebhoy K (1998) Taurolidine 2% as an antimicrobial lock solution for prevention of recurrent catheter-related bloodstream infections. JPEN J Parenter Enteral Nutr 22: 242–244.
17. Koldehoff M, Zakrzewski JL (2004) Taurolidine is effective in the treatment of central venous catheter-related bloodstream infections in cancer patients. Int J Antimicrob Agents 24: 491–495.
18. Simon A, Ammann RA, Wiszniewsky G, Bode U, Fleischhack G, et al. (2008) Taurolidine-citrate lock solution (TauroLock) significantly reduces CVAD-associated grampositive infections in pediatric cancer patients. BMC Infect Dis 8: 102.
19. Bradshaw JH, Puntis JW (2008) Taurolidine and catheter-related bloodstream infection: a systematic review of the literature. J Pediatr Gastroenterol Nutr 47: 179–186.
20. Liu Y, Zhang AQ, Cao L, Xia HT, Ma JJ (2013) Taurolidine lock solutions for the prevention of catheter-related bloodstream infections: a systematic review and meta-analysis of randomized controlled trials. PLoS One 8: e79417.
21. Betjes MG, van Agteren M (2004) Prevention of dialysis catheter-related sepsis with a citrate-taurolidine-containing lock solution. Nephrol Dial Transplant 19: 1546–1551.
22. Dumichen MJ, Seeger K, Lode HN, Kuhl JS, Ebell W, et al. (2012) Randomized controlled trial of taurolidine citrate versus heparin as catheter lock solution in paediatric patients with haematological malignancies. J Hosp Infect 80: 304–309.
23. Handrup MM, Moller JK, Schroder H (2013) Central venous catheters and catheter locks in children with cancer: a prospective randomized trial of taurolidine versus heparin. Pediatric Blood & Cancer 60: 1292–1298.
24. Solomon LR, Cheesbrough JS, Ebah L, Al-Sayed T, Heap M, et al. (2010) A randomized double-blind controlled trial of taurolidine-citrate catheter locks for the prevention of bacteremia in patients treated with hemodialysis. Am J Kidney Dis 55: 1060–1068.
25. Zwiech R, Adelt M, Chrul S (2013) A Taurolidine-Citrate-Heparin Lock Solution Effectively Eradicates Pathogens From the Catheter Biofilm in Hemodialysis Patients. Am J Ther.
26. Olthof ED, Guelich AF, Rijs AJ, Nijland R, Wanten G (2013) Microbiocidal effects of various taurolidine containing catheter lock-solutions United European Gastroenterology Journal1: A585.

27. Kaptanoglu L, Kucuk HF, Colak E, Kurt N, Bingul SM, et al. (2008) The effect of taurolidine on experimental thrombus formation. Eur J Pharmacol 578: 238–241.
28. Timsit JF, Farkas JC, Boyer JM, Martin JB, Misset B, et al. (1998) Central vein catheter-related thrombosis in intensive care patients: incidence, risks factors, and relationship with catheter-related sepsis. Chest 114: 207–213.
29. Tacconelli E, Smith G, Hieke K, Lafuma A, Bastide P (2009) Epidemiology, medical outcomes and costs of catheter-related bloodstream infections in intensive care units of four European countries: literature- and registry-based estimates. J Hosp Infect 72: 97–103.
30. Yoshida K, Sakurai Y, Kawahara S, Takeda T, Ishikawa T, et al. (2008) Anaphylaxis to polyvinylpyrrolidone in povidone-iodine for impetigo contagiosum in a boy with atopic dermatitis. Int Arch Allergy Immunol 146: 169–173.
31. Ge X, Cavallazzi R, Li C, Pan SM, Wang YW, et al. (2012) Central venous access sites for the prevention of venous thrombosis, stenosis and infection. Cochrane Database Syst Rev 3: CD004084.

21

National Trends in Main Causes of Hospitalization: A Multi-Cohort Register Study of the Finnish Working-Age Population, 1976–2010

Anne Kouvonen[1,2,3]*, Aki Koskinen[4], Pekka Varje[4,5], Lauri Kokkinen[4], Roberto De Vogli[6,7], Ari Väänänen[4]

1 Department of Social Research, University of Helsinki, Helsinki, Finland, **2** University of Social Sciences and Humanities, Faculty in Wroclaw, Wroclaw, Poland, **3** UKCRC Centre of Excellence for Public Health (Northern Ireland), Queen's University Belfast, Belfast, United Kingdom, **4** Finnish Institute of Occupational Health, Helsinki and Tampere, Finland, **5** Department of Philosophy, History, Culture and Art Studies, University of Helsinki, Helsinki, Finland, **6** Department of Public Health Sciences, School of Medicine, University of California Davis, Davis, United States of America, **7** Department of Epidemiology and Public Health, University College London, London, United Kingdom

Abstract

Background: The health transition theory argues that societal changes produce proportional changes in causes of disability and death. The aim of this study was to identify long-term changes in main causes of hospitalization in working-age population within a nation that has experienced considerable societal change.

Methodology: National trends in all-cause hospitalization and hospitalizations for the five main diagnostic categories were investigated in the data obtained from the Finnish Hospital Discharge Register. The seven-cohort sample covered the period from 1976 to 2010 and consisted of 3,769,356 randomly selected Finnish residents, each cohort representing 25% sample of population aged 18 to 64 years.

Principal Findings: Over the period of 35 years, the risk of hospitalization for cardiovascular diseases and respiratory diseases decreased. Hospitalization for musculoskeletal diseases increased whereas mental and behavioral hospitalizations slightly decreased. The risk of cancer hospitalization decreased marginally in men, whereas in women an upward trend was observed.

Conclusions/Significance: A considerable health transition related to hospitalizations and a shift in the utilization of health care services of working-age men and women took place in Finland between 1976 and 2010.

Editor: Tina Hernandez-Boussard, Stanford University School of Medicine, United States of America

Funding: This work was supported by the Academy of Finland (grant 67172). A. Kouvonen was supported by the Medical Research Council (MRC) (grant MR/K023241/1) and the Economic and Social Research Council (ESRC) (grant ES/L007509/1). R. De Vogli was supported by the Economic and Social Research Council (ESRC) (grant RES-070-27-0034). The funders had no role in study design, data collection and analysis, decision to publish, or preparation of the manuscript.

Competing Interests: The authors have declared that no competing interests exist.

* Email: anne.kouvonen@helsinki.fi

Introduction

Change in population-wide disease patterns is a major public health issue. Knowledge of the disease trends and changing burden of disease is essential for estimating the impact of primary prevention, defining public health priorities, and predicting future health care needs [1]. Information on sex-specific patterns is important as different strategies may be needed for women and men. Previous studies examining sex-specific trends in hospitalization have typically focused on specific diseases or diagnostic categories, including diabetes [2], stroke [3], heart failure [4,5], myocardial infarction [6–8], acute coronary syndromes [9], coronary heart disease [10], peripheral artery disease [11], asthma [12], chronic obstructive pulmonary disease [13], and carpal tunnel syndrome [14]. However, research on sex-specific national trends in all-cause hospitalization and hospitalization for main diagnostic categories is rare and information on long-term trends is lacking. In Germany, Nowossadeck [15] analyzed changing rates of hospitalization for individual diagnoses between 2000 and 2009 and found increased rates for congestive heart failure and diseases for spine and back; whereas the hospitalization rates for ischemic heart disease, cerebrovascular diseases and certain cancers decreased. The underlying trends were mainly similar for women and men. However, there were also notable differences; lung cancer hospitalizations decreased in men but sharply increased in women [15].

The individual research findings on shifts in the disease burden based on long follow-ups can be interpreted from the point of view of the health transition theory. This theory suggests that economic, social, cultural and political changes are likely to produce proportional changes in causes of disability and death [16,17]. It is surprising that – to the best of our best knowledge – there are no previous studies on national hospitalization trends examining long-term proportional changes in disease burden across main diagnostic groups. The present study was set out to investigate the health transition and changing burden of disease in working-age population in Finland; a country which experienced dramatic societal change between the mid-1970s and 2010. In the working-age population the societal shift was reflected in changes in the occupational structure (from agricultural and industrial occupations to service and knowledge-sector occupations) and job content (from physically demanding and chemically hazardous jobs to mentally, socially and cognitively intensive tasks), overall growth of highly-skilled work force, the emergence of late modern work organisations based on the use of information technologies and mobile networks, and considerable changes in leisure time activities [18,19]. As an indicator of severe health problems and the use of medical treatment we analysed the transition in all-cause hospitalizations and hospitalizations for the main diagnostic categories from 1976 to 2010 in seven representative cohorts of working-age men and women. Hospitalization was measured by the number of discharges rather than by the total number of inpatient days.

Materials and Methods

Study population

The total study period was divided into seven five-year time periods (1976–1980, 1981–1985, 1986–1990, 1991–1995, 1996–2000, 2001–2005, and 2006–2010). These seven independent cohorts were constructed by randomly selecting 25% of the 18 to 64-year-old Finns. In total, the study population included 3,769,356 working-age adults (52% men). Data on age and sex were obtained from a population database maintained by Statistics Finland in which every Finnish resident is registered. The dates of death, where applicable, were obtained from the National Death Register kept by Statistics Finland.

Hospitalization data

Hospitalization data were obtained from the Finnish Hospital Discharge Register that is maintained by the National Institute for Health and Welfare. The data consist of information on all cases of inpatient medical treatment in Finnish public sector hospitals. A recent systematic review showed that completeness and accuracy in this register varies from satisfactory to very good [20]. For each individual the diagnosis data were linked to Statistics Finland records by using national identification numbers. Outcomes were all-cause hospitalization and hospitalizations for the five main diagnostic categories: Diseases of the circulatory system (International Classification of Diseases, Eighth (ICD-8) and Ninth Revision (ICD-9) codes 390–459, International Classification of Diseases, Tenth Revision (ICD-10 codes I00–I99); Mental and behavioral disorders (ICD-8 and ICD-9 codes 291–319; ICD-10 codes F04–F99); Diseases of the musculoskeletal system and connective tissue (ICD-8 and ICD-9 codes 710–739; ICD-10 codes M00–M99); Diseases of the respiratory systems (ICD-8 and ICD-9 codes 460–519; ICD-10 codes J00–J99); and Neoplasms (ICD-8 and ICD-9 codes 140–208; ICD-10 codes C00–C97)). Since the vast majority of pregnancy-related hospitalizations relate to healthy deliveries and therefore do not indicate morbidity, we excluded pregnancy-related causes (ICD8-9 630–679 and ICD10 O00–O99) from the analyses.

The proportions of the hospitalizations for the five main categories of all first hospitalizations were as follows: musculoskeletal disorders 20%, cardiovascular diseases 15%, respiratory diseases 10%, mental and behavioral disorders 6%, and cancer 4%.

We followed-up the hospitalization data over a five year period in each of the seven cohorts. The follow-up began on 1st January at the beginning of each cohort and ended on the day the participant was hospitalized or died. For the rest of the participants, the follow-up period ended five years after it began, on 31st December.

All records/information was anonymized and de-identified prior to linkage and analysis. Ethical approval for the study was received from the Finnish Institute of Occupational Health.

Statistical analyses

Age-standardized incidence rates for all-cause and the five main diagnostic categories of hospitalization were calculated separately for men and women and are expressed as the annual number of cases per 10,000 persons in each five-year cohort. For every individual within each cohort, only the first hospitalization for the given diagnostic category was included and the individual was then removed from the risk population (as in the case of death). We did not exclude individuals' subsequent hospitalizations for other diagnostic categories. To detect time trends we applied Cox regression model, which produced age-adjusted sex-stratified proportional hazard ratios (HR) with 95% confidence intervals (95% CI) for all-cause hospitalization and hospitalization for the five main diagnostic categories for each five-year cohort between 1981 and 2010 in relation to the earliest cohort (1976–1980). Due to the random selection method the same individual could appear in several cohorts, but such cases could not be identified and in the analyses the cohorts were assumed to be independent.

All analyses were performed using the SAS 9.2 (SAS Institute, Cary, NC, USA) software.

Results

Altogether 1,453,190 hospitalizations in men and 1,918,936 hospitalizations in women were recorded in the study cohorts between 1976 and 2010. The mean follow-up time per cohort was 4.97 years.

Figure 1 presents the total number of hospitalizations by cohort in men and women and the mean age and the mean follow-up time in each cohort. Figures 2–7 present the age-standardized incidence rates per 10,000 individuals for all-cause hospitalization and the five main diagnostic categories in the seven cohorts. Compared to women, men had higher age-standardized rates of hospitalization for cardiovascular diseases and mental and behavioral disorders, whereas age-standardized incidence rates of musculoskeletal disorders and cancer were higher in women. Up until 2001–2005 men had considerably higher levels of hospitalization for respiratory diseases, but the gap has been narrowing and in 2006–2010 the difference was very small.

In men, the age-standardized incidence rate decreased in all main causes of hospitalization apart from musculoskeletal disorders where it rose from 87 in 1976–1980 to 161 in 1996–2000 and remained stable until 2006–2010 (overall increase 85%). In women the age-standardized incidence rate of hospitalizations for musculoskeletal diagnoses increased from 112 in 1976–2010 to

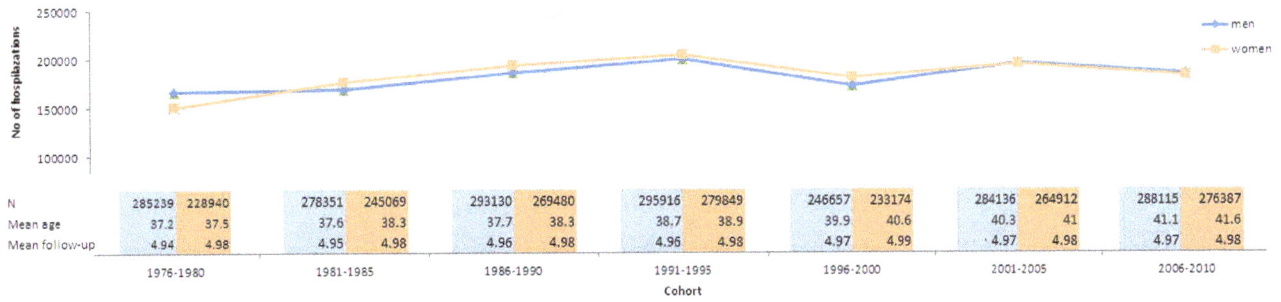

Figure 1. The total number of hospitalizations by cohort in men and women and the mean age and the mean follow-up time in each cohort, Finland 1976–2010.

174 in 2006–2010 (overall increase 55%). During the same period, the incidence rate of hospitalization for cardiovascular diseases decreased from 165 to 95 (overall decrease 42%) in men and from 165 to 66 (60%) in women. In a similar way, the incidence rate for respiratory diseases decreased, from 82 to 57 (30%) in men and from 66 to 51 (23%) in women. The incidence rate of hospitalizations for mental and behavioral disorders decreased from 45 to 30 (50%) in men and from 29 to 23 (21%) in women. In men the incidence rate for cancer-related hospitalizations decreased slightly from 31 to 28 (10%), whereas in women it increased from 29 to 44 in (52%). In men, cardiovascular diseases was the most common diagnostic category at the start of the study period, but was replaced by musculoskeletal disorders in 1996–2000. In women, musculoskeletal diagnoses overtook cardiovascular diagnoses as the largest diagnostic category already in 1986–1990.

Table 1 presents sex-stratified age-adjusted proportional risks of all-cause hospitalization and hospitalizations for the five main diagnostic categories among men and women in 1981–2010 using the first cohort (1976–1980) as the reference group. With the exception of cancer, the time trends were very similar in men and women. The risk of all-cause hospitalization remained relatively stable throughout the study period. The risk of hospitalization for cardiovascular diseases decreased systematically throughout the study period (HR 0.57; 95% CI: 0.56, 0.58 in 2006–2010 in men and HR 0.39; 95% CI: 0.38, 0.40 in 2006–2010 in women). The risk of hospitalization for musculoskeletal disorders increased, but the increase levelled off already in 1996–2000 (HR 1.83; 95% CI: 1.79, 1.88 in 2006–2010 in men and HR 1.52; 95% CI: 1.48, 1.55 in 2006–2010 women). The risk of hospitalization for mental and behavioral disorders decreased slightly (HR 0.63; 95% CI: 0.61, 0.66 in 2006–2010 in men and HR 0.81; 95% CI: 0.78, 0.85 in 2006–2010 in women).

The risk of hospitalization for respiratory diseases has declined both in men and women. The risk of cancer hospitalization has decreased very slightly in men, whereas in women a constant upward trend in the risk can be observed (HR 1.51; 95% CI: 1.45, 1.59 in 2006–2010).

Discussion

The present study examined incidence rates and proportional risks for all-cause hospitalization and for the five main diagnostic categories in seven representative consecutive cohorts of Finnish working-age men and women between 1976 and 2010. The findings show that musculoskeletal disorders have increased their proportion of the total of all five diagnostic categories that were included in this study whilst the proportion of cardiovascular diseases has decreased. The observed overall trends were very similar in men and women with the exception of cancer: these hospitalizations marginally decreased in men but increased in women. The findings provide new evidence which specifies the

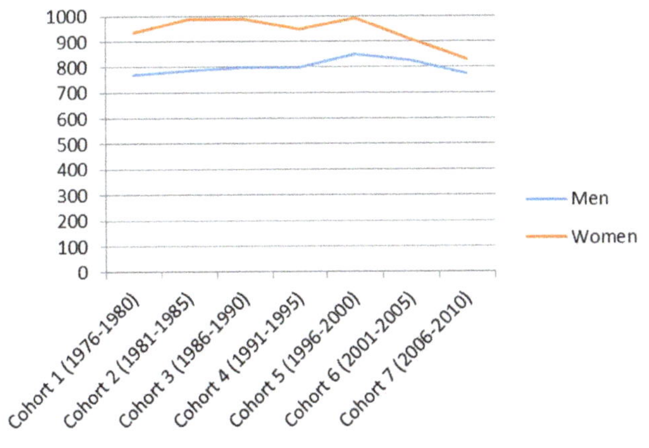

Figure 2. Age-standardized incidence rates per 10,000 individuals for all-cause hospitalizations in men and women, Finland 1976–2010.

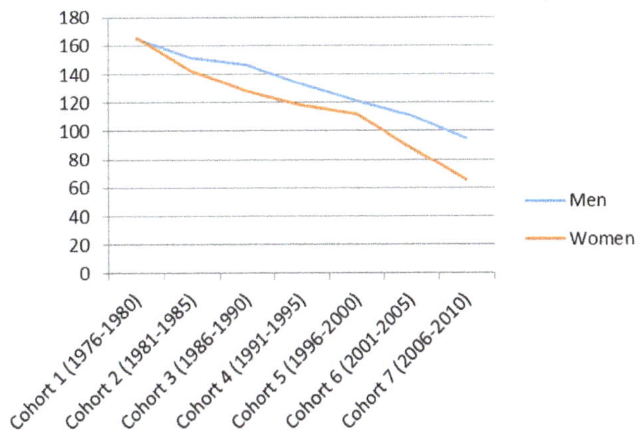

Figure 3. Age-standardized incidence rates per 10,000 individuals for hospitalizations for cardiovascular disease in men and women, Finland 1976–2010.

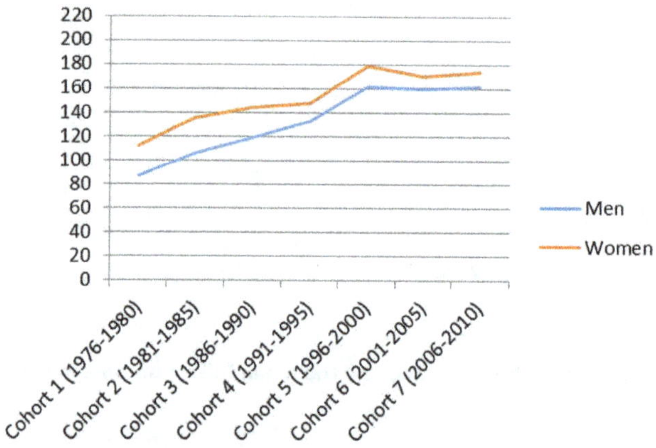

Figure 4. Age-standardized incidence rates per 10,000 individuals for hospitalizations for musculoskeletal disorders in men and women, Finland 1976–2010.

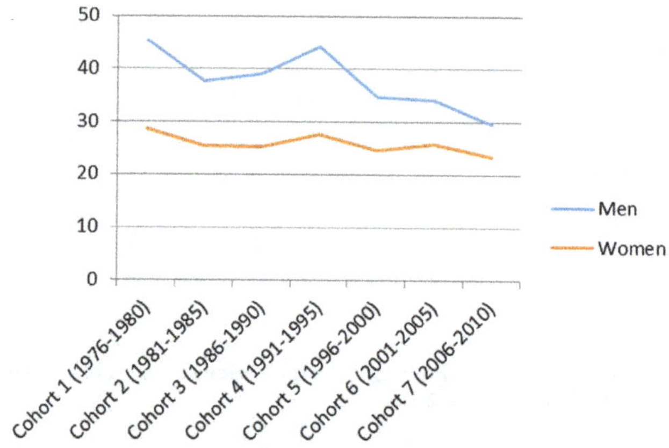

Figure 5. Age-standardized incidence rates per 10,000 individuals for hospitalizations for mental and behavioral disorders in men and women, Finland 1976–2010.

health transition theory. It seems that the general transition occurs in hospitalizations when the nation moves towards the late modern societal order but the pattern of the changes is partly different for women and men. The general secular shifts and sex-specific findings are probably related to notable changes in lifestyles and in living and working conditions but at the same time they also are likely to be connected to developments in health care, health promotion, and health policies.

Cardiovascular disease

Our findings demonstrate a declining incidence of hospitalization for cardiovascular diseases; the decrease being a slightly larger in women. Studies from other national samples show that age-adjusted coronary heart disease and cerebrovascular disease hospitalization rates have significantly decreased [21]. The role of widespread primary prevention and decreases in conventional risk factors have been highlighted as important contributors to these reductions; including decreases in smoking prevalence and population wide levels of systolic blood pressure as well as favorable lipid effects [22,23]. The widespread and increasing use of antihypertensive drugs as well as statins and other lipid-lowering drugs, has probably also contributed to these trends [24,25]. However, it has been predicted that increasing prevalence of overweight and obesity may be compromising favorable trends in the risk factors in the future [23].

Moreover, it is well known that trends in cardiovascular diseases may be set decades before the conditions become manifest [26], and that early-life poor socio-economic conditions are associated with a higher cardiovascular risk later in life [27]; an important part of this is their potential effect on development of conventional risk factors [28]. It is therefore plausible that population-wide improvements in childhood socio-economic environments have contributed to declining cardiovascular risk. In addition, decreases in cardiovascular risk factors relate to an upward shift in educational attainment; a substantially smaller proportion of the population than before is exposed to the risk associated with low education [28]. The contribution of educational shift has been shown to be somewhat stronger for women than for men. In addition, changes in policies, such as introduction of comprehensive smoke-free policy, may have helped to change social norms [29].

Musculoskeletal disorders

Our results show a clear increase in hospitalizations for musculoskeletal disorders. Indeed, musculoskeletal disorders have become the most common reason for claiming sickness allowance in Finland [30]. Hospitalization due to musculoskeletal disorders has also increased in Germany [15]. In the US health care utilisation for spine conditions, the prevalence of chronic impairing low back pain, and back and neck-related health expenditure have increased [31,32]. In Finland it has been noted that there have been improvements in diagnostic and therapeutic methods that reveal an increasing range of musculoskeletal disorders [33].

Increasing rates of musculoskeletal hospitalization may be attributable to changes in the nature of working life: the shift from manual types of jobs towards jobs involving more sedentary tasks such as more office-based and computer-based jobs. It is now acknowledged that for a large number of employees, lack of physical activity – both at work and on leisure time - is a major risk factor for musculoskeletal ill health [34]. At the same time, obesity, which is a risk factor for particularly certain musculoskeletal conditions [35], has rapidly increased.

Work-related psychosocial stress has also been linked to hospitalizations for musculoskeletal disorders [36]. Because of

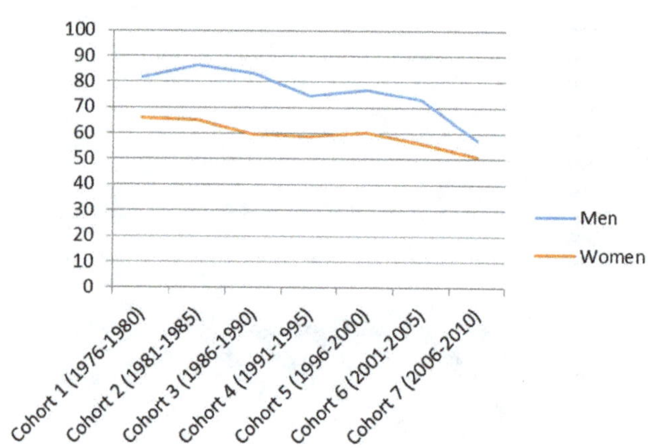

Figure 6. Age-standardized incidence rates per 10,000 individuals for hospitalizations for respiratory diseases in men and women, Finland 1976–2010.

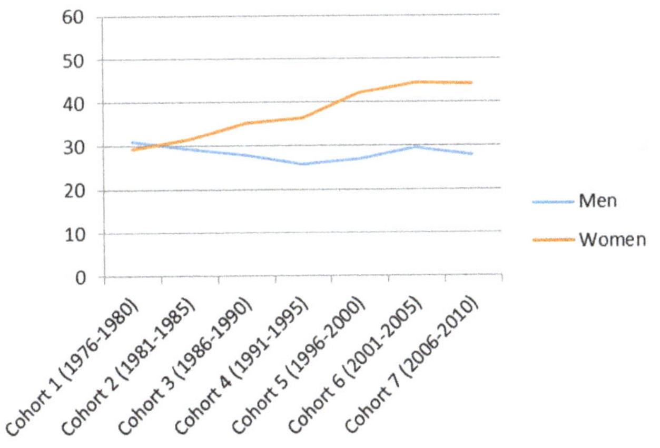

Figure 7. Age-standardized incidence rates per 10,000 individuals for hospitalizations for cancers in men and women, Finland 1976–2010.

the globalisation of work, widespread information technology and a growing pressure to increase productivity and more stressful psychosocial environments and working patterns are now affecting increasing proportions of both the male and female workforce [37].

Mental and behavioral disorders

The risk of psychiatric hospitalization decreased slightly. Mental disorders as a reason for sickness absence and disability pension have increased in recent decades in Finland [33]. As in most high income countries, mental health service in Finland has been dramatically transformed by an increase in ambulatory treatment and care. However, despite decrease in the total number of hospital beds, the annual number of psychiatric in-patients has remained largely unchanged over time; this is due to the decrease in average length of psychiatric hospital stay [38].

Respiratory diseases

Our data show that the risk of hospitalization for respiratory diseases has decreased. In a similar way, in Danish working population, the number of hospitalizations for chronic lower respiratory diseases has been reduced over time [39].

The decrease in hospitalizations both for cardiovascular and respiratory diseases can be partially explained by widespread smoke-free legislation, introduced in Finland from 1990s onwards. A recent meta-analysis showed that smoke-free legislation is associated for a lower risk of hospitalization for cardiac, cerebrovascular and respiratory diseases [40].

In addition, considerable regulatory measures have been taken to prevent the adverse health outcomes of hazardous substances, for example all asbestos usage has been banned and lead-exposed workers are being biologically monitored [41]. Occupational inhalation exposure to most chemical agents has decreased in Finland since 1970s and chemical exposures and related disease burden are expected to further decrease in the future [42].

Cancer

Our results showed that the risk of cancer hospitalization decreased marginally in men, whereas in women an upward trend in risk can be observed. An earlier study in the Finnish general population similarly showed that in men there have been only minor changes in the age-standardized total cancer incidence rates, whereas in women the total cancer morbidity has slightly increased since the 1950s [43].

A number of reasons may have contributed to increasing cancer rates in working-age women. First, the risk of breast cancer has continuously increased. The introduction of organised mammographic screening programme affects the breast cancer incidence rate in a population as the diagnosis is advanced in time [44]. In Finland national mammographic screening was introduced in 1987; in that year the incidence of breast cancer increased by about one-tenth [45]. An analysis of secular trends which corrected for the influence of screening showed that in Finland the breast cancer rates increased by 13% per 5-year period [44]. Another important contributing factor for the increased breast cancer risk relates to the increased use of postmenopausal hormone therapy (HT) [45]. A study examining the HT use and breast cancer risk in Nordic countries in 1995 showed that in three other Nordic countries (Sweden, Norway and Iceland) that had had a significant drop in HT use, the increasing trends of breast cancer incidences either experienced a down-turn or the increase declined whereas in Finland, with only a small decline in HT, this was less evident [46].

Second, strong and consistent increases in endometrial cancer have been reported over the last 50 years; the biggest increase has been seen in postmenopausal women but in the last decade the rates have also increased in younger women [47].

Third, in Finland smoking has systematically decreased in men already over several decades whereas in women smoking has started to decline only in recent years. As a consequence, the incidence of lung cancer has constantly increased in women and is projected to continue to increase [45].

Finally, obesity has strongly increased over the last three decades and it is well established that excess body adiposity is a risk factor for cancer development [48]. It has also been shown that both in relative and absolute terms, obesity-related cancer is a greater problem for women than men; and endometrial, breast and colorectal cancers have been identified as priorities for research and public health measures [48].

Strengths and limitations

A major strength of our study was that the hospitalization data were derived from a national hospital discharge register with proven good accuracy and coverage [20]. There was no loss to follow-up and the changes in International Classification of Diseases were recoded to correspond to the most recent classification. As far as we are aware, this was the first study to examine long-term national trends in main causes of hospitalization among working-age men and women.

Despite these strengths, it is also important to acknowledge potential limitations. First, we used hospitalization as a proxy for underlying morbidity. Hospitalization is considered to be a reliable indicator of the use of medical treatment [49]. However, the long-term shifts in the use of hospital services and proportional share of diagnoses related to hospitalizations within a population are also likely to reflect changes in treatments and options of health care. Moreover, over time changes in coding practices and diagnostic criteria may have affected hospitalization trends for some causes and proportional shares of main diagnostic categories.

Second, referral bias and differential access to hospital services might have affected the results [50]. Self-referral and referral by general practitioners may be influenced by a number of factors such as geography, employment status, age, education, and economic status [50]. There are significant differences in health care service provision between local authorities and significant

Table 1. Age-adjusted Proportional Hazard Ratios (HR) and their 95% Confidence Intervals for Hospitalization in Relation to the First Cohort in Seven Consecutive Cohorts, Finland, 1976–2010.

	Men			*Women*		
All-cause	N/Cases	HR	95% CI	N/Cases	HR	95% CI
1976–1980	285,239/81,164	1.00	reference	228,940/80,894	1.00	reference
1981–1985	278,351/80,108	1.03	1.02, 1.04	245,069/89,577	1.04	1.03, 1.05
1986–1990	293,130/86,562	1.06	1.05, 1.07	269,480/98,681	1.05	1.04, 1.06
1991–1995	295,916/88,868	1.05	1.04, 1.04	279,849/101,007	1.00	0.99, 1.01
1996–2000	246,657/79,058	1.13	1.12, 1.14	233,174/88,648	1.04	1.03, 1.05
2001–2005	284,136/90,563	1.10	1.09, 1.11	264,912/93,473	0.94	0.93, 0.95
2006–2010	288,115/88,795	1.02	1.01, 1.03	276,387/91,591	0.87	0.86, 0.88
	Cases	HR	95% CI	Cases	HR	95% CI
Cardiovascular diseases						
1976–1980	16,670	1.00	reference	15,500	1.00	reference
1981–1985	15,024	0.92	0.90, 0.94	14,505	0.85	0.83, 0.87
1986–1990	15,298	0.89	0.87, 0.91	14,256	0.76	0.74, 0.77
1991–1995	14,836	0.79	0.78, 0.81	14,194	0.70	0.68, 0.71
1996–2000	11,990	0.73	0.71, 0.74	11,903	0.66	0.64, 0.67
2001–2005	13,124	0.67	0.65, 0.74	10,775	0.52	0.50, 0.53
2006–2010	12,441	0.57	0.56, 0.58	8797	0.39	0.38, 0.40
Musculoskeletal disorders						
1976–1980	10,900	1.00	reference	10,965	1.00	reference
1981–1985	13,097	1.23	1.20, 1.26	14,230	1.20	1.17, 1.23
1986–1990	15,566	1.39	1.36, 1.42	16,631	1.28	1.25, 1.31
1991–1995	17,975	1.54	1.50, 1.57	18,470	1.31	1.28, 1.34
1996–2000	18,524	1.86	1.81, 1.90	19,416	1.57	1.53, 1.61
2001–2005	20,987	1.82	1.78, 1.86	20,953	1.48	1.45, 1.51
2006–2010	21,744	1.83	1.79, 1.88	22,673	1.52	1.48, 1.55
Mental and behavioral disorders						
1976–1980	6624	1.00	reference	3291	1.00	reference
1981–1985	5392	0.83	0.80, 0.86	3132	0.89	0.84, 0.93
1986–1990	5873	0.86	0.83, 0.89	3387	0.87	0.83, 0.91
1991–1995	6574	0.95	0.92, 0.98	3938	0.96	0.92, 1.01
1996–2000	4334	0.74	0.72, 0.95	2970	0.86	0.82, 0.91
2001–2005	4877	0.73	0.70, 0.76	3489	0.90	0.86, 0.94
2006–2010	4226	0.63	0.61, 0.66	3229	0.81	0.78, 0.85
Respiratory diseases						
1976–1980	11,326	1.00	reference	7449	1.00	reference
1981–1985	11,122	1.07	1.04, 1.09	7603	0.91	0.89, 0.94
1986–1990	11,343	1.04	1.01, 1.07	7611	0.96	0.93, 0.99
1991–1995	10,349	0.95	0.92, 0.97	8009	0.87	0.84, 0.90
1996–2000	8557	0.98	0.95, 1.01	6835	0.91	0.88, 0.94
2001–2005	9835	0.93	0.91, 0.96	7220	0.84	0.81, 0.87
2006–2010	7991	0.73	0.71, 0.75	6893	0.76	0.74, 0.79
Cancers						
1976–1980	3002	1.00	reference	2589	1.00	reference
1981–1985	2726	0.94	0.89, 0.99	3088	1.08	1.03, 1.14
1986–1990	2736	0.91	0.87, 0.96	3715	1.21	1.15, 1.27
1991–1995	2777	0.85	0.81, 0.89	4290	1.26	1.20, 1.33
1996–2000	2471	0.87	0.83, 0.92	4439	1.45	1.38, 1.52
2001–2005	3361	0.97	0.92, 1.02	5421	1.52	1.45, 1.59
2006–2010	3666	0.90	0.66, 0.95	5987	1.51	1.45, 1.59

socioeconomic and regional inequities in the provision of and access to health care services in Finland [33,51].

Third, we considered only the first hospitalization for any of the five diagnostic categories and excluded any subsequent hospitalizations for the same category.

Conclusions

The present study demonstrates that there have been significant secular shifts in main causes of hospitalization and consequently the content of disease burden requiring hospital treatment has considerably changed among the Finnish working-age population between 1976 and 2010. This study provides new evidence of the health transition in a nation that has moved towards the late modern spheres of life within a short period of time. Generally the main trend both in men and women was away from cardiovascular and respiratory diseases and towards musculoskeletal disorders. Interestingly, cancer treatments in hospitals decreased marginally in men but clearly increased in women. The exact reasons for the observed trends are not known. However, it is likely that two types of factors – health interventions and socio-economic and lifestyle changes - have affected these trends. Health interventions include better control of many cardiovascular risk factors and advances in medical treatments. Socio-economic and lifestyle changes beyond the health sector include changes in working life and in the occupational distribution of the labor force, higher educational levels, increased social mobility, increased use of digital technology, more sedentary work and lifestyles, and increasing obesity rates. The present findings can have significant policy implications. Awareness of sex-specific long-term temporal changes in main causes of hospitalizations can help to identify public health priorities and guide health care planning.

Author Contributions

Conceived and designed the experiments: A. Kouvonen A. Koskinen PV LK RDV AV. Analyzed the data: A. Koskinen. Wrote the paper: A. Kouvonen A. Koskinen PV LK RDV AV. Directed the implementation of the study and drafted the article: A. Kouvonen. Contributed to acquisition and interpretation of data and drafting and reviewing the article: A. Koskinen AV. Helped to conceptualize the ideas, interpret findings, and write and critically review drafts of the article: PV LK RDV.

References

1. Hoeymans N, Wong A, van Gool CH, Deeg DJH, Nusselder WJ, et al. (2012) The disabling effect of diseases: a study on trends in diseases, activity limitations, and their interrelationships. Am J Public Health 102: 163–170. doi:10.2105/AJPH.2011.300296.
2. Lee JM, Davis MM, Gebremariam A, Kim C (2010) Age and sex differences in hospitalizations associated with diabetes. J Womens Heal 19: 2033–2042.
3. Lewsey JD, Jhund PS, Gillies M, Chalmers JWT, Redpath A, et al. (2009) Age- and sex-specific trends in fatal incidence and hospitalized incidence of stroke in Scotland, 1986 to 2005. Circ Cardiovasc Qual Outcomes 2: 475–483. doi:10.1161/CIRCOUTCOMES.108.825968.
4. Haldeman GA, Croft JB, Giles WH, Rashidee A, Atlanta MS (1999) Congestive Heart Failure Hospitalization of patients with heart failure: National Hospital Discharge Survey, 1985 to 1995.
5. Schaufelberger M, Swedberga K, Koster M, Rosen M, Rosengren A (2004) Decreasing one-year mortality and hospitalization rates for heart failure in Sweden: Data from the Swedish Hospital Discharge Registry 1988 to 2000. Eur Heart J 25: 300–307.
6. Towfighi A, Markovic D, Ovbiagele B (2011) National gender-specific trends in myocardial infarction hospitalization rates among patients aged 35 to 64 years. Am J Cardiol 108: 1102–1107. doi:10.1016/j.amjcard.2011.05.046.
7. Wang OJ, Wang Y, Chen J, Krumholz HM (2012) Recent trends in hospitalization for acute myocardial infarction. Am J Cardiol 109: 1589–1593. doi:10.1016/j.amjcard.2012.01.381.
8. Schmidt M, Bonde J, Lash TL, Bøtker HE, Sørensen HT (2012) 25 year trends in first time hospitalisation for acute myocardial infarction, subsequent short and long term mortality, and the prognostic impact of sex and comorbidity: a Danish nationwide cohort study. BMJ 356: 1–12. doi:10.1136/bmj.e356.
9. Nedkoff LJ, Briffa TG, Preen DB, Sanfilippo FM, Hung J, et al. (2011) Age- and sex-specific trends in the incidence of hospitalized acute coronary syndromes in Western Australia. Circ Cardiovasc Qual Outcomes 4: 557–564. doi:10.1161/CIRCOUTCOMES.110.960005.
10. Briffa T, Nedkoff L, Peeters A, Tonkin A, Hung J, et al. (2011) Discordant age and sex-specific trends in the incidence of a first coronary heart disease event in Western Australia from 1996 to 2007. Heart 97: 400–404. doi:10.1136/hrt.2010.210138.
11. Inglis SC, Lewsey JD, Chandler D, Byrne DS, Lowe GDO, et al. (2012) Sex-specific time trends in first admission to hospital for peripheral artery disease in Scotland 1991–2007. Br J Surg 99: 680–687. doi:10.1002/bjs.8686.
12. Getahun D, Demissie K, Rhoads G (2005) Recent trends in asthma hospitalization and mortality in the United States. J Asthma 42: 373–378.
13. Lykkegaard J, Søndergaard J, Kragstrup J, Rømhild Davidsen J, Knudsen T, et al. (2012) All Danish first-time COPD hospitalisations 2002–2008: incidence, outcome, patients, and care. Respir Med 106: 549–556. doi:10.1016/j.rmed.2011.11.001.
14. Mattioli S, Baldasseroni A, Curti S, Cooke RMT, Bena A, et al. (2008) Incidence rates of in-hospital carpal tunnel syndrome in the general population and possible associations with marital status. BMC Public Health 8: 374. doi:10.1186/1471-2458-8-374.
15. Nowossadeck E (2012) Population aging and hospitalization for chronic disease in Germany. Dtsch Arztebl Int 109: 151–157. doi:10.3238/arztebl.2012.0151.
16. Frenk J, Bobadilla J, Stern C, Frejka T, Lozano R (1991) Elements for a theory of the health transition. Heal Transit Rev 1: 21–38.
17. Mesle F, Vallin J (2006) The health transition: trends and prospects. In: Caselli G, Vallin J, Wunsch G, editors. Demography, Analysis and Synthesis. A Treatise in Demography. New York: Elsevier. pp.247–602.
18. Hjerppe R, Jalava J (2006) Economic Growth and Structural Change: A Century and a Half of Catching-up. In: Ojala J, Eloranta J, Jalava J, editors. The Road to Prosperity: an Economic History of Finland. Helsinki: Suomalaisen Kirjallisuuden Seura.
19. Lehto A-M, Sutela H (2008) Työolojen kolme vuosikymmentä. Työolotutkimusten tuloksia 1977–2008 [Three decades of working conditions. Results from the Working Conditions Survey 1977–2008]. Helsinki: Tilastokeskus [Statistics Finland].
20. Sund R (2012) Quality of the Finnish Hospital Discharge Register: a systematic review. Scand J Public Health 40: 505–515. doi:10.1177/1403494812456637.
21. Liu L (2011) Changes in cardiovascular hospitalization and comorbidity of heart failure in the United States: findings from the National Hospital Discharge Surveys 1980–2006. Int J Cardiol 149: 39–45. doi:10.1016/j.ijcard.2009.11.037.
22. Luepker R V (2008) Decline in incident coronary heart disease: why are the rates falling? Circulation 117: 592–593. doi:10.1161/CIRCULATIONAHA.107.747477.
23. Ford ES, Ajani UA, Croft JB, Critchley JA, Labarthe DR, et al. (2007) Explaining the decrease in U.S. deaths from coronary disease, 1980–2000. N Engl J Med 356: 2388–2398. doi:10.1056/NEJMsa053935.
24. Danaei G, Finucane MM, Lin JK, Singh GM, Paciorek CJ, et al. (2011) National, regional, and global trends in systolic blood pressure since 1980: systematic analysis of health examination surveys and epidemiological studies with 786 country-years and 5·4 million participants. Lancet 377: 568–577. doi:10.1016/S0140-6736(10)62036-3.
25. Farzadfar F, Finucane MM, Danaei G, Pelizzari PM, Cowan MJ, et al. (2011) National, regional, and global trends in serum total cholesterol since 1980: systematic analysis of health examination surveys and epidemiological studies with 321 country-years and 3·0 million participants. Lancet 377: 578–586. doi:10.1016/S0140-6736(10)62038-7.
26. Ulmer H, Kelleher CC, Fitz-Simon N, Diem G, Concin H (2007) Secular trends in cardiovascular risk factors: an age-period cohort analysis of 698,954 health examinations in 181,350 Austrian men and women. J Intern Med 261: 566–576. doi:10.1111/j.1365-2796.2007.01779.x.
27. Galobardes B, Smith GD, Lynch JW (2006) Systematic review of the influence of childhood socioeconomic circumstances on risk for cardiovascular disease in adulthood. Ann Epidemiol 16: 91–104. doi:10.1016/j.annepidem.2005.06.053.
28. Harper S, Lynch J, Smith GD (2011) Social determinants and the decline of cardiovascular diseases: understanding the links. Annu Rev Public Health 32: 39–69. doi:10.1146/annurev-publhealth-031210-101234.
29. Thrasher JF, Boado M, Sebrié EM, Bianco E (2009) Smoke-free policies and the social acceptability of smoking in Uruguay and Mexico: findings from the International Tobacco Control Policy Evaluation Project. Nicotine Tob Res 11: 591–599. doi:10.1093/ntr/ntp039.
30. Kela [Social Insurance Institution] (2012) Statistical Yearbook of the Social Insurance Institution. Helsinki.
31. Freburger JK, Holmes GM, Agans RP, Jackman AM, Darter JD, et al. (2009) The rising prevalence of chronic low back pain. Arch Intern Med 169: 251–258. doi:10.1001/archinternmed.2008.543.

32. Martin BI, Deyo RA, Mirza SK, Turner JA, Comstock BA, et al. (2008) Expenditures and health status among adults with back and neck problems. JAMA 299: 656–664. doi:10.1001/jama.299.6.656.
33. Vuorenkoski L (2008) Finland: Health System Review. European Observatory on Health Systems and Policies.
34. Straker L, Mathiassen SE (2009) Increased physical work loads in modern work–a necessity for better health and performance? Ergonomics 52: 1215–1225. doi:10.1080/00140130903039101.
35. Wearing SC, Hennig EM, Byrne NM, Steele JR, Hills AP (2006) Musculoskeletal disorders associated with obesity: a biomechanical perspective. Obes Rev 7: 239–250. doi:10.1111/j.1467-789X.2006.00251.x.
36. Lincoln AE, Smith GS, Amoroso PJ, Bell NS (2002) The natural history and risk factors of musculoskeletal conditions resulting in disability among US Army personnel. Work 18: 99–113.
37. Schnall PL, Dobson M, Rosskam E, editors (2009) Unhealthy Work: Causes, Consequences, Cures. New York: Baywood Publishing.
38. Wahlbeck K, Westman J, Nordentoft M, Gissler M, Laursen TM (2011) Outcomes of Nordic mental health systems: life expectancy of patients with mental disorders. Br J Psychiatry 199: 453–458. doi:10.1192/bjp.bp.110.085100.
39. Tüchsen F, Hannerz H, Mølgaard EF, Brauer C, Kirkeskov L (2012) Time trend in hospitalised chronic lower respiratory diseases among Danish building and construction workers, 1981–2009: a cohort study. BMJ Open 2: 1–6. doi:10.1136/bmjopen-2012-001761.
40. Tan CE, Glantz SA (2012) Association between smoke-free legislation and hospitalizations for cardiac, cerebrovascular, and respiratory diseases: a meta-analysis. Circulation 126: 2177–2183. doi:10.1161/CIRCULATIONAHA.112.121301.
41. Nurminen M, Karjalainen A (2001) Epidemiologic estimate of the proportion of fatalities related to occupational factors in Finland. Scand J Work Environ Health 27: 161–213. doi:10.5271/sjweh.605.
42. Kauppinen T, Uuksulainen S, Saalo A, Mäkinen I (2013) Trends of Occupational Exposure to Chemical Agents in Finland in 1950–2020. Ann Occup Hyg 57: 593–609. doi:10.1093/annhyg/mes090.
43. Teppo L, Pukkala E, Sankila R (1999) Cancers. In: Koskinen S, Aromaa A, Huttunen J, Teperi J, editors. Health in Finland. Helsinki: National Public Health Institute KTL; National Research and Development Centre for Welfare and Health STAKES; Ministry of Social Affairs and Health.
44. Møller B, Weedon-Fekjaer H, Hakulinen T, Tryggvadóttir L, Storm HH, et al. (2005) The influence of mammographic screening on national trends in breast cancer incidence. Eur J Cancer Prev 14: 117–128.
45. Pukkala E, Sankila R, Rautalahti M (2013) Cancer in Finland. Helsinki: Cancer Society of Finland.
46. Hemminki E, Kyyrönen P, Pukkala E (2008) Postmenopausal hormone drugs and breast and colon cancer: Nordic countries 1995–2005. Maturitas 61: 299–304. doi:10.1016/j.maturitas.2008.09.022.
47. Lindemann K, Eskild A, Vatten LJ, Bray F (2010) Endometrial cancer incidence trends in Norway during 1953–2007 and predictions for 2008–2027. Int J Cancer 127: 2661–2668. doi:10.1002/ijc.25267.
48. Renehan AG, Soerjomataram I, Tyson M, Egger M, Zwahlen M, et al. (2010) Incident cancer burden attributable to excess body mass index in 30 European countries. Int J Cancer 126: 692–702. doi:10.1002/ijc.24803.
49. Alamgir H, Koehoorn M, Ostry a, Tompa E, Demers P (2006) An evaluation of hospital discharge records as a tool for serious work related injury surveillance. Occup Environ Med 63: 290–296. doi:10.1136/oem.2005.026047.
50. Tüchsen F, Andersen O, Olsen J (1996) Referral bias among health workers in studies using hospitalization as a proxy measure of the underlying incidence rate. J Clin Epidemiol 49: 791–794.
51. McCallum AK, Manderbacka K, Arffman M, Leyland AH, Keskimäki I (2013) Socioeconomic differences in mortality amenable to health care among Finnish adults 1992–2003: 12 year follow up using individual level linked population register data. BMC Health Serv Res 13: 3. doi:10.1186/1472-6963-13-3.

22

Influenza Vaccine Effectiveness in Preventing Influenza A(H3N2)-Related Hospitalizations in Adults Targeted for Vaccination by Type of Vaccine: A Hospital-Based Test-Negative Study, 2011–2012 A(H3N2) Predominant Influenza Season, Valencia, Spain

Joan Puig-Barberà[1,2]*, Juan García-de-Lomas[3], Javier Díez-Domingo[1], Alberto Arnedo-Pena[2], Montserrat Ruiz-García[2], Ramón Limón-Ramírez[4], Silvia Pérez-Vilar[4], José Luis Micó-Esparza[5], Miguel Tortajada-Girbés[6], Concha Carratalá-Munuera[7,8], Rosa Larrea-González[9], Juan Manuel Beltrán-Garrido[9], Maria del Carmen Otero-Reigada[10], Joan Mollar-Maseres[10], Patricia Correcher-Medina[11], Germán Schwarz-Chavarri[12], Vicente Gil-Guillén[8,13], for the Valencia Hospital Network for the Study of Influenza and Respiratory Virus Disease¶

1 Fundación para el Fomento de la Investigación Sanitaria y Biomédica de la Comunitat Valenciana (FISABIO), Valencia, Spain, **2** Centro de Salud Pública de Castellón, Castellón, Spain, **3** Instituto Valenciano de Microbiología, Valencia, Spain, **4** Hospital de la Plana, Vila-real, Spain, **5** Hospital Aranau de Vilanova, Valencia, Spain, **6** Hospital Doctor Peset, Valencia, Spain, **7** Hospital San Juan, Alicante, Spain, **8** Cátedra de Medicina de Familia, Departamento de Medicina Clínica, Universidad Miguel Hernández, San Juan, Alicante, Spain, **9** Hospital General de Castellón, Castellón, Spain, **10** Hospital Universitario y Politécnico La Fe, Valencia, Spain, **11** Hospital Lluis Alcanyis, Xativa, Spain, **12** Centro de Salud San Blas, Alicante, Spain, **13** Hospital de Elda, Elda, Spain

Abstract

Background: Most evidence of the effectiveness of influenza vaccines comes from studies conducted in primary care, but less is known about their effectiveness in preventing serious complications. Here, we examined the influenza vaccine effectiveness (IVE) against hospitalization with PCR-confirmed influenza in the predominant A(H3N2) 2011–2012 influenza season.

Methods: A hospital-based, test-negative study was conducted in nine hospitals in Valencia, Spain. All emergency admissions with a predefined subset of symptoms were eligible. We enrolled consenting adults age 18 and over, targeted for influenza vaccination because of comorbidity, with symptoms of influenza-like-illness within seven days of admission. We estimated IVE as (1-adjusted vaccination odds ratio)*100 after accounting for major confounders, calendar time and recruitment hospital.

Results: The subjects included 544 positive for influenza A(H3N2) and 1,370 negative for influenza admissions. Age was an IVE modifying factor. Regardless of vaccine administration, IVE was 72% (38 to 88%) in subjects aged under 65 and 21% (−5% to 40%) in subjects aged 65 and over. By type of vaccine, the IVE of classical intramuscular split-influenza vaccine, used in subjects 18 to 64, was 68% (12% to 88%). The IVE for intradermal and virosomal influenza vaccines, used in subjects aged 65 and over, was 39% (11% to 58%) and 16% (−39% to 49%), respectively.

Conclusions: The split-influenza vaccine was effective in preventing influenza-associated hospitalizations in adults aged under 65. The intradermal vaccine was moderately effective in those aged 65 and over.

Editor: Steven J. Drews, University of Calgary & ProvLab Alberta, Canada

Funding: The study was funded by contracts between FISABIO-Salud Publica (former CSISP) and Sanofi-Pasteur and FISABIO-Salud Pública (former CSISP) and Sanofi-Pasteur MSD. Sanofi-Pasteur and Sanofi-Pasteur MSD did not participate in the design or conduct of the study, collection, management, analysis, or interpretation of the data, writing of the manuscript, and the decision to submit the manuscript for publication.

Competing Interests: The authors have read the journal's policy and have the following conflicts: JPB and JDD work in FISABIO's Vaccines Research Area; FISABIO has received funding for GSK, Novartis, Pfizer, SanofiPasteur, Sanofi-Pasteur MSD for conducting epidemiological studies on infectious disease epidemiology, vaccine effectiveness, pharmacoeconomics, and safety studies. The Vaccines Research Area is and has been involved in various randomized clinical trials with GSK, Novartis, Pfizer and MSD vaccines. This specific study was funded by contracts between FISABIO-Salud Publica (former CSISP) and Sanofi-Pasteur and FISABIO-Salud Pública (former CSISP)and Sanofi-Pasteur MSD. There are no patents, products in development or marketed products to declare.

* Email: puig_joa@gva.es

¶ Membership of the Valencia Hospital Network for the Study of Influenza and Respiratory Virus Disease is provided in the Acknowledgments.

Introduction

Influenza runs on temperate zones as yearly seasonal epidemics [1]. These epidemics are associated with excess morbidity, hospitalizations and deaths [2–4]. Vaccination is considered the most effective strategy for preventing influenza and is recommended for individuals at high risk of serious complications [5].

Influenza vaccine effectiveness (IVE) varies seasonally depending on the antigenic proximity between the vaccine and circulating strains due to evolutionary drift [6–8] or altered antigenicity of the egg-derived strains in the vaccine [9–12]. IVE against laboratory-confirmed influenza in adults aged under 65 years old is described as moderate, whereas the evidence of protection in adults aged over 65 has been questioned [8]. Most evidence of the effectiveness of influenza vaccines comes from studies conducted in primary care, however, studies of the effectiveness in preventing serious complications, defined as admissions with influenza, are needed [13], as limited data on the effectiveness of the vaccines in preventing hospitalizations restrains advocacy for vaccination and the accuracy of estimates of the cost effectiveness of offering influenza vaccines [14].

The annual assessment of IVE against specific influenza-related outcomes is possible using real-time reverse transcription-polymerase chain reaction (rtRT-PCR) to ascertain influenza infection [15] and comparing the odds of being vaccinated among positive compared to negative for influenza admissions [16–20]. IVE estimates obtained from this test-negative approach are considered minimally biased, given that certain assumptions and conditions are met [20–22]. The test-negative study design has been used with consistent results [8].

The fact that for the 2011–2012 season three types of vaccine were offered free of charge to all inhabitants in Valencia (Spain) belonging to target groups for influenza vaccination [5,23], and the existence of the Valencia Hospital Network for the Study of Influenza and Respiratory Virus Disease (VAHNSI) [18], gave us the opportunity to estimate the IVE in preventing confirmed influenza hospitalizations by age group and type of vaccine.

Methods

Ethics Statement

The Ethics Research Committee of the Centro Superior de Estudios en Salud Pública (CSISP) approved the protocol of the study. All participants gave written informed consent before inclusion.

Study settings

We performed a prospective test-negative study. The study was conducted in nine health districts in Valencia, Spain. The hospitals in the participating districts, representing for the Valencia Hospital Network for the Study of Influenza and other Respiratory Virus Diseases (VAHNSI), provided health care services to 1,783,472 inhabitants, aged 18 years and over.

We considered that the influenza season began when two or more positive influenza hospitalizations were identified in two consecutive weeks and the season was considered to have ended in the week in which no identifications were observed for at least two consecutive weeks.

Three vaccines were acquired by public tender by the regional government and centrally distributed to be offered free of charge to groups targeted for influenza vaccination [23]: a split trivalent classical intramuscular vaccine (Gripavac, Sanofi Pasteur MSD, Lyon, France), a virosomal trivalent subunit vaccine (Inflexal-V, Crucell, Leiden, The Netherlands), and a split trivalent intradermal vaccine (Intanza 15 micrograms, Sanofi Pasteur MSD, Lyon, France). The split trivalent intramuscular (IM) influenza vaccine was offered to individuals belonging to groups targeted for influenza vaccination aged under 65 in all health districts. The virosomal vaccine was exclusively distributed in four health districts out of nine participating in the study and the intradermal vaccine was exclusively distributed in the other five districts. Both were aimed at individuals aged 65 or older.

From Monday to Saturday, study staff screened all previous 48-hour emergency admissions to identify eligible subjects because their indication for hospitalization could be related to influenza (Table S1) [17,18]. If the patient was considered eligible, the same study staff asked for written informed consent and collected all required data by means of a face-to-face interview, review of clinical records or by contacting the patient's physician. Finally, the same specifically trained study staff obtained a nasopharyngeal and a pharyngeal swab from each included patient. Samples were placed in vials with viral transport medium and kept at −20°C until sent to the reference laboratory (Text S1. Laboratory procedures).

Exclusion and inclusion criteria

Patients were excluded if they were institutionalized, non-residents in the healthcare district of enrollment, had severe egg allergy, a previous episode of laboratory-confirmed influenza in the current season or had been hospitalized in the previous 30 days.

Patients were included if they reported symptoms of influenza-like illness (ILI) [24], defined as at least one of four systemic symptoms (fever or feverishness, malaise, headache, myalgia) and one of three respiratory symptoms (cough, sore throat, shortness of breath) within 7 days of admission. Sudden onset of symptoms was not required for inclusion, and finally, patients were included if they belonged to targeted groups for influenza vaccination as defined in Valencia because of concurrent co-morbidity or age 60 and over [23].

Comparison groups and covariates

Influenza-positive admissions were compared with influenza-negative admissions [20–22]. Admissions were considered as influenza-positive or influenza-negative according to rtRT-PCR results (Text S1. Laboratory procedures).

Information was obtained on age, sex, eligibility criteria, hospitalization date, time from symptoms onset to hospitalization, time to swabbing, presence of major underlying medical conditions, long-term treatments, pregnancy status, number of physician encounters in the last three months, number of hospitalizations in the last year, prescription of antivirals, smoking habits, intensive care unit admission, death in hospital, length of stay, and three first recorded diagnoses at discharge or at death in hospital. The Barthel index was obtained in study subjects aged 65 or over [25]. Social class was assigned according to occupation [26,27].

Vaccination status

Reports of influenza vaccination were obtained by direct questioning and independently by a researcher blinded to patient characteristics through consultation of the Valencia population-based Vaccine Information System (Vaccine Information System), from which vaccination date, vaccine type, batch number, and manufacturer were ascertained. We obtained Vaccine Information System data on influenza vaccination for the 2010–2011 and

2009–2010 influenza seasons, monovalent 2009 pandemic, and 23 polysaccharide plain pneumococcal vaccine (23PPV).

A patient was considered immunized with the 2011–2012 influenza seasonal vaccine if the vaccine was recorded in the Vaccine Information System as administered more than 14 days before the date of the ILI onset or if the patients reported vaccination more than two weeks before symptoms onset.

Statistical analysis

We compared the differences in distribution using the Fisher exact test, Pearson chi square, Student's t-test or Kruskal-Wallis test, depending on the nature of the variable. We ascertained the contribution of covariates to the risk of laboratory confirmed influenza using the likelihood-ratio test (LRT).

We assessed confounding by considering biological and epidemiological plausibility and by analysis of the crude odds ratio of being a case and vaccinated compared to the same odds ratio when adjusted, one by one, by the collected covariates. We similarly estimated the LRT for departure from a linearity ($P<0.05$) in categorical ordered variables and the presence of interaction between potential confounders and current season vaccination. Evidence of clustering by enrollment site or epidemiological week was estimated by fitting random effects logistic regression models of the odds ratio of being influenza-positive and vaccinated.

Influenza vaccine effectiveness

IVE was defined as 100 x (1 - odds ratio). The odds ratio was estimated using a test-negative approach, comparing the odds of vaccination in admissions with confirmed influenza with the odds of vaccination in influenza-negative admissions [20–22]. The adjusted odds ratio (OR) was obtained with adjusted multivariate multilevel random effects logistic regression models, according to evidence on confounding, linearity, interaction, or clustering.

We defined six groups for IVE estimation: a) all subjects, b) subjects aged under 65, c) subjects aged 65 or older, d) subjects aged 65 or older targeted for vaccination with the intradermal vaccine, e) subjects aged 65 or older targeted for vaccination with the virosomal vaccine, and f) subjects aged under 65 targeted for vaccination with the classical IM split influenza vaccine.

The by type of vaccine estimates were restricted to subjects for whom vaccine type was ascertained through Vaccine Information System consultation. For groups "d" (intradermal) and "e" (virosomal) the analyses were restricted to residents of the health districts where the type of vaccine was distributed. Patients registered as vaccinated with vaccines not recommended in their district of residence or vaccinated with vaccines recommend for a different age group were not included in the analysis of IVE by type of vaccine.

All IVE analyses accounted for calendar time defined by epidemiological week of admission and hospital of enrollment, and were restricted to weeks in which at least two influenza-related admissions were observed. The same criteria were applied to the subgroup analyses. Given that this was a predominant A(H3N2) season and that only 5 out of 549 samples positive for influenza were not A(H3N2) we limited our analysis to the 544 samples positive for influenza A(H3N2).

All probabilities were 2-tailed; $P<0.05$ was considered significant. Associations were considered statistically significant when the 95% confidence interval (CI) of the OR did not include the unit. Analyses were performed with Stata 12.1 (StataCorp, College Station, TX).

Results

We identified 7,122 eligible admissions and included after consent 1,914 subjects who complied with the criteria for inclusion. A total of 544 (29%) were positive for influenza A(H3N2) and 1,370 (71%) were negative for influenza (Figure 1). The study period began on December 18, 2011, epidemiological week 51–2011, and ended on March 31, 2012, epidemiological week 13–2012 (Figure 2).

Subject characteristics and clinical outcomes according to PCR result for influenza

Influenza-positive subjects were admitted more often because of acute respiratory conditions (Table 1). Cough and fever were significantly more common in influenza-positive subjects than in negative subjects (Table 1). There were no differences in either length of stay or death while at hospital, and intensive care unit admission was slightly more frequent in negatives subjects (Table 1). Positive subjects did not differ from negative subjects on age, sex, body mass index or smoking habits. Partially skilled and unskilled employment types were overrepresented among positives (Table 2). The distribution of high-risk conditions was similar among positive and negative subjects (Table 2). Negative subjects consulted their general practitioner and had been hospitalized in the last 12 months more often than the positive subjects (Table 2). In subjects aged 65 or older moderate to severe functional impairment (Barthel score below 60) was more frequent in negative subjects compared with positive subjects (22% compared to 16%; $P=0.0133$).). Finally, we obtained swabs within seven days of ILI onset in 93% influenza-positive admissions compared to with 87% of negative admissions (Table 3) without evidence of a trend in positive results according to the elapsed days ($P=0.1764$).

Vaccination

The record of previous vaccination (influenza or other) in the Vaccine Information System was similar in both groups (Table 4). Overall, 1,086 (57%) subjects had a record of vaccination with the 2011–2012 seasonal influenza vaccine 15 or more days before symptoms onset, whereas 1,134 (59%) subjects reported being vaccinated for influenza two weeks or more before ILI symptoms onset. We considered as immunized 58% of influenza-positive and 62% of influenza-negative ($P=0.0585$) admissions (Table 4).

The mean (standard deviation) number of days from vaccination to onset of symptoms for influenza-positive subjects was 119 (21) compared with 109 (32) for influenza-negative subjects, with a significant trend for increasing risk ($P<0.0001$) of a positive influenza result in the unadjusted analysis considering days elapsed since vaccination to onset of symptoms (Table 4). This effect was no longer observed after adjusting by epidemiological week (Figure S1).

According to the Vaccine Information System similar proportions of positive and negative subjects were vaccinated with the influenza vaccine in the previous two seasons (2010–2011, 2009–2010) or with the monovalent pandemic 2009 H1N1vaccine (Table 4). The positive subjects were vaccinated with the 23PPV more often than negative subjects.

Type of vaccine

The intradermal vaccine was administered to 60% of influenza-positive and 70% of influenza-negative admissions aged 65 or over ($P=0.0080$). The virosomal vaccine was administered to 68% of influenza-positive and 68% of influenza-negative admissions aged 65 or over ($P=0.8970$). The split classical IM influenza vaccine

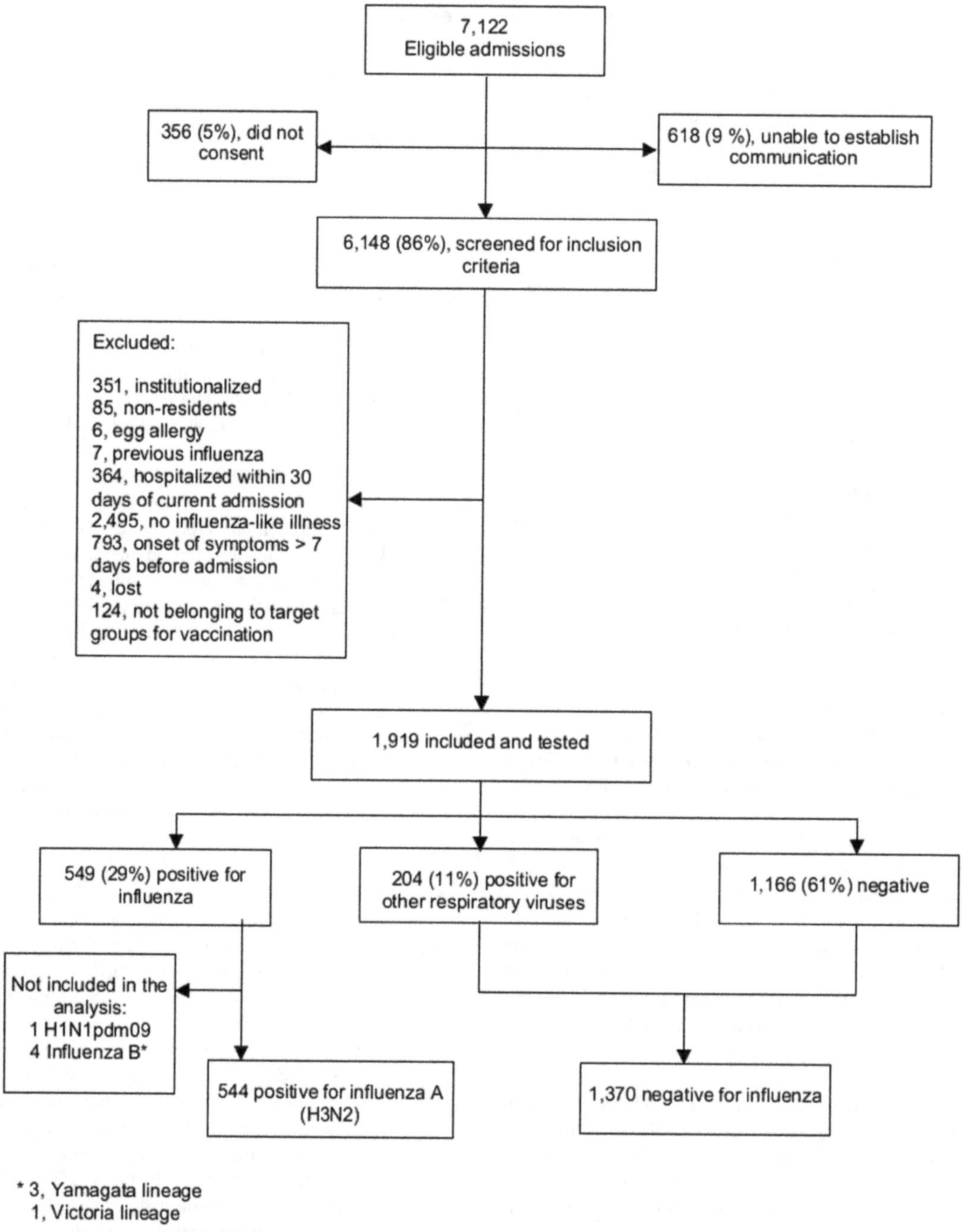

Figure 1. Flow diagram of study subjects.

was administered to 20% of the positive and 46% of the negative ($P = 0.0050$) subjects aged 18 to 64 (Table 5 and Table S3).

Effect modification, confounding and clustering

There was moderate evidence of age in deciles acting as an effect modifier, $P = 0.0540$ (Figure S2). Outpatient consultations in the preceding three months and previous vaccination with the 23PPV were associated with both being positive for influenza and current season influenza vaccination (Table 1, Table S4a and Table S4b). Overall, there was a strong ($P<0.0001$) clustering effect due to epidemiological week and to hospital.

Influenza vaccine effectiveness

The overall adjusted IVE against hospitalization with PCR-confirmed influenza was 31% (95%CI, 11% to 47%) (Table 6). The IVE estimate in subjects aged under 65 was 72% (38% to 88%) and 21% (−5% to 40%) for those aged 65 or older. Those estimates did not vary when we conducted sensitivity analyses taking into account how vaccination was defined (registry and recall, registry only, or recall only) or elapsed time from symptoms onset to swabbing (irrespective of elapsed time, seven days or less, or four days or less) (Figure 3). Overall the results were homogenous irrespective of how vaccination exposure was defined or the cut-off for days elapsed since symptoms onset to swabbing.

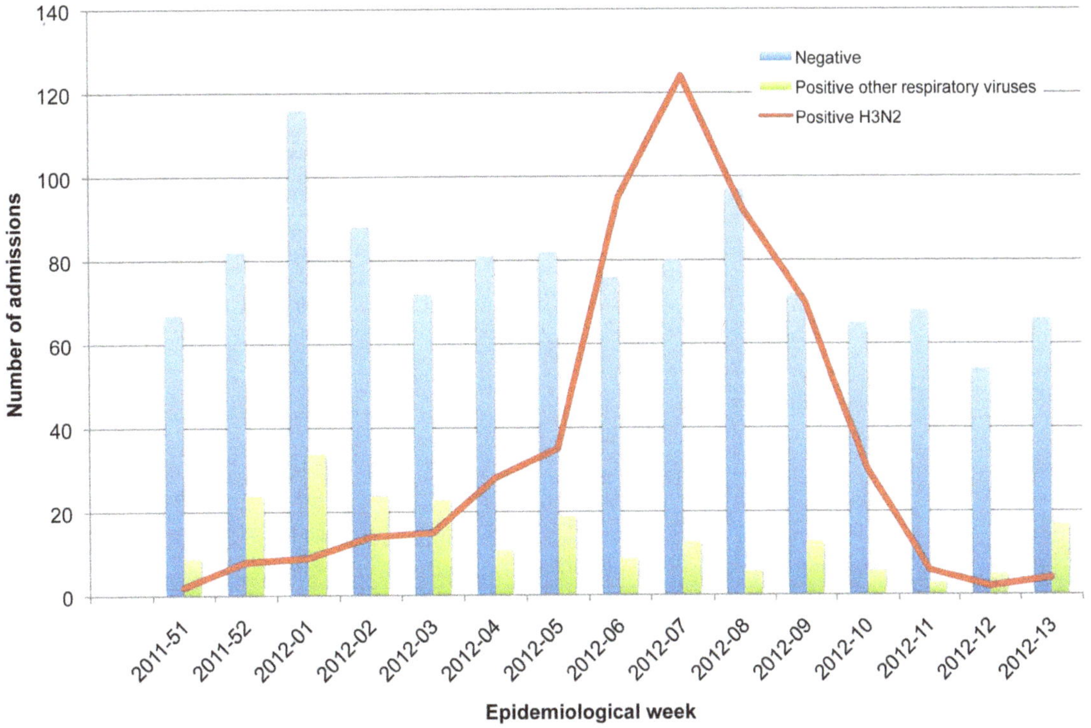

Figure 2. Admissions by epidemiological week and laboratory result.

There was strong evidence of heterogeneity (I-squared test, 74%) by age. The heterogeneity inside the groups shown in Figure 3 was 0%.

By type of vaccine, the split classical IM influenza vaccine used in those aged 18 to under 65 targeted for influenza had an adjusted IVE against hospitalization with PCR-confirmed influenza of 68% (12% to 88%). The intradermal vaccine, used in subjects aged 65 or older in five of the healthcare districts included in the study, had an adjusted IVE against hospitalization with PCR-confirmed influenza of 39% (11% to 58%); finally, for the virosomal vaccine, used in the remaining four healthcare districts studied, the adjusted IVE against hospitalization with PCR-confirmed influenza was 16% (−39% to 49%) effectiveness (Table 6).

Discussion

The overall adjusted estimate of IVE against laboratory-confirmed influenza A(H3N2) hospitalizations in adults targeted for vaccination in Valencia (Spain) of 31.1% (95% CI, 10.9% to 46.7%) suggested that vaccination may have prevented over 30% of the severe cases of influenza requiring hospitalization in vaccinated patients. These estimates of protection were larger in patients 18 to 64 years of age (72.4%, 95% CI, 37.7% to 87.8%) compared with patients of 65 years and older (20.6%, −5.1% to 40.0%). A classical IM vaccine used to vaccinate subjects aged under 65 displayed high IVE in preventing admissions related to influenza. In subjects aged 65 or older, the intradermal vaccine had a moderate effect in preventing admissions related to influenza. No effect was observed for the virosomal vaccine. To our knowledge, estimates on virosomal or intradermal vaccine in preventing confirmed influenza-related admissions in subjects aged 65 or older have not been published previously.

The results of observational studies are to be interpreted with caution because of the limitations related to unmeasured confounding, comparability of subjects, selection and classification bias or study design.

To take into consideration these limitations, we collected information on a comprehensive group of potential confounders that allowed us to account for frailty bias and confounding by indication [28–30]. Further, to improve comparability of vaccinated with unvaccinated subjects we constrained our analysis to subjects targeted for influenza vaccination.

Selection bias

Selection bias was minimized because we enrolled most eligible patients (Figure 1), and eligibility criteria were applied with no knowledge of vaccination or influenza infection. The test-negative study design minimized selection bias, as positive and negative subjects were similar in their healthcare-seeking behavior and chances of being identified and included in the study (Text S2. Bias due to design).

Misclassification

Vaccination status. Vaccination status established by interviews and by consulting vaccination records can be improved and misclassification reduced if both sources of information are combined (unpublished data). In the sensitivity analysis comparing IVE with vaccination ascertained by Vaccine Information System, by recall or with both methods combined, we obtained overlapping estimates. In the analysis by vaccine type we only included subjects with records in the Vaccine Information System information system.

Influenza status. We have used an endpoint of laboratory-confirmed influenza. Although it can be argued that we may have missed those influenza cases that were PCR negative at admission

Table 1. Main complaint at admission, influenza-like-illness symptoms within seven days to admission and clinical outcomes in influenza positive compared to influenza negative admissions

		Positive for influenza A(H3N2)	Negative for influenza	Crude odds ratio	P-value
		n = 544	n = 1370	(95% CI)	(LR test)
		Number (%)	Number (%)		
Main complaint at admission					
	Respiratory	446 (82)	1019 (74)	1.6 (1.2–2.0)	0.0003
	Cardiovascular	10 (2)	85 (6)	0.3 (0.4–0.6)	<0.0001
	Sepsis, SIRS, metabolic failure	86 (16)	238 (17)	0.9 (0.7–1.2)	0.4081
	Confusion, convulsion	1 (0.2)	13 (1)	0.2 (0.0–1.5)	0.0448
	Myalgias	1 (0.2)	15 (1)	0.2 (0.0–1.3)	0.0239
Influenza-like-illness symptoms		Number (%)	Number (%)		
	Sudden onset	328 (60)	792(58)	1.1 (0.9–1.4)	0.3192
	Fever	468 (86)	1030(75)	2.0 (1.6–2.7)	<0.0001
	Myalgia-malaise or headache	425 (78)	1064 (78)	1.0 (0.8–1.3)	0.8267
	Cough	508 (93)	1180 (86)	2.3 (1.6–3.3)	<0.0001
	Sore throat	178 (33)	416 (30)	1.1 (0.9–1.4)	0.3164
	Dyspnea	496 (91)	1270 (93)	0.8 (0.6–1.2)	0.2659
Length of stay (days), mean (SD)		7.3 (5.6)	7.3 (6.0)		0.9278
Intensive care unit admission					
	No	535 (98)	1325 (97)	1.0	0.0408
	Yes	9 (2)	45 (3)	0.5 (0.2–1.0)	
Died during hospital stay					
	No	513 (94)	1289 (94)	1.0	0.8569
	Yes	31 (6)	81 (6)	1.0 (0.6–1.5)	

CI Confidence Interval. LR Likelihood ratio. SD (standard deviation).
SIRS: Systemic inflammatory response syndrome.
Metabolic failure: hyperglycemic or hypoglycemic commas, acute renal failure, and disorders of fluid, electrolyte and acid-base balance.

[15]. PCR-confirmed influenza is likely to be more specific than hospitalization with clinically diagnosed ILI, as the majority of these cases are likely to be due to other co-circulating pathogens. Mathematical modeling has suggested that false positives may lower the IVE estimates, and therefore, the use of less-specific outcomes, such as clinical ILI, may generate even less accurate IVE estimates than PCR-confirmed influenza outcome [19].

We choose not to exclude subjects according to time to swab to preserve the information provided by true influenza-positive admissions and to avoid unknown misclassification bias [31]. Supporting our decision was the absence of a trend in the percentage of positives according to the days elapsed since symptoms onset and the overlapping IVE estimates obtained in the sensitivity analysis.

Vaccine effectiveness

Comparisons on the consistency of IVE estimates obtained in different influenza seasons or even for the same season but in different geographical locations are to be made cautiously, as IVE estimates are affected by season-to-season differences in virulence of circulating strains, levels of population immunity, healthcare-seeking behavior, matching of the vaccine recommended antigenic composition with the circulating strains, and different types of vaccines used in different settings.

Several additional reasons may explain the differences observed in point estimates of IVE (and the variability in confidence intervals) against medically attended outcomes with laboratory-confirmed H3N2 in our study compared with other test-negative studies performed during the same season [32–37].

First, the baseline characteristics of the patients included in the mentioned studies are different from ours in terms of risk factors that consistently affect IVE in regression analyses, as age distribution, presence of comorbidities, hospitalizations within the previous 12 months and percentage vaccinated.

In general, patients from primary-care surveillance systems, included in all of the above-mentioned studies, are younger, more likely to be free of comorbidities, and less likely to have been vaccinated or hospitalized within the previous 12 months compared with inpatients from hospital-based surveillance systems. In one study [32], patients were ascertained both at GP consultation and in hospital wards, but less than 10% of the study patients were inpatients.

Although the studies considered were performed in the northern hemisphere, differences in past exposure to H3N2 infection, infectious challenge, and vaccination policies, which are likely to vary geographically, may all underlie differences in vaccine effects across regions [38,39].

Finally, limited sample size or sub-group analyses lead to low precision around point estimates and random highs and lows.

Despite all of these limitations, for patients aged under 65 years (Figure S3a), in terms of the confidence intervals of our results, 72% (38% to 88%) overlap with those reported in Navarre [32],

Table 2. Characteristics of study subjects according to PCR result.

	Positive for influenza A(H3N2) n = 544 Number (%)	Negative for influenza n = 1370 Number (%)	Crude odds ratio (95% CI)	P-value (LR test)
Age (in years) group				
18–49	23 (4)	64 (5)	1.0	0.0908
50–64	63 (12)	187 (14)	0.9 (0.5–1.6)	
65–74	107 (20)	302 (22)	1.0 (0.6–1.7)	
75–79	122 (22)	247 (18)	1.4 (0.8–2.3)	
80–84	109 (20)	232 (17)	1.3(0.8–2.2)	
>=85	120 (22)	338 (25)	1.0 (0.6–1.7)	
Sex				
Male	317 (58)	753 (55)	1.0	0.1880
Female	227 (42)	617 (45)	0.9 (0.7–1.1)	
Number of high-risk conditions				
None	76 (14)	157 (12)	1.0	0.1476
One	199 (37)	475 (35)	0.9 (0.6–1.2)	
Two or more	269 (50)	738 (54)	0.8 (0.6–1.0)	
Body mass index				
<18.5	6 (1)	24 (2)	0.71 (.3–1.8)	
18.5 to 24.9	150 (28)	427 (31)	1.0	0.1329
25 to 29.9	234 (43)	512 (37)	1.3 (1.0–1.7)	
30 to 39.9	139 (26)	368 (27)	1.1 (0.8–1.4)	
>=40	15 (3)	39 (3)	1.1 (0.0-2-0)	
Smoker				
Never	253 (47)	620 (45)	1.0	0.1450
Ex-smoker	211 (39)	586 (43)	0.9 (0.7–1.1)	
Current smoker	80 (15)	164 (12)	1.2 (0.9–1.6)	
Socioeconomic class				
Professional to skilled manual	108 (20)	339 (25)	1.0	0.0210
Partially skilled to unskilled	436 (80)	1031 (75)	1.3 (1.0–1.7)	
Outpatient visits last three months				
None	132 (24)	292 (21)	1.0	0.0117
One	131 (24)	269 (20)	1.1 (0.8–1.4)	
Two or more	281 (52)	809 (59)	0.8 (0.6–1.0)	
Number of hospitalization previous 12 months				
None	376 (69)	870(64)	1.0	0.0008
One	123 (23)	298 (22)	1.0 (0.7–1.2)	
Two	26 (5)	100 (7)	0.6 (0.4–0.9)	
Three or more	19 (3)	102 (7)	0.4 (0.3–0.7)	

PCR real-time reverse transcription-polymerase chain reaction. CI Confidence Interval. LR Likelihood ratio.

44% (−11% to 72%). For I-MOVE [33], the number is 63% (26%–82%); and for Canada [36], the number is 44%(−41% to 78%). Those results are statistically homogenous, with a pooled IVE estimate of 56%(42% to 71%). A similar result is obtained when heterogeneity among IVE estimates against laboratory-confirmed influenza is explored in IVE estimates for subjects over 50 to over 65 (Figure S3b), depending on the study [32–36], with a pooled IVE estimate of 30% (14 to 46%); or among studies reporting overall IVE estimates (Figure S3c) against laboratory confirmed H3N2 for the 2011–2012 season [32–37] with a pooled IVE estimate of 35% (26% to 44%). In summary, we report similar overall moderate to low IVE results as those reported by others for the same 2011–2012 season, with an overall better IVE in young adults belonging to target groups for vaccination and an overall lower response in the elderly.

Table 3. Time since symptom onset to swabbing according to PCR result.

	Positive for influenza A(H3N2)	Negative for influenza	Crude odds ratio	P-value [a]
	n = 544	n = 1370	(95% CI)	
	Number (%)	Number (%)		
Onset to swab (days)				
1 to 2	77 (14)	271 (20)	1.0	<0.1764
3 to 4	237 (44)	440 (32)	1.9 (1.4–2.6)	
5 to 7	194 (36)	486 (35)	1.4 (1.0–1.9)	
>7	36 (7)	173 (13)	0.7 (0.5–1.1)	

PCR real-time reverse transcription-polymerase chain reaction. CI Confidence Interval.
a: Score test for trend of odds.

Table 4. Vaccination according to PCR result.

	Positive for influenza A(H3N2)	Negative for influenza	Crude odds ratio	P-value
	n = 544	n = 1370	(95% CI)	(LR test)
	Number (%)	Number (%)		
Included in Vaccine Information System [a]				
No	73 (13)	218 (16)	1.0	0.1662
Yes	471 (87)	1,152 (84)	1.2 (0.9–1.6)	
Immunized with current 2011–2012 season influenza vaccine [b]				
No	230 (42)	515 (38)	1.00	0.0585
Yes	314 (58)	855 (62)	0.82 (0.67–1.01)	
Days since vaccination to onset of symptoms [c]				
Mean (s.d.)	119 (21)	109 (32)		<0.0001
14 to 89	25 (9)	243 (31)	1.0	<0.0001
90 to 119	105 (37)	358 (32)	4.0 (2.5–6.3)	
120–184	158 (55)	297 (37)	5.2 (3.3–8.2)	
Vaccinated on previous seasons				
Seasonal, 2010–2011				
No	239 (44)	558 (41)	1.0	0.2003
Yes	305 (56)	812 (59)	0.9 (0.7–1.1)	
Seasonal, 2009–2010				
No	223 (41)	547 (40)	1.0	0.6682
Yes	321 (59)	823 (60)	1.0 (0.8–1.2)	
Pandemic, 2009–2010				
No	377 (69)	964 (70)	1.0	0.6473
Yes	167 (31)	406 (30)	1.1 (0.9–1.3)	
23 polysaccharide pneumococcal vaccine				
No	392 (72)	1,067 (78)	1.0	0.0076
Yes	152 (28)	303 (22)	1.4 (1.1–1.7)	

PCR real-time reverse transcription-polymerase chain reaction. CI Confidence Interval. LR Likelihood ratio.
[a]Any vaccination ever recorded in the Vaccine Information System.
[b.]A patient was considered immunized with the 2011–2012 influenza seasonal vaccine if the vaccine was recorded in the Vaccine Information System as administered more than 14 days before the date of the ILI onset or if the patients reported vaccination more than two weeks before symptoms onset.
[c]Data from 1,086 (288 positive and 798 negative) patients vaccinated 15 or more days before onset of symptoms according to the information in the Vaccine Information System out of 1,169 classified as immunized because of information retrieved from the Vaccine Information System or by patient's recall of vaccination two weeks before symptoms onset.

Table 5. Influenza vaccines recorded as administered by type of vaccine, age group, and PCR result.

Type of vaccine [a]	PCR result for influenza						P value
	Positive		Negative		Total		
	n	%	n	%	n	%	
Intradermal (subjects>=65 years of age) [b]							
No	82	40.0	136	29.6	218	32.8	
Yes	123	60.0	324	70.4	447	67.2	*P*=0.0080
Total	205	100.0	460	100.0	665	100.0	
Virosomal (subjects>=65 years of age) [b]							
No	60	32.4	102	31.9	162	32.1	
Yes	125	67.6	218	68.1	343	67.9	*P*=0.8970
Total	185	100.0	320	100.0	505	100.0	
Split conventional (subjects 18 to <65 years of age) [c]							
No	39	79.6	30	53.6	69	65.7	
Yes	10	20.4	26	46.4	36	34.3	*P*=0.0050
Total	49	100.0	56	100.0	105	100.0	

PCR real-time reverse transcription-polymerase chain reaction.

[a] Recorded vaccinations in the Vaccine Information System only (see Table 4 for the percentage of patients included in the Vaccine Information System). The percentages reported over all participants included in the Vaccine Information System and with any vaccination ever recorded in the Vaccine Information System.

[b] Encompassing epidemiological weeks 52 to 12, with influenza related admissions identified in>=65 years subjects. This was the age group targeted to receive this type of vaccine.

[c] Encompassing epidemiological weeks 4 to 10, with influenza related admissions identified in <65 years old subjects. This was the age group targeted to receive this type of vaccine.

Table 6. Influenza vaccine effectiveness in preventing admissions related to H3N2 influenza.

Considered groups	Vaccinated positives (n)/all positives (N)		Vaccinated negatives (n)/all negatives (N)		IVE (IC95%)		IVE (95% CI)	
	n/N (%)		n/N (%)		Non-adjusted		Adjusted	
Overall	314/544	(58)	855/1370	(62)	17.8	(−0.7 to 32.8)	31.1	(10.9 to 46.7) [a]
By age group, cut-point at 65 years of age								
<65	20/82	(24)	50/102	(49)	66.5	(35.1 to 82.6)	72.4	(37.7 to 87.8) [b]
>=65	294/457	(64)	705/1054	(67)	10.7	(−12.4 to 29.1)	20.6	(−5.1 to 40.0) [a]
By vaccine type, recommended age group								
Split classical IM, <65	10/49	(20)	26/56	(46)	70.4	(26.5 to 88.1)	67.5	(11.8 to 88.1) [c]
Split intradermal, ≥ 65	123/205	(60)	324/460	(70)	37.0	(11.0 to 55.5)	38.9	(10.8 to 58.1) [d]
Subunit virosomal, ≥65	125/185	(68)	218/320	(68)	2.5	(−43.6 to 33.9)	15.7	(−39.0 to 48.8)[e]

Positives admissions with influenza confirmed influenza by real time reverse transcription polymerase chain reaction (rtRT-PCR). Negatives admissions with a negative rtRT-PCR result for influenza. IVE influenza vaccine effectiveness. CI Confidence Interval.

a Strong evidence ($P<0.002$) of between hospital and between epidemiological week variability. Hospital and epidemiological week included as random effect parameters in the multilevel analysis to estimate influenza vaccine effectiveness adjusted by age (deciles), sex, number of outpatient consultations in the last three months, and previous administration of plain 23 polysaccharide pneumococcal vaccine.

b Moderate evidence of between hospital variability ($P=0.045$) and of between epidemiological week variability ($P=0.015$). Hospital and epidemiological week included as a random effect parameter in the multilevel analysis to estimate influenza vaccine effectiveness in this group, adjusted as in (a).

c Weak evidence of between hospital variability ($P>0.05$). Strong evidence ($P=<0.001$) of between epidemiological week variability. Epidemiological week included as a random effect parameter in the multilevel analysis to estimate split conventional influenza vaccine effectiveness in this age group, adjusted as in (a) with hospital included in the model as an indicator variable.

d Weak evidence of between hospital variability ($P=0.497$). Strong evidence ($P=<0.001$) of between epidemiological week variability. Epidemiological week included as a random effect parameter in the multilevel analysis to estimate influenza vaccine effectiveness in this group, adjusted as in (a) with hospital included in the model as an indicator variable.

e Moderate evidence ($P=0.042$) of between hospital variability and strong evidence ($P=<0.001$) of between epidemiological week variability. Hospital and epidemiological included as random effect parameters in a multilevel analysis to estimate influenza vaccine effectiveness adjusted as in (a).

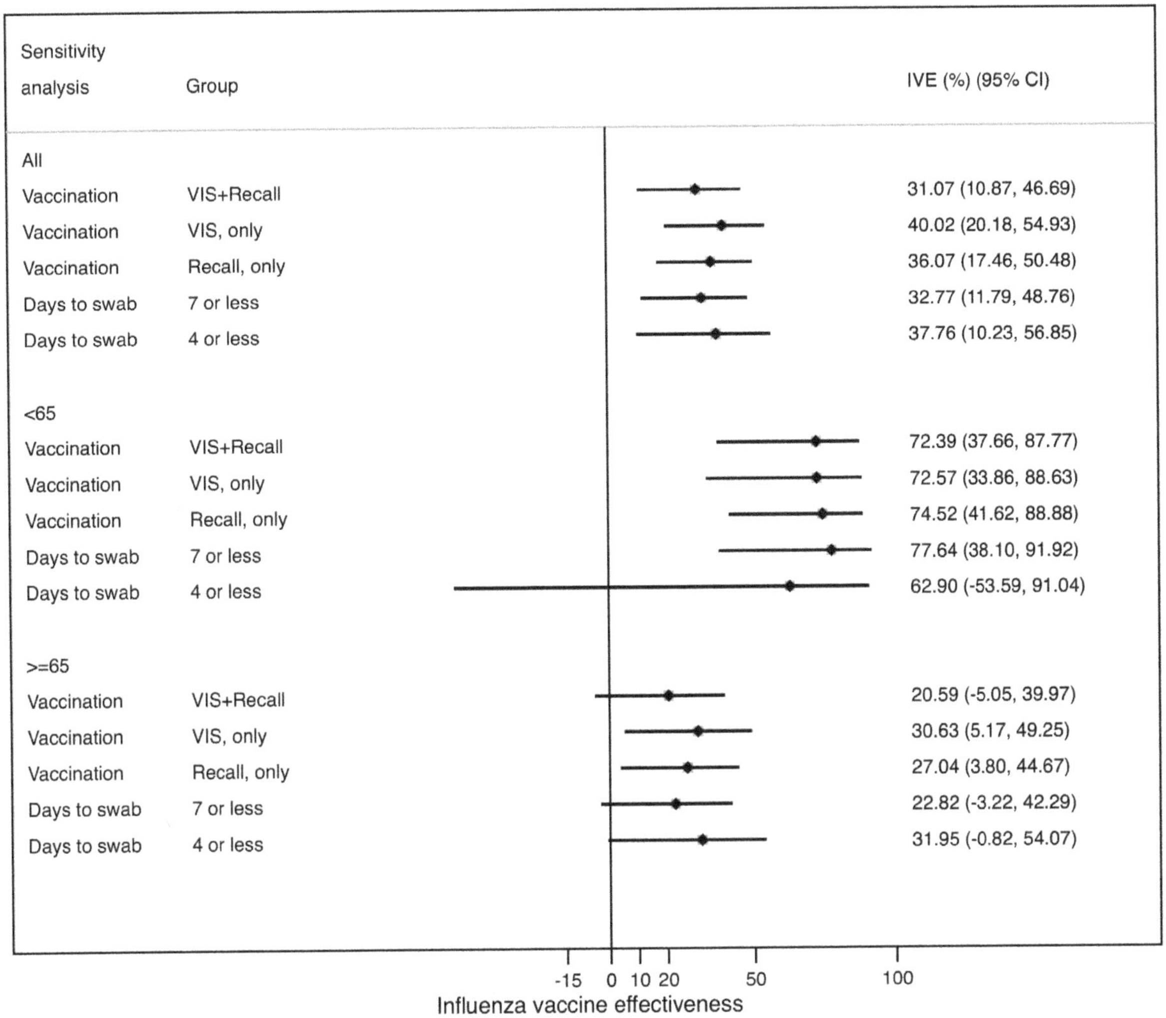

Figure 3. Sensitivity analysis of adjusted influenza vaccine effectiveness. Adjusted influenza vaccine effectiveness (IVE) assessed for all ages, <65 and>=65, and by: a) vaccination ascertainment method: Vaccine Information System (VIS), as reported by the patient (recall) and both combined; b) days to swab: seven or less, four or less. Reference category for all analyses includes all patients irrespective of time elapsed to swab and vaccination according to VIS or recall. OR: adjusted odds ratio. OR adjusted as reported in footnotes in Table 6.

Our estimates add to the evidence indicating a significant IVE against hospitalization with laboratory-confirmed influenza during the 2011–2012 season [33,40–44]. However, these estimates vary widely across studies, which used different criteria to select the group of patients to be included in the IVE sub-group analyses. Furthermore, caution is needed because of the limited sample size usually associated with sub-group analyses, which may have led to low precision around point estimates and random highs and lows, making comparisons across studies difficult. Our moderate-low overall estimate of IVE against hospitalization for 2011–2012 is very similar to that reported by others. It has been suggested that antigenically different circulating A(H3N2) from that of the vaccine strain in Europe may explain the low effectiveness reported in Europe [45].

Influenza A (H3N2) viruses circulating in Spain during the 2011–2012 season were distributed in three genetic groups that displayed evidence of antigenic diversity regarding the A/Perth/16/2009 vaccine strain [46,47]. The results we report for those aged 65 and over are consistent with those reported previously for the elderly in seasons with poor matching between vaccine and circulating strains [8,48,49].

Although we do not have information to support that mutations in the egg-passaged A/Perth/16/2009 (H3N2) NYMC X-187 derived from the A/Victoria/210/2009 strains used in the 2011–2012 vaccines could explain the moderate influenza vaccine effectiveness we have found, we cannot disregard that egg passage could have a similar effect in the immunogenic capability of the 2011–2012 vaccine as the one described for the H3N2 egg-passaged strain in the 2012–2013 seasonal vaccine [12,45,50].

Conclusions

In this season we observed relevant influenza vaccine effectiveness in adults aged 18 to 64 years old in contrast to a low and non-significant vaccine effectiveness in subjects aged 65 and over.

Most of the variability in IVE estimates observed by us in the studied season could be explained by age.

The significant effect of the intradermal vaccine, recommended for subjects aged 65 and over, in a season with a questionable match between the circulating and vaccine strain, could be interpreted as a proof of concept of the opportunities of the intradermal approach to protect those more at risk because of advancing age.

The year-by-year drift of the influenza virus and the variable protection conferred by different influenza vaccine formulations, combined with the interaction of those factors with age and other risk conditions, justify the year-by-year active surveillance of severe cases of influenza and of IVE in preventing severe influenza-related outcomes as the one performed in the Valencia Hospital Network for the Study of Influenza and Respiratory Virus Disease.

Supporting Information

Figure S1 Risk of being influenza-positive according to time elapsed since vaccination to onset of symptoms (vaccination waning immunity effect) when not adjusting for calendar time and after adjusting for calendar time.

Figure S2 Odds ratio of being positive for influenza if vaccinated by age in deciles.

Figure S3 a. Comparative analysis of influenza vaccine effectiveness estimates published by various groups in preventing medically attended influenza-like illness or admissions with H3N2-confirmed influenza for the 2011–2012 season in subjects aged less than 65 years of age. **b.** Comparative analysis of influenza vaccine effectiveness estimates published by various groups in preventing medically attended influenza-like illness or admissions with H3N2-confirmed influenza for the 2011–2012 season in subjects aged at least over 50 years of age. **c.** Comparative analysis of influenza vaccine effectiveness estimates published by various groups in preventing medically attended influenza-like illness or admissions with H3N2-confirmed influenza for the 2011–2012 season, all age groups.
(PDF)

Table S1 Eligibility criteria: list of admission diagnoses possibly associated with an influenza infection.

Table S2 Influenza vaccination as recorded in the Vaccine Information System for the 2011–2012 influenza season. Vaccine type and healthcare district/hospital.

Table S3 a. Characteristics of unvaccinated and vaccinated subjects (i); demographic, socioeconomic, smoking habits, body mass index, and number of risk factors. **b**. Characteristics of unvaccinated and vaccinated subjects (ii): use of healthcare services, previous vaccination, length of stay, intensive care unit admission and in-hospital death.

Acknowledgments

The authors thank the staff of Hospital General de Castelló in Castellón; La Plana, in Vila-real; Arnau de Vilanova, in Valencia; La Fe, in Valencia; Lluis Alcanyis, in Xàtiva; San Juan, in Alicante; Hospital General de Alicante, in Alicante; and Hospital de Elda, in Elda. We also thank all the study participants and their families.

Contributors

The members of the Valencia Hospital Network for the Study of Influenza and Respiratory Virus Disease (VAHNSI) are: Main contact: Joan Puig-Barberà (puig_joa@gva.es). Group members: Juan Manuel Beltrán-Garrido, Hospital General de Castellón, Castellón; Concha Carratalá-Munuera, Hospital San Juan de Alicante; Patricia Correcher-Medina, Hospital Lluis Alvanyís, Xàtiva; Vicente Gil-Guillén, Hospital de Elda, Elda; Rosa Larrea-González, Hospital General de Castellón, Castellón; Ramón Limón-Ramírez, Hospital La Plana, Vila-real; José Luis Micó-Esparza, Hospital Arnau de Vilanova, Valencia; Joan Mollar-Maseres, Hospital La Fe, Valencia; Maria del Carmen Otero-Reigada, Hospital la Fe, Valencia; Germán Schwarz-Chavarri, Hospital General de Alicante; Miguel Tortajada-Girbés, Hospital Dr. Peset, Valencia.

Author Contributions

Conceived and designed the experiments: JPB. Analyzed the data: JPB AAP. Contributed reagents/materials/analysis tools: JGL. Wrote the paper: JPB JDD AAP JGL. Conception and design: MRG RLR SPV JLME MTG CCM RLG JMBG MCOR JMM PCM GSC VGG. Acquisition of data: MRG RLR SPV JLME MTG CCM RLG JMBG MCOR JMM PCM GSC VGG. Interpretation of data: MRG RLR SPV JLME MTG CCM RLG JMBG MCOR JMM PCM GSC VGG. Reviewed article or revised it critically for important intellectual content: MRG RLR SPV JLME MTG CCM RLG JMBG MCOR JMM PCM GSC VGG.

References

1. Bloom-Feshbach K, Alonso WJ, Charu V, Tamerius J, Simonsen L, et al. (2013) Latitudinal variations in seasonal activity of influenza and respiratory syncytial virus (RSV): a global comparative review. PLoS One 8: e54445.
2. Olson DR, Heffernan RT, Paladini M, Konty K, Weiss D, et al. (2007) Monitoring the impact of influenza by age: emergency department fever and respiratory complaint surveillance in New York City. PLoS Med 4: e247.
3. Zhou H, Thompson WW, Viboud CG, Ringholz CM, Cheng PY, et al. (2012) Hospitalizations associated with influenza and respiratory syncytial virus in the United States, 1993–2008. Clin Infect Dis 54: 1427–1436.
4. Thompson WW, Shay DK, Weintraub E, Brammer L, Cox N, et al. (2003) Mortality associated with influenza and respiratory syncytial virus in the United States. JAMA 289: 179–186.
5. World Health Organization (2012) Vaccines against influenza WHO position paper – November 2012. Wkly Epidemiol Rec 87: 461–476.
6. Carrat F, Flahault A (2007) Influenza vaccine: the challenge of antigenic drift. Vaccine 25: 6852–6862.
7. Belongia EA, Kieke BA, Donahue JG, Greenlee RT, Balish A, et al. (2009) Effectiveness of inactivated influenza vaccines varied substantially with antigenic match from the 2004–2005 season to the 2006–2007 season. J Infect Dis 199: 159–167.
8. Osterholm MT, Kelley NS, Sommer A, Belongia EA (2011) Efficacy and effectiveness of influenza vaccines: a systematic review and meta-analysis. Lancet Infect Dis 12: 36–44.
9. Katz JM, Webster RG (1989) Efficacy of inactivated influenza A virus (H3N2) vaccines grown in mammalian cells or embryonated eggs. J Infect Dis 160: 191–198.
10. Rocha EP, Xu X, Hall HE, Allen JR, Regnery HL, et al. (1993) Comparison of 10 influenza A (H1N1 and H3N2) haemagglutinin sequences obtained directly from clinical specimens to those of MDCK cell- and egg-grown viruses. J Gen Virol 74 (Pt 11): 2513–2518.
11. Ndifon W, Wingreen NS, Levin SA (2009) Differential neutralization efficiency of hemagglutinin epitopes, antibody interference, and the design of influenza vaccines. Proc Natl Acad Sci U S A 106: 8701–8706.
12. Skowronski DM, Janjua NZ, De Serres G, Sabaiduc S, Eshaghi A, et al. (2014) Low 2012–13 influenza vaccine effectiveness associated with mutation in the egg-adapted H3N2 vaccine strain not antigenic drift in circulating viruses. PLoS One 9: e92153.
13. Puig-Barberà J, Natividad-Sancho A, Launay O, Burtseva E, Ciblak MA, et al. (2014) 2012–2013 Seasonal Influenza Vaccine Effectiveness against Influenza Hospitalizations: Results from the Global Influenza Hospital Surveillance Network. PLoS One 9: e100497.
14. Maciosek MV, Edwards NM, Coffield AB, Flottemesch TJ, Nelson WW, et al. (2006) Priorities among effective clinical preventive services: methods. Am J Prev Med 31: 90–96.
15. Lee N, Chan PK, Hui DS, Rainer TH, Wong E, et al. (2009) Viral loads and duration of viral shedding in adult patients hospitalized with influenza. J Infect Dis 200: 492–500.

16. Rothman KJ, Greenland S, Lash TL (2008) Case-Control Studies. In: Rothman KJ, Greenland S, Lash TL, editors. Modern epidemiology. Philadelphia: Wolters Kluwer Health/Lippincott Williams & Wilkins. pp. 111–127.
17. Puig-Barberà J, Arnedo-Pena A, Pardo-Serrano F, Tirado-Balaguer MD, Pérez-Vilar S, et al. (2010) Effectiveness of seasonal 2008-2009, 2009–2010 and pandemic vaccines, to prevent influenza hospitalizations during the autumn 2009 influenza pandemic wave in Castellón, Spain. A test-negative, hospital-based, case-control study. Vaccine 28: 7460–7467.
18. Puig-Barberà J, Diez-Domingo J, Arnedo-Pena A, Ruiz-García M, Pérez-Vilar S, et al. (2012) Effectiveness of the 2010–2011 seasonal influenza vaccine in preventing confirmed influenza hospitalizations in adults: A case-case comparison, case-control study. Vaccine 30: 5714–5720.
19. Orenstein EW, De Serres G, Haber MJ, Shay DK, Bridges CB, et al. (2007) Methodologic issues regarding the use of three observational study designs to assess influenza vaccine effectiveness. Int J Epidemiol 36: 623–631.
20. De Serres G, Skowronski DM, Ambrose C (2013) The test-negativee design: validity, accuracy and precision of vaccine efficacy estimates compared to the gold standard of randomised placebo-controlled clinical. Eurosurveillance 18: pii = 20585.
21. Jackson ML, Nelson JC (2013) The test-negative design for estimating influenza vaccine effectiveness. Vaccine 31: 2165–2168.
22. Foppa IM, Haber M, Ferdinands JM, Shay DK (2013) The case test-negative design for studies of the effectiveness of seasonal influenza vaccine. Vaccine 31: 3104–3109.
23. Portero-Alonso A, Pastor-Villalba E, Martín-Ivorra R, Alguacil-Ramos AM, López-Maside A, et al. (2012) Prevención y vigilancia de la gripe en la Comunitat Valenciana. Temporada 2011–2012. Informe 135. Conselleria de Sanitat. Dirección General de Investigación y Salud Pública. Available: http://www.sp.san.gva.es/biblioteca/publicacion_dgsp.jsp?cod_pub_ran=709064217&tacc=15. Accessed 2013 May 10.
24. European Influenza Surveillance Network (EISN) website. Influenza case definitions. Clinical criteria. Influenza-like illness (ILI). European Centre for Disease Prevention and Control (ECDC) 2005–22012. Available: http://ecdc.europa.eu/en/activities/surveillance/EISN/surveillance/Pages/influenza_case_definitions.aspx. Accessed: 2012 Nov 2.
25. Puig-Barberà J, Diez-Domingo J, Pérez Hoyos S, Belenguer Varea A, González Vidal D (2004) Effectiveness of the MF59-adjuvanted influenza vaccine in preventing emergency admissions for pneumonia in the elderly over 64 years of age. Vaccine 23: 283–289.
26. Benach J, Amable M (2004) [Social classes and poverty]. Gac Sanit 18 Suppl 1: 16–23.
27. Regidor E, Grupo de Trabajo de la SEE (2001) The Goldthorpe Social Class Classification: reference framework for a proposal for the measurement of social class by the Working Group of the Spanish Society of Epidemiology. Rev Esp Salud Publica 75: 13–22.
28. Jackson LA, Jackson ML, Nelson JC, Neuzil KM, Weiss NS (2006) Evidence of bias in estimates of influenza vaccine effectiveness in seniors. Int J Epidemiol 35: 337–344.
29. Jackson LA, Nelson JC, Benson P, Neuzil KM, Reid RJ, et al. (2006) Functional status is a confounder of the association of influenza vaccine and risk of all cause mortality in seniors. Int J Epidemiol 35: 345–352.
30. Nelson JC, Jackson ML, Weiss NS, Jackson LA (2009) New strategies are needed to improve the accuracy of influenza vaccine effectiveness estimates among seniors. J Clin Epidemiol 62: 687–694.
31. Greenland S, Robins JM (1985) Confounding and misclassification. Am J Epidemiol 122: 495–506.
32. Castilla J, Martinez-Baz I, Martinez-Artola V, Reina G, Pozo F, et al. (2013) Decline in influenza vaccine effectiveness with time after vaccination, Navarre, Spain, season 2011/12. Euro Surveill 18: pii:20388.
33. Kissling E, Valenciano M, Larrauri A, Oroszi B, Cohen J, et al. (2013) Low and decreasing vaccine effectiveness against influenza A(H3) in 2011/12 among vaccination target groups in Europe: results from the I-MOVE multicentre case-control study. Euro Surveill 18: pii = 20390.
34. Ohmit SE, Thompson MG, Petrie JG, Thaker SN, Jackson ML, et al. (2014) Influenza vaccine effectiveness in the 2011–2012 season: protection against each circulating virus and the effect of prior vaccination on estimates. Clin Infect Dis 58: 319–327.
35. Pebody R, Andrews N, McMenamin J, Durnall H, Ellis J, et al. (2013) Vaccine effectiveness of 2011/12 trivalent seasonal influenza vaccine in preventing laboratory-confirmed influenza in primary care in the United Kingdom: evidence of waning intra-seasonal protection. Euro Surveill 18: pii: 20389.
36. Skowronski DM, Janjua NZ, Sabaiduc S, De Serres G, Winter AL, et al. (2014) Influenza A/subtype and B/lineage effectiveness estimates for the 2011–12 trivalent vaccine: cross-season and cross-lineage protection with unchanged vaccine. J Infect Dis 210: 126–137.
37. Jiménez-Jorge S, de Mateo S, Delgado-Sanz C, Pozo F, Casas I, et al. (2013) Effectiveness of influenza vaccine against laboratory-confirmed influenza, in the late 2011–2012 season in Spain, among population targeted for vaccination. BMC Infect Dis 13: 441.
38. Smith DJ, Forrest S, Ackley DH, Perelson AS (1999) Variable efficacy of repeated annual influenza vaccination. Proc Natl Acad Sci U S A 96: 14001–14006.
39. Skowronski DM, Janjua NZ, De Serres G, Purych D, Gilca V, et al. (2012) Cross-reactive and Vaccine-Induced Antibody to an Emerging Swine-Origin Variant of Influenza A Virus Subtype H3N2 (H3N2v). J Infect Dis 206: 1852–1861.
40. Talbot HK, Zhu Y, Chen Q, Williams JV, Thompson MG, et al. (2013) Effectiveness of Influenza Vaccine for Preventing Laboratory-Confirmed Influenza Hospitalizations in Adults, 2011–2012 Influenza Season. Clin Infect Dis 56: 1774–1777.
41. Bonmarin I, Belchior E, Le Strat Y, Levy-Bruhl D (2012) First estimates of influenza vaccine effectiveness among severe influenza cases, France, 2011/12. Euro Surveill 17.
42. Turner N, Pierse N, Bissielo A, Huang QS, Baker MG, et al. (2014) The effectiveness of seasonal trivalent inactivated influenza vaccine in preventing laboratory confirmed influenza hospitalisations in Auckland, New Zealand in 2012. Vaccine.
43. Thomas HL, Andrews N, Green HK, Boddington NL, Zhao H, et al. (2014) Estimating vaccine effectiveness against severe influenza in England and Scotland 2011/2012: applying the screening method to data from intensive care surveillance systems. Epidemiol Infect 142: 126–133.
44. Cheng AC, Brown S, Waterer G, Holmes M, Senenayake S, et al. (2013) Influenza epidemiology, vaccine coverage and vaccine effectiveness in sentinel Australian hospitals in 2012: the Influenza Complications Alert Network (FluCAN). Commun Dis Intell Q Rep 37: E246–E252.
45. World Health Organization (2013) Review of the 2012–2013 winter influenza season, northern hemisphere. Wkly Epidemiol Rec 88: 225–232.
46. Delgado-Sanz C, Jiménez-Jorge S, López-Perea N, Pozo F, Gómez-Barroso D, et al. (2013) Vigilancia de la gripe en España. Temporada 2011–12 (desde la semana 40/2011 hasta la semana 20/2012). Boletín Epidemiológico Semanal 20: 153–167.
47. World Health Organization (2012) Recommended composition of influenza virus vaccines for use in the 2012–2013 northern hemisphere influenza season. Wkly Epidemiol Rec 87: 83–95.
48. Legrand J, Vergu E, Flahault A (2006) Real-time monitoring of the influenza vaccine field effectiveness. Vaccine 24: 6605–6611.
49. McElhaney JE, Beran J, Devaster JM, Esen M, Launay O, et al. (2013) AS03-adjuvanted versus non-adjuvanted inactivated trivalent influenza vaccine against seasonal influenza in elderly people: a phase 3 randomised trial. Lancet Infect Dis 13: 485–496.
50. World Health Organization (2013) Recommended composition of influenza virus vaccines for use in the 2013–2014 northern hemisphere influenza season. Wkly Epidemiol Rec 88: 101–114.

23

LAT Software Induced Savings on Medical Costs of Alcohol Addicts' Care - Results from a Matched-Pairs Case-Control Study

Mihajlo Jakovljevic[1]*, Mirjana Jovanovic[2], Nemanja Rancic[3], Benjamin Vyssoki[4], Natasa Djordjevic[5]

1 Department of Pharmacology and Toxicology; The Faculty of Medical Sciences, University of Kragujevac, Kragujevac, Serbia, **2** Department of Psychiatry; The Faculty of Medical Sciences, University of Kragujevac, Kragujevac, Serbia, **3** Centre for Clinical Pharmacology; Medical Faculty Military Medical Academy, University of Defense, Belgrade, Serbia, **4** Department of Psychiatry and Psychotherapy; Medical University of Vienna, Vienna, Austria, **5** Department of Pharmacology and Toxicology; The Faculty of Medical Sciences, University of Kragujevac, Kragujevac, Serbia

Abstract

Lesch Alcoholism Typology (LAT) is one of the most widely used clinical typologies of alcohol addiction. Study tested whether introduction of LAT software in clinical practice leaded to improved outcomes and reduced costs. Retrospective matched-pairs case-control cost comparison study was conducted at the Regional Addiction Center of the University Clinic in Serbia involving 250 patients during the four-year period. Mean relapse frequency followed by outpatient detoxification was 0.42±0.90 vs. 0.70±1.66 (LAT/non-LAT; p = 0.267). Adding relapses after inpatient treatment total mean-number of relapses per patient was 0.70±1.74 vs. 0.97±1.89 (LAT/non-LAT; p = 0.201). However, these relapse frequency differentials were not statistically significant. Total hospital costs of Psychiatry clinic based non-LAT addicts' care (€54,660) were significantly reduced to €36,569 after initiation of LAT. Mean total cost per patient was reduced almost by half after initiation of LAT based treatment: €331±381 vs. €626±795 (LAT/non-LAT; p = 0.001). Mean cost of single psychiatry clinic admission among non-LAT treatment group was €320±330 (CI 95% 262–378) and among LAT €197±165 (CI 95% 168–226) (p = 0.019). Mean LAT software induced net savings on psychiatric care costs were €144 per patient. Total net savings on hospital care including F10 associated somatic co-morbidities amounted to €295 per patient. More sensitive diagnostic assessment and sub-type specific pharmacotherapy and psychotherapy following implementation of LAT software lead to significant savings on costs of hospital care.

Editor: Helge Bruns, University Hospital Oldenburg, Germany

Funding: The Ministry of Education, Science and Technological Development of the Republic of Serbia through OI Grant N° 175014, has fully financed this study. The funder had no role in study design, data collection and analysis, decision to publish, or preparation of the manuscript.

Competing Interests: The authors have declared that no competing interests exist.

* Email: jakovljevicm@medf.kg.ac.rs

Introduction

Due to its high prevalence [1] and chronic clinical course [2], alcohol dependence represents a heavy burden for health care systems across the globe [3]. National health budgets are becoming increasingly constrained and therefore effortis put into assessment of cost-effectiveness of specificmedical treatment strategies, such as addiction specific psychotherapy techniques [4,5] or anticraving medication for relapse prevention [6–8]. Theseresults contributed to more efficient care and evidence based allocation of resources [9]. However, the impactof distinct medical typologies that contain clinical practice guidelines on medical costs have not been researched thoroughly [10–13]. There are several typologies of alcohol dependence [14–16] which are widely adopted in the published literature.

Through the course of past century over a dozen of distinct clinical typologies of alcoholic dependence have been developed with Cloninger, Jellinek's, Babor's, LAT being only some of the most famous and broadly adopted. Lesch Alcoholism Typology (LAT), introduced in 1991, is regarded particularly helpful in terms of providing treatment recommendations grounded in patient's age of onset, family history, co-morbidity, and alcohol-related disabilities. The LAT typology is applied in clinical practice as a clinician's oriented software. It has been translated in 12 languages and validated in many countries, offering essential recommendations for pharmacological treatment of withdrawal and relapse prevention [17–21]. As to our best knowledge, so far there have been no attempts to assess the impact of clinical typologies implementation to the overall costs of alcohol addicts' medical care in a clinical trial. In this study we therefore want to evaluate the impact of a newly introduced sub-type specific treatment program, the LAT, on the cost of medical treatment in alcohol dependent patients.

Materials and Methods

Ethics Statement

The study was conducted according to Helsinki Declaration; current positive legislature on good clinical practice and guidelines on retrospective database analysis. Ethical committee approval was granted by the Ethical Committee of University Clinical Center Kragujevac, Serbia – Submission N° 01/11639 date 30. October 2013; Decision reached on 18. November 2013; N° 01-12299. Patient data were handled anonymously during the study. Patient records/information was anonymized and de-identified prior to analysis.

Setting

Since January 2012, LAT typology and software, translated and administered in Serbian language, was introduced to the clinical practice in seven regional addiction centers throughout Serbia [22,23]. The Regional Addiction Center Kragujevac provides services for up to 400 alcohol dependent patients per year and belongs to the Psychiatry Clinic of the single largest tertiary care university hospital in Central Serbia region with 1300 beds capacity (www.kc-kg.rs). Southeastern European country of Serbia has an upper middle income post-socialist transitional economy [9]. It's healthcare system is marked with typical strengths and weaknesses familiar to the most Eastern European economies including post-2004 EU members [22,23]. Therefore, Serbia can be regarded representative of a wider regional setting. Its substantial national deficit of budget allocation to combat huge alcohol dependency burden emphasizes urgent need for effective resource allocation in this field [24]. So far, health economics principles were not part of routine policy making on reimbursement of antic raving medicines, detoxification procedures or psychotherapy techniques indicated in alcohol addiction treatment [25].

Data

Study sample was selected out of 813 alcohol dependent cases being either outpatients or inpatients within the institutional framework of the Regional Addiction Center of the University Clinical Center Kragujevac, Serbia during the period 2010–2013. One hundred and twenty five case-control pairs were selected based on their clinically confirmed diagnosis of alcohol dependence according to ICD-10 and DSM-IV-TR, age and gender. There were no other grounds for patient selection except the possibility of close clinical matching so this was the maximum of available patient couples for comparison. LAT patients' medical services utilization was observed during 2012–2013 period, while non-LAT processed alcohol addicts were observedin2010–2011 period. Economic data on resource use and costs were extracted out of the University Clinical Center electronic registry of discharge invoices. Observed clinical setting was state owned not-for-profit hospital which is generally charging governmental budget subsidized prices to the citizens. Therefore this database presents reliable insight into the actual costs of care. Although individual periods while these costs accrued slightly varied, complete symmetry was obeyed in duration of the observation among cases coupled. That means that medical and resource use history for each single case was extracted either for one or for two years (depending on his/her actual physician visits and admissions) duration while his/her counterpart from control pool, was observed during equally long period of time (either one or two years). Clinical outcomes data accessible was individual frequency of relapse events followed by either outpatient detoxification or hospital admission. According to availability these relapses were evidenced for 2012–2013 observation time, in equal duration between patient pairs. Resource use and costs accrued due to alcohol dependence diagnostics, treatment and rehabilitation were observed separately within institutional frameworks of Psychiatry Clinic, Internal Medicine Clinic and Neurology Clinic for each case.

Analysis

It is rather difficult to assess trends in clinical decision making and resource use patterns among alcohol addicts due to high clinical heterogeneity of patient's backgrounds [26]. Therefore, in the present study, matched-pairs case control retrospective study design was employed in a cost comparison analysis framework [27]. This approach, previously applied in clinical trials on addiction disorders [26–29], allows reliable elimination of statistical bias impact to the study results. Grounds for choosing such methodology was lying in the fact that medical services utilization patterns and associated costs otherwise might have been affected with differences between groups in clinical background, disease course and treatment response [30].

Costs were converted from national currency – Republic of Serbian Dinar (RSD) to Euro (€) in line with mean official exchange rates of the National Bank of Serbia in the respective years (www.nbs.rs). This way the effect of slight devaluation of domestic currency was avoided. There were no sudden swifts in pricing policy or significant changes in medical service charges related to alcoholism treatment during this period of time. Therefore chronological gap between experimental and control group (before and after LAT intervention) had rather minor impact to the price levels 2010–2013. Foreign currency (€) based prices remained stable.

Statistics

Complete statistical analysis was carried out using Statistical Software PASW Statistics 18 and Microsoft Office Excel 2007. Cases and controls were matched according to sex, age and diagnosis. After pairing patients, cost analysis has done, during one-year or two-year period, between controls observed before and cases observed after implementation of LAT software - guidelines. Categorical variables were presented as frequencies of certain categories, while statistical significance of differences was tested using Chi-square test. Continuous variables were summarized as mean, standard deviation, range and 95% confidence interval. Continuous variables were compared using the Student's *t* test for independent samples and the Mann-Whitney U test, while nonparametric Kruskal Wallis H test was used to test the statistical significance among continuous variables with three or more categories. Analysis of money spending was done by nonparametric tests (the large standard deviations). Multiple regression analysis was performed on both LAT and non-LAT patients, while dependent variable were total hospital costs. Two models (LAT and non-LAT) were developed indicating key predictors of costs of care. All the analyses were estimated at $p<0.05$ level of the statistical significance.

Results

Number of relapses

Mean number of relapses followed by outpatient detoxification was 0.42 ± 0.90 vs. 0.70 ± 1.66 (LAT/non-LAT) ($p=0.267$) (see Table 1). Frequency of relapses followed by hospital admission was 0.28 ± 1.10 vs. 0.26 ± 0.58 (LAT/non-LAT) ($p=0.339$). Thus we come to the average rate of total relapses of 0.70 ± 1.74 vs. 0.97 ± 1.89 (LAT/non-LAT) while this difference was not statistically significant ($p=0.201$).

Inpatient and outpatient care

Total number of Psychiatry Clinic hospital admissions was 155 vs. 156 while there were 6 vs. 26 Internal Medicine Clinic admissions (Chi square test; $p=0.0016$) and 5 vs. 6 Neurology Clinic admissions (Chi square test; $p=0.8415$) (LAT/non-LAT)

Table 1. Demography and resource use patterns among alcohol dependent matched patient pairs, LAT vs. non-LAT comparison.

	LAT (n = 125)	Non-LAT (n = 125)	p value**
ICD-10 codes#	F.10.0–F10.9	F.10.0–F10.9	N/A
Age (M ± SD)	48.26±10.51	48.20±10.49	p = 0.966
Gender (male/female)	120/5	120/5	N/A
Relapses followed by hospital admission	0.28±1.10	0.26±0.58	p = 0.339
Relapses followed by outpatient detoxification	0.42±0.90	0.70±1.66	p = 0.267
Total relapse rates (2012–2013)	0.70±1.74	0.97±1.89	p = 0.201
Outpatient physician consultations	10.45±9.09	10.29±12.50	**p = 0.050***
Inpatient physician consultations	7.19±57.81	2.95±9.37	p = 0.777
Mean N° Hospital admissions per patient - Psychiatry Clinic	1.24±1.42	1.25±1.42	p = 0.986
Hospital admissions N° - Internal Medicine Clinic (due to F10)	0.05±0.31	0.21±0.65	**p = 0.008***
Hospital admissions N° - Neurology clinic (due to F10)	0.04±0.20	0.05±0.33	p = 0.491
Mean admissions N° (Internal + Neurology)	1.44±1.73	1.59±1.54	p = 0.151
Mean N° of all hospital admissions (M ± SD)	0.94±1.27	0.92±0.74	p = 0.855
Duration of Hospital admissions (M ± SD)	12.49±14.77	10.80±11.52	p = 0.315
Total hospital admissions – Psychiatry	155	156	N/A
Total N° of all hospital admissions – Internal Clinic	6	26	**p = 0.0016***
Total N° of all hospital admissions – Neurology Clinic	5	6	p = 0.8415
Total joint Internal Medicine Clinic and Neurology Clinic hospital admissions	11	32	**p = 0.0047***
Typology according to Lesch (type I/II/III/IV)	10/27/57/31	N/A	N/A

#All resource use at the Internal Medicine Clinic and Neurology Clinic were accounted exclusively for medical services consumed in relation to alcohol dependence diagnostics, treatment and rehabilitation (ICD-10 F10 diagnostic code group); p value- statistical signifiance of difference;
**- Mann-Whitney U test; !- Chi square test;
*- p<0.05; M ± SD- mean ± standard deviation.

(see Table 1). Total joint Internal Medicine Clinic and Neurology Clinic hospital admissions frequency was 11 vs. 32 (LAT/non-LAT) (Chi square test; p = 0.0047). Mean Internal Medicine Clinic admissions frequency was significantly higher in non-LAT group 0.05±0.31 vs. 0.21±0.65 (p = 0.008).

Mean hospital costs per patient due to joint Internal Medicine Clinic and Neurology Clinic admissions were higher among non-LAT patients €38±238 vs. €189±623 (LAT/non-LAT; p = 0.102) (see Table 2). Total costs of hospital care in all clinics were substantially lower in LAT group, €41,331 compared to €78,226 in non-LAT patients (p = 0.001) (see Table 2 and Fig. 1). Average net savings on direct medical costs of psychiatric hospital care highly likely attributable to the LAT software implementation were €144 per patient. Average net savings in total costs of hospital care for F10 associated mental and somatic disorders across all clinics were €295 per patient.

Mean number of hospital admissions per patient to the Psychiatry Clinic, during the examined time period was 1.24±1.42/1.25±1.42 (LAT/non-LAT) (p = 0.986). Mean total duration of hospital admissions was 12.49±14.77/10.80±11.52 days (LAT/non-LAT) (p = 0.315). Attending psychiatrists delivered on average 10.69±9.06/12.81±16.06 sessions of social therapy, including implementation of psychotherapeutic techniques (LAT/non-LAT) (p = 0.200). Total Psychiatry Clinic hospital costs of non-LAT addicts' care amounted to €54,660, which were significantly reduced (€36,569, p = 0.008) after initiation of LAT (see Fig. 1). Mean cost of psychiatric care per patient decreased after initiation of LAT based treatment (€293±308 (CI 95%- 239-347) *vs.* €437±415 (CI 95%- 364-510) €), and the decrease was significant (p = 0.008). Mean per patient values of all cost domains in the non-LAT controls were higher than among LAT cases but only some of these findings were statistically significant (see Table 2; Fig. 2).

Lesch Alcoholism Typology- Subtypes

Mean costs of care per LAT subtypes differed significantly (Kruskal Wallis H test; p = 0.005) and amounted to: LAT I – €326±88 (CI 95% 271–380) €, LAT II – €256±304 (CI 95% 141–370) €, LAT III – €256±295 (CI 95% 180–333) € and LAT IV – €381±368 (CI 95% 251–511) € among LAT classified patients. Mean cost of single hospital admission among non-LAT treatment group was €320±330 (CI 95% 262–378) € and among LAT €197±165 (CI 95% 168–226) € (Mann-Whitney U test; p = 0.019).

Multiple regression analysis was conducted using value of total hospital cost as dependent variable. It showed that model developed for LAT treated patients significantly better explaines costs variance compared to non-LAT ($R^2 = 0.517$ vs. $R^2 = 0.132$) (see Table 3 and Table 4). Variables exposing strongest impact to total cost of care among LAT cases were: age, duration of hospital admissions and outpatient physician consultations, while among non-LAT controls there were no such predictors with significant impact to the total cost of care.

Discussion

The impact of good clinical practice guidelines implementation to the clinicians' prescription patterns and their economic awareness was previously assessed and reported in recent studies [24]. Our study is the first to evaluate the impact of a newly introduced, sub-type specific alcohol dependency classification system on economic and clinical outcomes.

Table 2. Costs of hospital medical care; LAT vs. non-LAT comparison (€).

Cost domain (total values per group)[#]	LAT (n = 125)	Non-LAT (n = 125)	p value**
Psychiatry Clinic			
Outpatient Care	11,113	12,598	p = 0.773
Inpatient Care	25,456	42,062	**p = 0.008***
Total costs of hospital care	36,569	54,660	**p = 0.008***
Main Cost Domains			
Physician Consultations	6,132	7,942	p = 0.966
Outpatient physician consultations	5,074	4,785	p = 0.382
Inpatient physician consultations	1,058	3,157	p = 0.757
Psychotherapeutic Interventions	5,726	7,235	p = 0.720
Hospital admission	18,604	18,765	p = 0.430
General Medical Care	929	5,438	**p<0.001***
Laboratory Analysis	2,044	6,794	**p<0.001***
Imaging Diagnostics	887	2,976	**p = 0.044***
Pharmaceuticals	2,246	5,510	p = 0.081
Other Clinics			
Internal Medicine Clinic	3,562	20,161	**p = 0.008***
Neurology clinic	1,200	3,405	p = 0.497
Total somatic ward costs (Internal + Neurology Clinic)	4,762	23,566	p = 0.102
Total Hospital costs	**41,331**	**78,226**	**p = 0.001***
Mean cost per patient – Psychiatry (M ± SD)	293±308	437±415	**p = 0.008***
Mean cost per patient - Somatic wards/clinics (M ± SD)	38±238	189±623	p = 0.102
Mean total hospital costs per patient (M ± SD)	**331±381**	**626±795**	**p = 0.001***

[#]All admission costs to the Internal Medicine Clinic and Neurology Clinic were accounted exclusively for medical services consumed in relation to alcohol dependence diagnostics, treatment and rehabilitation (ICD-10 F10 diagnostic code group); p value- statistical signifiance of difference;
**- Mann-Whitney U test;
*- p<0.05; M ± SD- mean ± standard deviation.

LAT cases exposed statistically significantly higher demand for outpatient physician consultations. On the opposite, Internal Medicine Clinic admissions were significantly more frequent among non-LAT controls. All other resource use differentials between the two groups were not statistically significant. With regards to costs of care, statistical significance in favor of LAT cases (substantially lower cost of care) was proved on numerous cost domains: Inpatient Care, Total costs of hospital care and Internal Medicine Clinic costs. Besides these aforementioned domains, LAT cases exhibited significantly lower costs of care

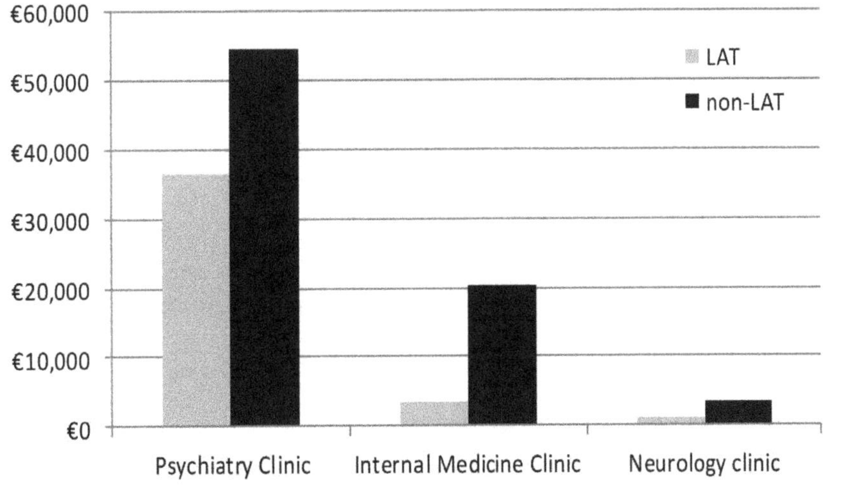

Figure 1. Costs of hospital care, inter-clinic differentials; total amounts per group; comparison LAT vs. non-LAT matched pairs (Y axis presents € values).

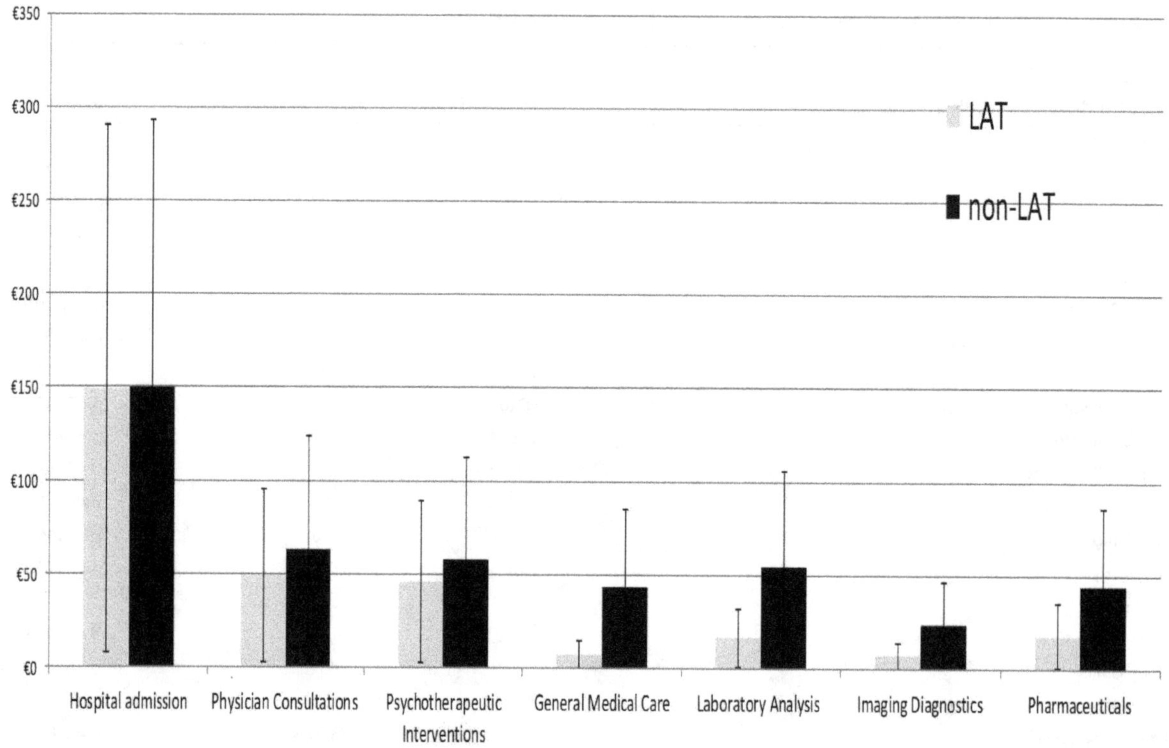

Figure 2. Cost domains; Mean values per patient presented with CI 95% range; comparison LAT vs. non-LAT matched pairs (Y axis presents € values).

compared to non-LAT controls in terms of mean cost per patient treated at Psychiatry Clinic as well as ultimately total hospital costs per patient. Noticed cost saving trend after LAT software and guidelines implementation in clinical practice was also statistically significant in consecutive domains: Laboratory analysis and Imaging diagnostics and General Medical (dominantly nursing) Care. An explanation for this phenomenon was overutilization of CTs and NMR imaging of the brain which was wide spreaded clinicans' practice before LAT introduction. Demands to perform blood tests covering too broad variety of targeted medical conditions (substance addiction, infections etc.) were also more frequent in 2010–2011. Cost savings on nursing care among LAT patients are partly attributable to more frequent outpatient visits to the attending psychiatrists recommended by LAT software acting as substitute for more costly hospital treatment being quite effective in controlling disease.

Resource use patterns exhibited in this trial point to the opportunity of reshaping clinician's behavior with evidence based guidelines [32]. We could observe frequency of outpatient visits to the attending psychiatrist and frequency of hospital admissions as an indirect sign of occasional relapses that these patients commonly experience [25].

LAT patients tended to consume less nursing care, laboratory analysis, imaging diagnostics and pharmaceuticals (see Table 2

Table 3. The impact of independent variables on total hospital cost among non-LAT treated patients (multiple regression analysis).

Model non-LAT	b	SE-b	beta	Pearson r
Constant	58.480	535.195		
Age	5.523	6.812	0.073	0.048
Gender	−15.258	328.707	−0.004	−0.007
Number of hospital admissions	265.450	140.739	0.246	0.316
Duration of hospital admissions	4.429	9.620	0.064	0.296
Outpatient physician consultations	−1.858	5.545	−0.029	−0.016
Inpatient physician consultations	11.342	8.243	0.134	0.211
Relapses followed by hospital admission	65.125	123.029	0.048	0.035
Relapses followed by outpatient detoxification	−9.298	43.931	−0.019	−0.066

Note: The dependent variable was Total hospital cost. $R^2 = 0.132$, Adjusted $R^2 = 0.072$.

Table 4. The impact of independent variables on total hospital cost among LAT treated patients (multiple regression analysis).

Model LAT	b	SE-b	beta	Pearson r
Constant	442.672	213.732		
Age*	−4.862	2.445	**−0.134**	−0.206
Gender	−94.649	130.726	−0.049	−0.109
Number of hospital admissions	66.641	40.408	0.221	0.645
Duration of hospital admissions*	11.905	3.450	**0.461**	0.675
Type of LAT	−16.626	29.024	−0.038	0.036
Outpatient physician consultations*	5.608	2.798	**0.134**	0.138
Inpatient physician consultations	0.233	0.442	0.035	0.159
Relapses followed by hospital admission	28.232	27.235	0.081	0.027
Relapses followed by outpatient detoxification	−26.307	33.150	−0.062	−0.087

Note: The dependent variable was Total hospital cost. $R^2 = 0.517$, Adjusted $R^2 = 0.480$; $p < 0.05$*.

and Fig. 2). Interestingly, recently published trial testing efficiency of sodium oxibate in maintaining alcohol abstinence among addicts showed that anticraving medicines could prove themselves useful regardless of actual LAT type of patient. This finding might support lack of significant differences between LAT and non-LAT cases in drug acquisition costs [31]. Lower demand for diagnostic services by the attending psychiatrists is attributable to the precise and focused clinical tools provided by interactive LAT software. These are allowing for earlier diagnostic recognition of patient type based on accurate anamnesis and examination criteria.

Statistically significant cost differentials among four stages of alcoholism clinical evolution according to LAT confirms broadly recognized LAT sensitivity for distinct recognition of patients with profoundly different drinking patterns and treatment needs [16–18,21].

Non-LAT cases were more frequently treated at the Internal Clinic (Gastrointestinal and Hepatology wards) and Neurology Clinic due to alcohol related somatic disorders such as liver cirrhosis, polyneuritis and others. These wards demand much more expensive imaging examinations and blood tests compared to Psychiatry clinic [33]. Cost-reduction observed among LAT patients, probably happened due to their less severe somatic complications compared to respective non-LAT couples during the investigated time period consecutively somatic disorders worsened by occasional heavy drinking episodes were rather seldom among LAT cases. Authors believe that patient rambling among specialty Internal Medicine Clinic and Neurology Clinic delayed alcoholism type recognition and was additional underlying reason for their more demanding and expensive hospital care.

The hot issue of cost containment remains high on the agenda of regional health policy makers due to Western Balkan's difficulties in provision of sustainable health care funding, triggered by worldwide economic crisis [22,23]. Cost saving procedures are considered by many experts a trade off with quality of medical services [34,35]. In this particular alcohol addicted population, authors assumed that patients experienced clinical improvement because of more efficient diagnostic algorithm leading to the more targeted, individually adjusted treatment and weaker demand for health care. As a consequence, it appears that they needed less frequent outpatient physician consultations and consumed less resources which is the phenomena well described in literature [30]. Range of costs reported in upper-middle income Serbia is rather modest compared to high-income settings [24,25]. Regardless of some evidenced intra-European differences in LAT sub-type structure across ethnicities [36], LAT associated savings should be expected elsewhere. Observed resource use patterns will likely cause decrease in overall costs of medical care for somatic symptoms, in other countries as well.

Limitations

Matching of patients into couples with highly similar clinical background should have eliminated the potential bias and external validity issues in the study, which might have been affected by medical heterogeneity of samples in other similar clinical trials [26]. Regardless of few minor setbacks in this study design it provides high statistical reliability for generalizations of conclusions [37].

University Clinical Center Kragujevac electronic database of discharge invoices was used as a source of data on medical services utilization costs. Tight internal and external control of accounting offices of respective Clinics is conducted due to the fact that these invoices serve as grounds for negotiations on reimbursement with republican Health Insurance fund representatives. Therefore, these data should be regarded of satisfactory reliability and quality. Sample size is rather modest, due to the fact that authors had no access to other addiction centers throughout the country or abroad. According to authors' opinion this would probably be the core weakness of the study. Nevertheless, matching of patient pairs forms an appropriate control group allowing for the generalizability of conclusions. Deeper insight into indirect costs of lost productivity would be very helpful and would allow for more inclusive insight into the costs of care [38], as, due to adopting payer's perspective, these were rather out of scope of present trial. Clinical background data relied on relapse rates only. In real world clinical setting, there is no efficient way to assess any relapses that did not lead to additional treatment, so frequency of relapses marked as "total relapse rates" in this article, actually presents clinically visible fraction of them. Lack of an in-depth assessment of other clinical outcomes such as abstinence duration, was the another key weakness of this trial. The prospective approach would certainly provide deeper insight into the clinical efficiency of LAT based treatments.

Conclusions

In conclusion, the significant medical savings documented by this matched-pair case-control study are anticipated consequence of more targeted therapeutic approach. Here we explain that noticed cost savings induced by LAT typology, and LAT software introduction the core underlying cost driver was higher rate of hospital admissions to the Internal Medicine wards due to severe somatic symptoms among non-LAT patients. Likely clinical improvements among LAT patients are believed to be achieved due to proper LAT type recognition and decreased need for physicians' consultations, detoxifications, fewer and shorter hospital admissions and lower drug acquisition costs. The present study is one of the pioneering assessments of health economic justifications for systematic relying on common typologies in clinical practice. These are promising signs of delivering more efficient and cost saving care to alcohol addicts based on LAT in Southeastern Europe. Such evidence should be regarded a stimuli for further research on guidelines impact on the costs of addiction disorders medical care. Applied health economics research in increasingly prevalent addiction disorders could bring partial release to the constrained national health care budgets. Finding alternative ways to deliver cost-effective medical care for alcohol dependents bears particularly heavy policy impact among aging nations of northern hemisphere. Vast economic consequences for the community are particularly evident in these disorders affecting young population. Various substance addictions bring huge opportunity cost due to long lasting decreased working ability, absenteeism and premature mortality. Dissemination of good clinical practice guidelines recommending cost-effective diagnostics and treatment options could be highly effective policy tool for the future of addiction medicine.

Author Contributions

Conceived and designed the experiments: M. Jakovljevic BV M. Jovanovic ND NR. Performed the experiments: M. Jakovljevic M. Jovanovic. Analyzed the data: M. Jakovljevic ND NR. Contributed reagents/materials/analysis tools: M. Jakovljevic ND. Wrote the paper: M. Jakovljevic BV M. Jovanovic ND NR.

References

1. Shield KD, Rylett M, Gmel G, Gmel G, Kehoe-Chan TA, et al. (2013) Global alcohol exposure estimates by country, territory and region for 2005–a contribution to the comparative risk assessment for the 2010 Global Burden of Disease Study. Addiction 108: 912–922.
2. Ando B, Rozsa S, Kurgyis E, Szkaliczki A, Demeter I, et al. (2013) Direct and Indirect Symptom Severity Indicators of Alcohol Dependence and the Personality Concept of the Biosocial Model. Subst Use Misuse.
3. Chisholm D, Rehm J, Van Ommeren M, Monteiro M (2004) Reducing the global burden of hazardous alcohol use: a comparative cost-effectiveness analysis. J Stud Alcohol 65: 782–793.
4. Neighbors CJ, Barnett NP, Rohsenow DJ, Colby SM, Monti PM (2010) Cost-effectiveness of a motivational intervention for alcohol-involved youth in a hospital emergency department. J Stud Alcohol Drugs 71: 384–394.
5. Wutzke SE, Shiell A, Gomel MK, Conigrave KM (2001) Cost effectiveness of brief interventions for reducing alcohol consumption. Soc Sci Med 52: 863–870.
6. Palmer AJ, Neeser K, Weiss C, Brandt A, Comte S, et al. (2000) The long-term cost-effectiveness of improving alcohol abstinence with adjuvant acamprosate. Alcohol Alcohol 35: 478–492.
7. Rychlik R, Siedentop H, Pfeil T, Daniel D (2003) Cost-effectiveness of adjuvant treatment with acamprosate in maintaining abstinence in alcohol dependent patients. Eur Addict Res 9: 59–64.
8. Walters D, Connor JP, Feeney GF, Young RM (2009) The cost effectiveness of naltrexone added to cognitive-behavioral therapy in the treatment of alcohol dependence. J Addict Dis 28: 137–144.
9. Jakovljevic M, Jovanovic M, Lazic Z, Jakovljevic V, Djukic A, et al. (2011) Current efforts and proposals to reduce healthcare costs in Serbia. Ser J Exp Clin Res 12: 161–163.
10. Ciaranello AL, Perez F, Engelsmann B, Walensky RP, Mushavi A, et al. (2013) Cost-effectiveness of World Health Organization 2010 guidelines for prevention of mother-to-child HIV transmission in Zimbabwe. Clin Infect Dis 56: 430–446.
11. Drozda JP (2013) Physician specialty society clinical guidelines and bending the cost curve: comment on "Cost consideration in the clinical guidance documents of physician specialty societies in the United States". JAMA Intern Med 173: 1097–1099.
12. French MT, Salome HJ, Sindelar JL, McLellan AT (2002) Benefit-cost analysis of addiction treatment: methodological guidelines and empirical application using the DATCAP and ASI. Health Serv Res 37: 433–455.
13. Picon PD, Beltrame A, Banta D (2013) National guidelines for high-cost drugs in Brazil: achievements and constraints of an innovative national evidence-based public health policy. Int J Technol Assess Health Care 29: 198–206.
14. Babor TF, Dolinsky ZS, Meyer RE, Hesselbrock M, Hofmann M, et al. (1992) Types of alcoholics: concurrent and predictive validity of some common classification schemes. Br J Addict 87: 1415–1431.
15. Cloninger CR, Bohman M, Sigvardsson S (1981) Inheritance of alcohol abuse. Cross-fostering analysis of adopted men. Arch Gen Psychiatry 38: 861–868.
16. Lesch WC, Celuch KG (1991) Females' use of alcoholic beverages: a study in context. J Health Soc Policy 2: 23–38.
17. Lesch OM, Walter H (1996) Subtypes of alcoholism and their role in therapy. Alcohol Alcohol Suppl 1: 63–67.
18. Bleich S, Bayerlein K, Reulbach U, Hillemacher T, Bonsch D, et al. (2004) Homocysteine levels in patients classified according to Lesch's typology. Alcohol Alcohol 39: 493–498.
19. Kiefer F, Helwig H, Tarnaske T, Otte C, Jahn H, et al. (2005) Pharmacological relapse prevention of alcoholism: clinical predictors of outcome. Eur Addict Res 11: 83–91.
20. Leggio L, Kenna GA, Fenton M, Bonenfant E, Swift RM (2009) Typologies of alcohol dependence. From Jellinek to genetics and beyond. Neuropsychol Rev 19: 115–129.
21. Lesch OM, Walter H, Wetschka C, Hesselbrock M, Hesselbrock V (2011) Alcohol and tobacco. Medical and sociological aspects of use, abuse and addiction.Vienna, Austria, Springer-Verlag.
22. Jakovljevic M, Rankovic A, Rancic N, Jovanovic M, Ivanovic M, et al. (2013) Radiology services costs and utilization patterns estimates in Southeastern Europe - a retrospective analysis from Serbia. Value in health regional issues 2: 218–225.
23. Jakovljevic MB (2013) Resource allocation strategies in Southeastern European health policy. Eur J Health Econ 14: 153–159.
24. Jovanovic M, Jakovljevic M (2011) Inpatient detoxification procedure and facilities: financing considerations from an Eastern European perspective. Alcohol Alcohol 46: 364–365.
25. Jakovljevic M, Jovanovic M, Nikic K, Radovanovic A, Pirkovic I, et al. (2011) Inpatient detoxification and law enforcement costs following acute drinking event, in typical eastern European upper – middle income, health care setting. Health Behavior & Public Health 1: 1–7.
26. Pedrero Perez E, Rojo Mota G (2008) [Personality differences between substance addicts and general population. Study of clinical cases with matched controls using Cloninger's TCI-R]. Adicciones 20: 251–261. Spanish.
27. Westermeyer J, Specker S (1999) Social resources and social function in comorbid eating and substance disorder: a matched-pairs study. Am J Addict 8: 332–336.
28. Johnson RS, Tobin JW, Cellucci T (1992) Personality characteristics of cocaine and alcohol abusers: more alike than different. Addict Behav 17: 159–166.
29. Westermeyer J, Peng G (1977) Opium and heroin addicts in Laos. II. A study of matched pairs. J Nerv Ment Dis 164: 351–354.
30. Stockwell T (1998) Towards guidelines for low-risk drinking: quantifying the short- and long-term costs of hazardous alcohol consumption. Alcohol Clin Exp Res 22: 63S–69S.
31. Caputo F, Del Re A, Brambilla R, Grignaschi A, Vignoli T et al. (2014). Sodium oxybate in maintaining alcohol abstinence in alcoholic patients according to Lesch typologies: A pilot study. Journal of Psychopharmacology, 28(1), 23–30.
32. Djordjevic ND, Jankovic SM (2006) Characteristics of decision-making process during prescribing in general practice. Vojnosanit Pregl 63: 279–285.
33. Rankovic A, Rancic N, Jovanovic M, Ivanovic M, Gajovic O, et al. (2013) Impact of imaging diagnostics on the budget–are we spending too much? Vojnosanit Pregl 70: 709–711.
34. Jakovljevic M, Vukovic M, Chia-Ching C, Yamada T, Antunovic M, et al. (2013) Do policy measures impact cost consciousness of healthcare professionals? Value in Health 16: A542, doi:10.1016/j.jval.2013.08.1376.
35. Haas L, Stargardt T, Schreyoegg J, Schlosser R, Klapp BF, et al. (2013) The trade-off between costs and quality of care in the treatment of psychosomatic patients with somatoform pain disorder. Appl Health Econ Health Policy 11: 359–368.
36. Jakovljevic M, Riegler A, Jovanovic M, Djordjevic N, Patek K, et al. (2013) Serbian and Austrian alcohol-dependent patients: a comparison of two samples regarding therapeutically relevant clinical features. Alcohol Alcohol 48: 505–508.

37. Hussey AM, Koch G, Preisser JS, Saville RB (2013) Analysis of matched studies with dichotomous outcomes using nonparametric randomization-based analysis of covariance. Statistics in Biopharmaceutical Research, 5.

38. Zweifel P (2012) The Grossman model after 40 years. Eur J Health Econ 13: 677–682.

The Effects of Pharmacist Intervention on Emergency Department Visits in Patients 80 Years and Older: Subgroup Analyses by Number of Prescribed Drugs and Appropriate Prescribing

Anna Alassaad[1,2]*, Maria Bertilsson[3], Ulrika Gillespie[2], Johan Sundström[1,3], Margareta Hammarlund-Udenaes[4], Håkan Melhus[1]

1 Department of Medical Sciences, Uppsala University, Uppsala, Sweden, 2 Uppsala University Hospital, Uppsala, Sweden, 3 Uppsala Clinical Research Center, Uppsala, Sweden, 4 Department of Pharmaceutical Sciences, Uppsala University, Uppsala, Sweden

Abstract

Background: Clinical pharmacist interventions have been shown to have positive effect on occurrence of drug-related issues as well as on clinical outcomes. However, evidence about which patients benefiting most from the interventions is limited. We aimed to explore whether pharmacist intervention is equally effective in preventing emergency department (ED) visits in patients with few or many prescribed drugs and in those with different levels of inappropriate prescribing.

Methods: Patient and outcome data from a randomized controlled trial exploring the clinical effects of a ward-based pharmacist intervention in patients, 80 years and older, were used. The patients were divided into subgroups according to the number of prescribed drugs (<5 or ≥5 drugs) and the level of inappropriate prescribing [using the Screening Tool Of Older People's potentially inappropriate Prescriptions (STOPP) and the Screening Tool to Alert doctors to Right Treatment (START) with a score of ≥2 (STOPP) and ≥1 (START) as cutoff points]. The effect of the intervention on the number of times the different subgroups visited the ED was analyzed.

Results: The pharmacist intervention was more effective with respect to the number of subsequent ED visits in patients taking <5 drugs on admission than in those taking ≥5 drugs. The rate ratio (RR) for a subsequent ED visit was 0.22 [95% confidence interval (CI) 0.09–0.52] for <5 drugs and 0.70 (95% CI 0.47–1.04) for ≥5 drugs (p = 0.02 for the interaction). The effect of intervention did not differ between patients with high or low STOPP or START scores.

Conclusion: In this exploratory study, the pharmacist intervention appeared to be more effective in preventing visits to the ED for patients who were taking fewer drugs before the intervention. Our analysis of STOPP and START scores indicated that the level of inappropriate prescribing on admission had no effect on the outcomes of intervention with respect to ED visits.

Editor: Alfonso Carvajal, Universidad de Valladolid, Spain

Funding: The study was funded by the non-profit organization Swedish Academy for Pharmaceutical Sciences (one PhD student via scholarship). Uppsala University funded biostatistic consulting. The University Hospital of Uppsala and Uppsala University co-funded the study by letting involved physician and pharmacists participate in meetings during work hours. The funders had no role in study design, data collection and analysis, decision to publish, or preparation of the manuscript.

Competing Interests: The authors have declared that no competing interests exist.

* Email: anna.alassaad@medsci.uu.se

Introduction

The increased possibility of pharmacologically treating chronic illnesses has resulted in the prescription of a high number of drugs to many individual older patients with complex co-morbidities. This increases the potential for drug-disease and drug-drug interactions [1]. A high number of prescribed drugs for any one individual has also been associated with an increased risk of inappropriate prescribing [2–5], medication errors [6,7], and non-compliance with treatment [8]. The administration of ≥5 drugs at once is a common definition of polypharmacy [9]. In Sweden, all patients ≥75 years of age who are prescribed ≥5 drugs are, according to national guidelines [1], subject to an annual mandatory medication review by a general practitioner, pharmacist or nurse; similarly, in Australia, the use of ≥5 regular drugs is one of the criteria for determining a patient's eligibility for home medicines review [10]. However, more important than the actual number of prescribed drugs, is the quality of the prescribed drug treatment [11]. Inappropriate, or suboptimal, prescribing may be prescribing of more drugs than are clinically needed (overprescribing) or prescribing drugs incorrectly by prescribing the wrong drug, dose or frequency (misprescribing), but it may also be a failure to prescribe drugs that are needed (underprescribing) [9,11–13]. In fact, the issue of underprescribing is often overlooked and the underuse of medications is common in patients, whether they are taking few or many medications [2]. There are a number of validated and well-studied tools for measuring the quality of prescribing. Two examples are the Screening Tool Of Older People's potentially inappropriate Prescriptions (STOPP) and the Screening Tool to Alert doctors to Right Treatment (START) [14–16]. These comprise sets of criteria for identification of over- or misprescribing (STOPP) and underprescribing (START).

Pharmacists, when integrated in the health care team, can help promote appropriate prescribing, and clinical pharmacist interventions have shown positive effects on overprescribing as well as mis- and underprescribing in hospitalized patients [17–20]. However, to our knowledge, differences in the effects of clinical pharmacist intervention on clinical outcomes between patients taking few or many drugs, or between those with a high or low level of inappropriate prescribing have not been analyzed. Our research group has previously demonstrated that the addition of a pharmacist to the health-care team at an acute internal medicine hospital ward reduces visits to the emergency department (ED) by 47%, revisits to hospital by 16%, and drug-related readmissions by 80% for patients aged ≥80 years [21]. Determination of which patients gain most benefit from pharmacist intervention, and further analysis of the elements of the intervention will allow rational designing and targeting of future interventions.

The primary aim of this study was to explore whether pharmacist intervention is equally effective in preventing subsequent visits to the ED for patients who are receiving few (<5) or many (≥5) prescribed drugs on admission. In addition, the study explored whether the effect of the intervention was consistent for patients with a high or low level of inappropriate prescribing (as measured with STOPP and START). The secondary aim was to describe the impact of the pharmacist intervention on the quality of prescribing in the <5 and ≥5 subgroups.

Methods

Ethics statement

Each study participant has given their written informed consent, and the study protocol was approved by the Uppsala regional ethics committee. Trial Registration: clinicaltrials.gov Identifier: NCT00661310.

Pharmacist intervention

This study was a post-hoc subgroup analysis of patient and outcome data from a prospective, randomized, controlled study (RCT) [21] that compared patients receiving standard (non-pharmacist; control) care with those receiving enhanced, more comprehensive services where a pharmacist was part of the health-care team (intervention). The RCT has been described in detail elsewhere [21]. Briefly, 400 consecutive patients, aged 80 years or older, admitted to the acute internal medicine wards at Uppsala University Hospital were included and randomly assigned to intervention or control groups. The main elements of the intervention were medication reconciliation on admission and at discharge, a thorough medication review where drug-related problems were identified and recommendations were orally communicated to the physician in charge, patient counseling throughout the hospital stay, communication of the treatment plan to the primary care physician, and a follow-up phone call to the patients two months after discharge from hospital. The medication review was structured but none of the available tools for assessing appropriate prescribing (e.g. STOPP and START) was used prospectively. The patients were followed for 12 months after discharge from hospital and the number of revisits to hospital (ED visits and readmissions) was recorded. The number of revisits to hospital was the primary endpoint of the study. The clinical pharmacists had postgraduate clinical knowledge and training and had hospital work experience. The health-care team (for the intervention and control groups) included nurses, physicians, physiotherapists, dieticians and occupational therapists. Specialists, e.g. geriatricians, were involved as consultants when needed.

Quality of prescribing

STOPP and START were chosen to assess the quality of the prescribing. STOPP consists of 65 criteria to identify drug-disease interactions, i.e. drugs that should be avoided in certain conditions in older people. The START criteria identify drug omissions; they contain 22 diagnoses where drug treatment should always be initiated if no contraindication is present [14]. The criteria for both STOPP and START are arranged in categories according to the relevant physiological system and each criterion can generate one point. The scores are not weighted. A high number of points, i.e. a high score, indicates a high level of inappropriate prescribing. A clinical pharmacist applied the tools to the RCT dataset retrospectively; each patient's drug therapy was assessed on the first day of the hospital stay (before the pharmacists had made any recommendations to the physician) and again on the day of discharge. The total STOPP and START score on admission and at discharge were calculated for each patient. Information required for the assessment was obtained from the patients' medication administration records [19].

Outcome assessment

The clinical outcome variable for the primary aim in the present study was the number of visits to the ED during the 12-month follow-up period. This outcome was chosen because this was the endpoint on which the pharmacist intervention had the largest impact in the main study [21]. For the secondary aim, the changes in STOPP and START scores from admission to discharge were used to describe the effects of pharmacist intervention on the quality of prescribing for the different subgroups. In addition, the number, type and acceptance rate of the pharmacists' recommendations generated by the medication review were used to illustrate the outcomes of medication review. The types of recommendations included discontinuation of drug(s), initiation of drug therapy, changes to the drug/dosage/route, and patient counseling.

Subgroup assignment

The patients were divided into subgroups according to the number of medications prescribed for them on admission to hospital (main analysis) and the quality of the prescriptions. The patients' regular medications, as well as the p.r.n. (as required) medications used at least once the past six months, were included. Only products with an active ingredient were considered as medications, i.e. steroid creams were included while moisturizing creams were not. In the main subgroup analysis, ≥5 drugs on admission was used as the cut-off point. This cut-off point was chosen because ≥5 drugs is a common definition for polypharmacy. Since the subgroups receiving <5 drugs and ≥5 drugs were not well balanced in size, a sensitivity analysis using the median number of drugs (eight) as the cut-off point was performed. The differential effect of the intervention between patients with a high and low level of inappropriately prescribed drugs on admission was also explored. The cut-off points used in these analyses were based on the median scores for STOPP (≥2) and START (≥1), where a higher score indicated a higher level of inappropriate prescribing.

Statistical analysis

The baseline characteristics of the participants were summarized using frequencies for categorical variables and means with standard deviations for continuous variables. Poisson regression models, with group (intervention/control), subgroup factor, and the interaction between group and subgroup factor as independent variables, using the logarithm of time spent outside the hospital as an offset, were used for the subgroup analyses of the number of ED visits. Analyses of changes from admission to discharge in STOPP and START scores in the <5 and ≥5 drugs subgroups were performed using rank analysis of covariance [22,23], with group (intervention/control) as a factor and score on admission as a covariate. Unpaired two-sample t-tests were used to compare the number of pharmacist recommendations between subgroups. The Chi-square test was used for categorical data (comparisons of the rate of acceptance of the pharmacist recommendations). A p-value of <0.05 was regarded as statistically significant. No adjustments for multiplicity were made, as all tests were considered to be exploratory. All analyses were carried out using SAS software (version 9.3, SAS Institute, Cary, North Carolina) and Microsoft® Excel® 2008.

Results

Ninety patients were receiving <5 drugs and 278 were receiving ≥5 drugs on admission. The patients receiving <5 drugs on admission, irrespective of their assignment to control or intervention group, had on average fewer diagnoses and were less likely to live in nursing homes than the patients receiving a higher number of drugs. The groups did not differ substantially in any other perspective, including age (Table 1).

The effect of pharmacist intervention on the number of ED visits differed significantly between the subgroups defined by the number of drugs on admission (Table 2). The patients receiving < 5 drugs (main analysis) benefited more [relative rate reduction 78%; rate ratio (RR) 0.22 (95% CI 0.09–0.52)] from pharmacist intervention in this respect than those receiving ≥5 drugs (30%; RR 0.70 (95% CI 0.47–1.04)). The overall rate reduction was 47%. The sensitivity analysis confirmed our findings that the intervention was more effective for the patients receiving a lower number of drugs (RR 0.21 (95% CI 0.11–0.40) for the subgroup of patients receiving <8 drugs and 1.11 (95% CI 0.68–1.82) for those receiving ≥8 drugs).

The effect of pharmacist intervention on the number of ED visits was not altered by the level of inappropriate prescribing on admission, as measured by START and STOPP (Table 2).

On admission, the intervention <5 and ≥5 drugs subgroup, had on average 0.35 and 1.70 STOPP scores respectively, and 0.38 and 0.37 START scores respectively. The control group subgroups had on average 0.55 and 1.82 STOPP scores, and 0.23 and 0.50 START scores (<5 drugs and ≥5 drugs subgroups respectively) on admission. During the hospital stay, the mean STOPP score decreased (−0.7) for the intervention group patients receiving ≥5 drugs on admission but was essentially unchanged (0.1) for the intervention group patients receiving <5 drugs. The mean START scores decreased for the intervention group (across subgroups) but were unchanged for the control group (across subgroups) during the hospital stay (Table 3).

For the subgroups receiving <5 drugs, across intervention/control groups, the mean number of drugs increased during the hospital stay (change from admission: 2.1 (SD = 2.3) for the intervention group and 1.8 (SD = 2.0) for the control group).

The STOPP category that generated most points (n = 248; 47% of total STOPP criteria) on admission was "drugs that adversely affect fallers" and in this category the criteria "prescribing of benzodiazepines" (n = 118) was the most common. A patient was in this assessment considered a faller if he/she had experienced a fall during the past year. The category of STOPP criteria for which the intervention group patients had the most relative improvement, was "musculoskeletal system"; the prescribing of non-steroidal anti-inflammatory drugs (NSAIDs) was discontinued for all intervention group patients with a history of peptic ulcer disease, moderate-to-severe hypertension, heart failure and/or chronic renal failure except for two patients (17 points on admission and 2 points at discharge). In contrast, the control group had 16 points on admission and 12 points at discharge. On admission, the START criteria category "cardiovascular diseases" generated more scores than any other category (67% of total START scores), and this was also the category in which the intervention group patients had the largest improvement (intervention group: 46 points on admission and 10 points at discharge; control group: 51 points on admission and 59 points at discharge). The individual START criterion yielding most scores was omission of an ACE inhibitor for patients with chronic heart failure (intervention group: 15 points on admission and 4 points at discharge; control group: 20 points on admission and 26 points at discharge).

The pharmacist made a total of 49 recommendations for 24 of the 37 (65%) patients in the subgroup receiving <5 drugs (no recommendations were made for the remaining 13 patients in this subgroup). The mean number of recommendations for these patients was 2.0 (SD = 1.2) and the acceptance rate (i.e. the percentage of suggested actions carried out by the physician) was 86%. For the subgroup of patients receiving ≥5 drugs (n = 145), 481 recommendations were made for 130 of the 145 (90%) patients; the mean number of suggestions was 3.2 (SD = 1.7) and the acceptance rate was 73%. The mean number of recommendations per patient was lower in the subgroup receiving fewer drugs (p = 0.001 [t = 3.29; df = 152]) and the acceptance rate appeared to be higher (p = 0.057 [χ^2 = 3.61; df = 1]). The most common recommendations for the patients receiving <5 drugs were initiation of new drug therapy (n = 21, 43% of the total number of suggestions) and discontinuation of current drug therapy (n = 7, 14% of the total number of suggestions). For the patients receiving ≥5 drugs, the most frequent recommendations were discontinuation of current drug therapy (n = 132, 32%), initiation of new drug therapy (n = 71, 17%) and dose reduction (n = 71, 17%). The overall acceptance rate of the pharmacists' suggestions did not differ between the recommendations (p = 0.45 [χ^2 = 0.57; df = 1], 74% for discontinuation and 70% for initiation).

Discussion

This subgroup analysis from a randomized controlled intervention study showed that it was patients receiving a lower number of drugs who benefited most from the clinical pharmacist intervention. Since a large number of drugs often is associated with an increased risk of drug-related issues [2–8], the conclusion often reached, although it is not evidence-based, is that patients receiving a high number of drugs are in most need for drug-use quality improvement efforts and should be prioritized. The results from this study were therefore unexpected. Further, the analysis of the STOPP and START subgroup results found no differences in the effects of pharmacist intervention on ED visits between patients with a high and low level of inappropriate prescribing on admission to the hospital.

Table 1. Baseline characteristics for the patients in the <5 drugs and ≥5 drugs subgroups.

Baseline characteristics	Patients with <5 drugs (n = 90)	Patients with ≥5 drugs (n = 278)
Age, mean (SD), years	87.4 (4.08)	86.5 (4.09)
Female, No (%)	48 (53.3)	168 (60.4)
Body weight, mean (SD), kg		
Women	58.6 (12.6)	62.1 (13.5)
Men	68.8 (12.3)	72.3 (12.6)
Laboratory values, mean (SD)		
Creatinine clearance, mL/min/1.73 m^2	43.5 (19.6)	39.3 (18)
Sodium level, mEq/L	137.7 (5.3)	137.5 (4.5)
Potassium level, mEq/L	3.9 (0.7)	4.1 (0.6)
Social support, No (%)		
Spouse or partner	25 (27.8)	79 (28.4)
Residential home	7 (7.8)	21 (21.6)
None	58 (64.4)	139 (50.0)
Number of diagnoses, mean (SD)	1.5 (1.07)	2.9 (1.48)
Medical history, No (%)		
Heart failure	13 (14.4)	128 (46.0)
Diabetes	6 (6.7)	82 (29.5)
Chronic obstructive pulmonary disease	5 (5.6)	40 (14.4)
Arrhythmia	18 (20.0)	124 (44.6)
Malignancy	18 (20.0)	43 (15.5)
Ischemic heart disease	9 (8.9)	106 (38.1)
Cerebral vascular lesion	15 (16.7)	57 (20.5)
Myocardial infarct	15 (16.7)	83 (29.9)
Hypertension	21 (23.3)	126 (45.3)
Dementia	16 (17.8)	35 (12.6)

For the intervention <5-drugs subgroup, the number of drugs increased during the hospital stay; however, the START scores also improved for these patients. This indicates that the drugs that were added were appropriate, i.e. drugs that the patient had an indication for and that were previously omitted. Importantly, the number of drugs taken by the control <5-drugs subgroup also increased during their hospital stay, although without an improvement in START scores. This was possibly because drug therapy changes for this group during the hospital stay were mainly focused on the reason for admission, with limited attention paid to other diseases and medications, thus the overall quality of prescribing was not improved. The so-called treatment-risk paradox suggests that doctors are more unwilling to prescribe drugs to patients with polypharmacy [24]. A thorough medication review evaluates the need for new drugs and re-evaluates the need for current drugs. As it aims to avoid medications without a valid indication (even if they do not pose a risk for the patient), it decreases the incidence of unnecessary drug prescriptions that could prevent the initiation of useful drugs.

A plausible explanation to why the intervention <5-drugs subgroup did not have an improvement in STOPP, is that the number of STOPP scores in this groups was very small on admission, and a reduction therefore was difficult to obtain.

The pharmacists made more recommendations for optimizing drug therapy (both a higher frequency of recommendations, and for a larger proportion of the patients) for patients receiving ≥5 drugs on admission than for those receiving fewer drugs, but with a lower acceptance rate. This suggests that the intervention was more effective for the patients receiving fewer drugs than for those receiving more drugs in improving quality of prescribing.

The subgroup of patients who were receiving fewer drugs on admission had a lower number of co-morbidities and lower levels of social support. It has previously been demonstrated that patients living in nursing homes (i.e. has a high level of social support) generally have a higher number of drugs [25,26] and are less involved in their drug therapy [27]. Presumably, the study patients in the <5-drugs subgroup were engaged in their drug therapy to a higher degree, and were therefore more accepting of the parts of the pharmacist intervention that aimed to improve patient knowledge and compliance to drug therapy. In addition, these patients were probably more able to communicate any perceived drug therapy issues, which would improve the quality and efficacy of the intervention. It is possible, therefore, that these patients had greater potential for benefiting from pharmacist intervention. The involvement of more primary care nurses and/or caretakers in information collection and drug counseling could thus improve the pharmacist intervention experience for patients dwelling in nursing homes, who are less involved in their own drug therapy. An alternative explanation of the results, is that patients with a high number of drugs has a greater co-morbidity burden which may limit the potential effect of a pharmacist intervention on the clinical outcome.

The pharmacists did not use STOPP and START prospectively during the medication review. Because some of the STOPP and

Table 2. Subgroup analyses for the number of ED-visits.

	INTERVENTION GROUP				CONTROL GROUP					
Variable	**Patients (n)**	**Person years (n)**	**ED Visits (n)**	**Rate**	**Patients (n)**	**Person years (n)**	**ED Visits (n)**	**Rate**	**RR (95% CI)[a]**	**P-value interaction[a]**
Overall effect	182	140.9	49	0.35	186	141.0	93	0.66	0.53 (0.37–0.75)	-
Number of drugs										0.0175
<5	37	31.9	6	0.19	53	45.7	39	0.85	0.22 (0.09–0.52)	
≥5	145	109.0	43	0.39	133	95.2	54	0.57	0.70 (0.47–1.04)	
Number of drugs										<0.0001
<8	74	62.1	11	0.18	96	78.8	66	0.84	0.21 (0.11–0.40)	
≥8	108	78.8	38	0.48	90	62.2	27	0.43	1.11 (0.68–1.82)	
STOPP score										0.9051
<2	109	86.7	31	0.36	110	85.5	59	0.69	0.52 (0.34–0.80)	
≥2	73	54.2	18	0.33	76	53.4	34	0.64	0.54 (0.31–0.96)	
START score										0.2020
<1	133	102.4	43	0.42	126	95.9	70	0.73	0.58 (0.39–0.84)	
≥1	49	38.5	6	0.16	60	45.0	23	0.51	0.31 (0.12–0.75)	

[a]Rate ratios, 95% confidence intervals and p-values from poisson regression models with group, subgroup factor and their interaction as independent variables.

Table 3. Change in STOPP and START from admission to discharge for <5- and ≥5-drugs subgroups.

	STOPP		
	Change from admission[a]		
	INTERVENTION (n = 182)	CONTROL (n = 186)	p-value[b]
<5 drugs (n = 37+53), mean (SD)	0.1 (0.6)	0.3 (0.6)	0.0089
<5 drugs (n = 37+53), median (min-max)	0 (−1, 2)	0 (−1, 2)	
≥5 drugs (n = 145+133), mean (SD)	−0.7 (1.03)	0.2 (0.8)	0.0001
≥5 drugs (n = 145+133), median (min-max)	−1 (−4, 2)	0 (−3, 3)	
All patients (n = 182+186), mean (SD)	−0.5 (1.01)	0.2 (0.7)	
All patients (n = 182+186), median (min-max)	0 (−4, 2)	0 (−3, 3)	
	START		
	Change from admission[a]		
	INTERVENTION (n = 182)	**CONTROL (n = 186)**	**p-value[b]**
<5 drugs (n = 37+53), mean (SD)	−0.4 (0.9)	0.04 (0.3)	0.0002
<5 drugs (n = 37+53), median (min-max)	0 (−4, 0)	0 (−1, 2)	
≥5 drugs (n = 145+133), mean (SD)	−0.3 (0.5)	0.04 (0.4)	<0.0001
≥5 drugs (n = 145+133), median (min-max)	0 (−2, 0)	0 (−1, 1)	
All patients (n = 182+186), mean (SD)	−0.3 (0.6)	0.04 (0.4)	
All patients (n = 182+186), median (min-max)	0 (−4, 0)	0 (−1, 2)	

SD, Standard deviation.
[a]Change from admission calculated as STOPP/START Score at discharge - STOPP/START Score on admission.
[b]p-values from rank analysis of covariance for the effect of group (Intervention or Control) on change from admission, adjusted for the score on admission.

START criteria depart from Swedish guidelines and established practice, the scores do not entirely capture the content of the medication review as performed in the study. An example is the STOPP criteria "bensodiazepines for patients with recurrent falls". In Sweden, the bensodiazepine derivate zopiclone is the recommended drug for patients with sleeping disorders in need for medical treatment. Therefore, the pharmacists often suggested a change from a long-acting benzodiazepine (that poses a higher risk for falls and other adverse drug reactions in older people) to zopiclone; which is considered a quality improvement in prescribing, however not reflected in the STOPP scores. It should also be emphasized that drugs listed as potentially inappropriate in explicit criteria (e.g. STOPP and START) may be inappropriate for most older people but the best drug of choice for others, and drugs considered as generally appropriate can be inappropriate in certain patients and in certain situations. By mainly focusing on drugs that are listed as potentially inappropriate, the potential risk of the patient's other drugs can be underestimated [28,29]. Explicit criteria are also often criticized for not taking the patients' co-morbidities into account [30]. The clinical pharmacists' medication reviews are based on general consensus about appropriateness of prescribing, but the recommendations are altered depending on the characteristics, health status and preferences of the individual patient. This results in a more individualized assessment. To describe the effects of the intervention in this study more accurately, a record was kept of the number, type and acceptance rate of the pharmacists' actual recommendations. Still, the strength of STOPP and START is their status as validated methods of assessing the quality of prescribing. STOPP and START also have the advantage of taking a broad view of inappropriate prescribing into account (as they estimate the level of overprescribing as well as underprescribing), which makes them superior to other available tools used to analyze inappropriate prescribing in this context. All the process assessment methods used in this study (START and STOPP assessments, and pharmacist recommendations) only reflected parts of the pharmacist intervention in the main study, i.e. the medication review. Changes in the elements of the intervention that aimed to improve patient safety and compliance and increase patients' understanding of their drug therapy were not measured and the outcomes can only be surmised.

This is a post-hoc subgroup analysis of a RCT, the trial was not powered for interaction tests and no adjustments for multiplicity were undertaken. The results should therefore be considered primarily as hypothesis generating. It should also be noted that the number of patients in each subgroup is relatively small, and therefore comparisons between the subgroups, e.g. evaluation of the impact of the pharmacist intervention, should be interpreted with caution. Yet, the subgroup effects identified in this study are clinically important; the analyses were based on a rational indication and the studied variables are valid for all hospitalized older people.

Drug-related issues, e.g. inappropriate prescribing, occur in patients irrespective of low or high numbers of prescribed drugs. Accordingly, patients receiving fewer drugs on admission to hospital should not be automatically dismissed when prioritizing who should be targeted for efforts to improve the quality of drug treatment. Our study suggests, in fact, that these patients benefit more from a clinical pharmacist intervention. Further, the results of this study do not support prioritization of patients with inappropriate prescribing (as measured with STOPP and START) for comprehensive pharmacist intervention. Future studies to test this hypothesis in patients in another age group (e.g. ≥65 years) are warranted. The elements of a ward-based pharmacist intervention that are most effective in different subgroups of patients also need to be further explored.

Conclusions

Unexpectedly, the pharmacist intervention appeared to be more effective in preventing future visits to the ED for patients who were receiving fewer drugs on admission to hospital. Based on our analysis of STOPP and START scores, there was no difference in effect between the patients with higher and lower levels of inappropriate prescribing. The overall quality of prescribing was improved for the intervention <5 and ≥ 5 drugs subgroups, compared to the control group.

Author Contributions

Conceived and designed the experiments: AA MB UG JS HM. Performed the experiments: AA MB. Analyzed the data: AA MB UG JS MHU HM. Wrote the paper: AA MB UG JS MHU HM.

References

1. Socialstyrelsens föreskrifter och allmänna råd (SOSFS 2000:1) om läkemedelshantering i hälso- och sjukvården (n.d.). Available: http://www.socialstyrelsen.se/sosfs/2000-1/. Accessed 18 June 2013.
2. Steinman MA, Landefeld CS, Rosenthal GE, Berthenthal D, Sen S, et al. (2006) Polypharmacy and prescribing quality in older people. J Am Geriatr Soc 54: 1516–1523. doi:10.1111/j.1532-5415.2006.00889.x.
3. Fialová D, Topinková E, Gambassi G, Finne-Soveri H, Jónsson PV, et al. (2005) Potentially inappropriate medication use among elderly home care patients in Europe. JAMA J Am Med Assoc 293: 1348–1358. doi:10.1001/jama.293.11.1348.
4. Cahir C, Fahey T, Teeling M, Teljeur C, Feely J, et al. (2010) Potentially inappropriate prescribing and cost outcomes for older people: a national population study. Br J Clin Pharmacol 69: 543–552. doi:10.1111/j.1365-2125.2010.03628.x.
5. Gallagher PF, Barry PJ, Ryan C, Hartigan I, O'Mahony D (2008) Inappropriate prescribing in an acutely ill population of elderly patients as determined by Beers' Criteria. Age Ageing 37: 96–101. doi:10.1093/ageing/afm116.
6. Coleman EA, Smith JD, Raha D, Min S (2005) Posthospital medication discrepancies: prevalence and contributing factors. Arch Intern Med 165: 1842–1847. doi:10.1001/archinte.165.16.1842.
7. Alassaad A, Gillespie U, Bertilsson M, Melhus H, Hammarlund-Udenaes M (2013) Prescription and transcription errors in multidose-dispensed medications on discharge from hospital: an observational and interventional study. J Eval Clin Pract 19: 185–191. doi:10.1111/j.1365-2753.2011.01798.x.
8. Parkin DM, Henney CR, Quirk J, Crooks J (1976) Deviation from prescribed drug treatment after discharge from hospital. Br Med J 2: 686–688.
9. Scott I, Jayathissa S (2010) Quality of drug prescribing in older patients: is there a problem and can we improve it? Intern Med J 40: 7–18. doi:10.1111/j.1445-5994.2009.02040.x.
10. Home Medicines Review (HMR) - Medicare Australia (n.d.). Available: http://www.medicareaustralia.gov.au/provider/pbs/fourth-agreement/hmr.jsp. Accessed 19 November 2013.
11. Patterson SM, Hughes C, Kerse N, Cardwell CR, Bradley MC (2012) Interventions to improve the appropriate use of polypharmacy for older people. Cochrane Database Syst Rev Online 5: CD008165. doi:10.1002/14651858.CD008165.pub2.
12. Simonson W, Feinberg JL (2005) Medication-related problems in the elderly: defining the issues and identifying solutions. Drugs Aging 22: 559–569.
13. Hanlon JT, Schmader KE, Ruby CM, Weinberger M (2001) Suboptimal prescribing in older inpatients and outpatients. J Am Geriatr Soc 49: 200–209.
14. Gallagher P, Ryan C, Byrne S, Kennedy J, O'Mahony D (2008) STOPP (Screening Tool of Older Person's Prescriptions) and START (Screening Tool to Alert doctors to Right Treatment). Consensus validation. Int J Clin Pharmacol Ther 46: 72–83.
15. Gallagher P, Baeyens J-P, Topinkova E, Madlova P, Cherubini A, et al. (2009) Inter-rater reliability of STOPP (Screening Tool of Older Persons' Prescriptions) and START (Screening Tool to Alert doctors to Right Treatment) criteria amongst physicians in six European countries. Age Ageing 38: 603–606. doi:10.1093/ageing/afp058.
16. Barry PJ, Gallagher P, Ryan C, O'mahony D (2007) START (screening tool to alert doctors to the right treatment)–an evidence-based screening tool to detect prescribing omissions in elderly patients. Age Ageing 36: 632–638. doi:10.1093/ageing/afm118.
17. Hellström LM, Bondesson A, Höglund P, Midlöv P, Holmdahl L, et al. (2011) Impact of the Lund Integrated Medicines Management (LIMM) model on medication appropriateness and drug-related hospital revisits. Eur J Clin Pharmacol 67: 741–752. doi:10.1007/s00228-010-0982-3.
18. Spinewine A, Swine C, Dhillon S, Lambert P, Nachega JB, et al. (2007) Effect of a collaborative approach on the quality of prescribing for geriatric inpatients: a randomized, controlled trial. J Am Geriatr Soc 55: 658–665. doi:10.1111/j.1532-5415.2007.01132.x.
19. Gillespie U, Alassaad A, Hammarlund-Udenaes M, Mörlin C, Henrohn D, et al. (2013) Effects of pharmacists' interventions on appropriateness of prescribing and evaluation of the instruments' (MAI, STOPP and STARTs') ability to predict hospitalization–analyses from a randomized controlled trial. PloS One 8: e62401. doi:10.1371/journal.pone.0062401.
20. Kaboli PJ, Hoth AB, McClimon BJ, Schnipper JL (2006) Clinical pharmacists and inpatient medical care: a systematic review. Arch Intern Med 166: 955–964. doi:10.1001/archinte.166.9.955.
21. Gillespie U, Alassaad A, Henrohn D, Garmo H, Hammarlund-Udenaes M, et al. (2009) A comprehensive pharmacist intervention to reduce morbidity in patients 80 years or older: a randomized controlled trial. Arch Intern Med 169: 894–900. doi:10.1001/archinternmed.2009.71.
22. Koch GG, Amara IA, Davis GW, Gillings DB (1982) A review of some statistical methods for covariance analysis of categorical data. Biometrics 38: 563–595.
23. Stokes M., Davis CG, Koch GG (n.d.) Categorical data analysis using the SAS system. Second edition. Cary, NC: SAS Institute Inc. 2000.
24. Lee DS, Tu JV, Juurlink DN, Alter DA, Ko DT, et al. (2005) Risk-treatment mismatch in the pharmacotherapy of heart failure. JAMA J Am Med Assoc 294: 1240–1247. doi:10.1001/jama.294.10.1240.
25. Gordon AL, Franklin M, Bradshaw L, Logan P, Elliott R, et al. (2013) Health status of UK care home residents: a cohort study. Age Ageing. doi:10.1093/ageing/aft077.
26. Olsson J, Bergman A, Carlsten A, Oké T, Bernsten C, et al. (2010) Quality of drug prescribing in elderly people in nursing homes and special care units for dementia: a cross-sectional computerized pharmacy register analysis. Clin Drug Investig 30: 289–300. doi:10.2165/11534320-000000000-00000.
27. Hughes CM, Goldie R (2009) "I just take what I am given": adherence and resident involvement in decision making on medicines in nursing homes for older people: a qualitative survey. Drugs Aging 26: 505–517. doi:10.2165/00002512-200926060-00007.
28. Budnitz DS, Lovegrove MC, Shehab N, Richards CL (2011) Emergency hospitalizations for adverse drug events in older Americans. N Engl J Med 365: 2002–2012. doi:10.1056/NEJMsa1103053.
29. Dormann H, Sonst A, Müller F, Vogler R, Patapovas A, et al. (2013) Adverse drug events in older patients admitted as an emergency: the role of potentially inappropriate medication in elderly people (PRISCUS). Dtsch Ärztebl Int 110: 213–219. doi:10.3238/arztebl.2013.0213.
30. Spinewine A, Schmader KE, Barber N, Hughes C, Lapane KL, et al. (2007) Appropriate prescribing in elderly people: how well can it be measured and optimised? Lancet 370: 173–184. doi:10.1016/S0140-6736(07)61091-5.

25

Acid Sphingomyelinase Serum Activity Predicts Mortality in Intensive Care Unit Patients after Systemic Inflammation: A Prospective Cohort Study

Matthias Kott[1*], Gunnar Elke[1], Maike Reinicke[1,2], Supandi Winoto-Morbach[2], Dirk Schädler[1], Günther Zick[1], Inéz Frerichs[1], Norbert Weiler[1], Stefan Schütze[2]

1 Department of Anesthesiology and Intensive Care Medicine, University Medical Center Schleswig-Holstein, Campus Kiel, Kiel, Germany, 2 Institute of Immunology, University Medical Center Schleswig-Holstein, Campus Kiel, Kiel, Germany

Abstract

Introduction: Acid sphingomyelinase is involved in lipid signalling pathways and regulation of apoptosis by the generation of ceramide and plays an important role during the host response to infectious stimuli. It thus has the potential to be used as a novel diagnostic marker in the management of critically ill patients. The objective of our study was to evaluate acid sphingomyelinase serum activity (ASM) as a diagnostic and prognostic marker in a mixed intensive care unit population before, during, and after systemic inflammation.

Methods: 40 patients admitted to the intensive care unit at risk for developing systemic inflammation (defined as systemic inflammatory response syndrome *plus* a significant procalcitonin [PCT] increase) were included. ASM was analysed on ICU admission, before (PCT_{before}), during (PCT_{peak}) and after (PCT_{low}) onset of SIRS. Patients undergoing elective surgery served as control (N = 8). Receiver-operating characteristics curves were computed.

Results: ASM significantly increased after surgery in the eight control patients. Patients from the intensive care unit had significantly higher ASM on admission than control patients after surgery. 19 out of 40 patients admitted to the intensive care unit developed systemic inflammation and 21 did not, with no differences in ASM between these two groups on admission. In patients with SIRS and PCT peak, ASM between admission and PCT_{before} was not different, but further increased at PCT_{peak} in non-survivors and was significantly higher at PCT_{low} compared to survivors. Survivors exhibited decreased ASM at PCT_{peak} and PCT_{low}. Receiver operating curve analysis on discrimination of ICU mortality showed an area under the curve of 0.79 for ASM at PCT_{low}.

Conclusions: In summary, ASM was generally higher in patients admitted to the intensive care unit compared to patients undergoing uncomplicated surgery. ASM did not indicate onset of systemic inflammation. In contrast to PCT however, it remained high in non-surviving ICU patients after systemic inflammation.

Editor: Lyle L. Moldawer, University of Florida College of Medicine, United States of America

Funding: This study was funded by a restricted grant of the Christian-Albrechts University Kiel, Germany and in part supported by a grant of the Deutsche Forschungsgemeinschaft (SCHU 733/9-2) given to S. Schütze. The funders had no role in study design, data collection and analysis, decision to publish, or preparation of the manuscript.

Competing Interests: The authors have declared that no competing interests exist.

* Email: matthias.kott@uksh.de

These authors contributed equally to this work.

Introduction

Despite advances in critical care, systemic inflammatory response syndrome (SIRS) and sepsis syndrome with subsequent multi-organ failure still contribute to overall mortality in critically ill patients, equalling the number of deaths caused by acute myocardial infarction [1]. Besides specific treatment of the underlying cause of systemic inflammation, early diagnosis based on clinical findings and laboratory testing is of paramount importance to enable successful therapy [2]. The kinetics of biomarkers reflecting changes in the inflammatory condition can be helpful to identify patients at high risk for complications.

At present, procalcitonin (PCT) is regarded as the best available laboratory tool for the diagnosis of infection and systemic inflammation in combination with clinical symptoms [3,4] and has been introduced as a variable in the diagnostic criteria for sepsis in the recently updated Surviving Sepsis Campaign guidelines [5]. PCT has the advantage of an earlier peak level upon infection, a better specificity and correlation to disease severity and clinical outcome as compared to routine biomarkers such as white blood cell count or C-reactive protein (CRP) [6–9].

Activation of acid sphingomyelinase, a C-type phosphodiesterase leads to generation of ceramide from biological inert sphingomyelin derived from the cell membrane. Generation of ceramide at the outer leaflet of cell membranes induces changes in composition and spatial arrangement in terms of forming ceramide-enriched membrane lipid rafts, leading to receptor clustering and apoptosis signalling and modification of the cellular response to stress stimuli [10,11]. Clinical data concerning the potential role of acid sphingomyelinase serum activity (ASM) is infrequent. In a retrospective study of 12 patients with severe sepsis, Claus et al. showed that elevated ASM levels can be observed after the onset of sepsis, and that a further increase may be associated with worse outcome [12]. On the other hand, recent animal studies suggest a protective role of ASM secretion during the early host response as a first line of defence [13]. Due to its pathophysiological properties in the early host response, determination of ASM may also be used as an early diagnostic marker before the onset of systemic inflammation. The aim of our pilot study was to evaluate the role of ASM in a mixed intensive care unit (ICU) population at risk for the development of systemic inflammation. We hypothesized that ASM a) increases before the onset of systemic inflammation, and b) may be used as a prognostic marker of outcome.

Materials and Methods

Study design and patients

This single-center prospective cohort study was conducted in two surgical intensive care units of a tertiary medical center (University Medical Center Schleswig-Holstein, Campus Kiel, Kiel, Germany) with the approval of the local ethics committee of the Christian-Albrechts University Kiel, Germany. Written informed consent was obtained from each patient or the legal representative, respectively.

We prospectively included patients (age≥18 years) who were admitted to the ICU and deemed to be at high risk for the development of systemic inflammation (ICU group). High risk criteria were defined as the following ICU admission diagnoses: extended surgery, polytrauma, respiratory insufficiency, and patients with an expected length of ICU stay >3 days. Patients were evaluated on a daily basis for new onset of systemic inflammatory response syndrome (SIRS) fulfilling two or more of the defined clinical criteria according to the ACCP/SCCM recommendations [14] *plus* an increase in PCT. This PCT peak was defined as a two-fold increase in PCT concentration compared to the value of the preceding day and exceeding a

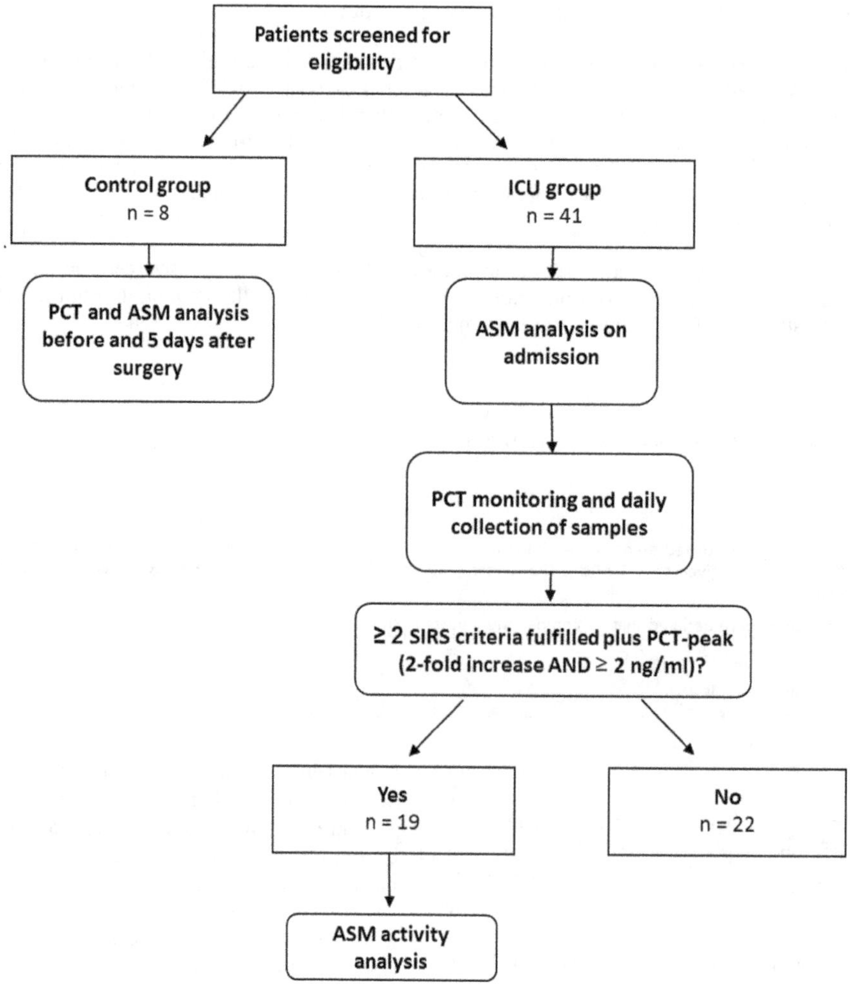

Figure 1. Study flow chart.

Table 1. Baseline patient characteristics and outcomes.

	Total	ICU Group			Control
		Total	SI	No SI	
Number	48	40	19	21	8
Age, median, years	69	69	69	69	65
Gender, male, n (%)	30 (62.5)	25 (63.4)	12 (63.2)	13 (66.6)	5 (62.5)
Mortality, n (%)	15 (31.2)	15 (36.6)	9 (47.4)	6 (27.3)	0
Main diagnosis, n (%)					
Abdominal surgery	22 (45.8)	14 (34.1)	8 (42.1)	6 (28.6)	8 (100)
Liver failure	1 (2.4)	1 (2.4)	1 (5.3)	-	-
Major bleeding	2 (4.9)	2 (4.9)	-	2 (9.5)	-
Major trauma	3 (7.3)	3 (7.3)	1 (5.3)	2 (9.5)	-
Mesenterial ischemia	2 (4.9)	2 (4.9)	-	2 (9.5)	-
Pancreatitis	2 (4.9)	2 (4.9)	2 (10.5)	-	-
Pneumonia	6 (14.6)	6 (14.6)	2 (10.5)	4 (19)	-
Soft tissue infection	3 (7.3)	3 (7.3)	-	3 (14.3)	-
Thoracic surgery	7 (17)	7 (17)	5 (26.3)	2 (9.5)	-

Systemic inflammation was defined as new onset of systemic inflammatory response syndrome plus a two-fold increase in PCT concentration compared to the value of the preceding day or exceeding a minimum of >2 ng/ml. PCT: procalcitonin, ICU: intensive care unit; SI: systemic inflammation.

minimum of >2 ng/ml. Exclusion criteria were diseases associated with hyperprocalcitoninaemia like small-cell lung cancer or C-cell carcinoma and administration of PCT inducing agents (Anti-Thymocyte globulin or OKT3 antibodies). Events with PCT elevations following re-operation during the ICU stay and patients receiving ASM inhibiting medications (amlodipin, sertralin, imipramin, desipramin, or steroids) were also excluded [15]. ASM was consecutively analysed at four time points: I), on ICU admission, II), the day before new onset of SIRS in combination with a PCT peak were detected (PCT_{before}), III), the first day of new onset of SIRS and a PCT peak (PCT_{peak}), and IV), on the first day when the PCT level was below 0.5 ng/ml or declined to a nadir with less than 30% of the PCT_{peak} concentration (PCT_{low}).

Patients undergoing uncomplicated elective major abdominal surgery were used as a control group to assess the peri-operative kinetics of ASM. In these patients, ASM was also determined before surgery to determine the influence of the surgical trauma on ASM. Serum samples for the analysis of ASM were collected

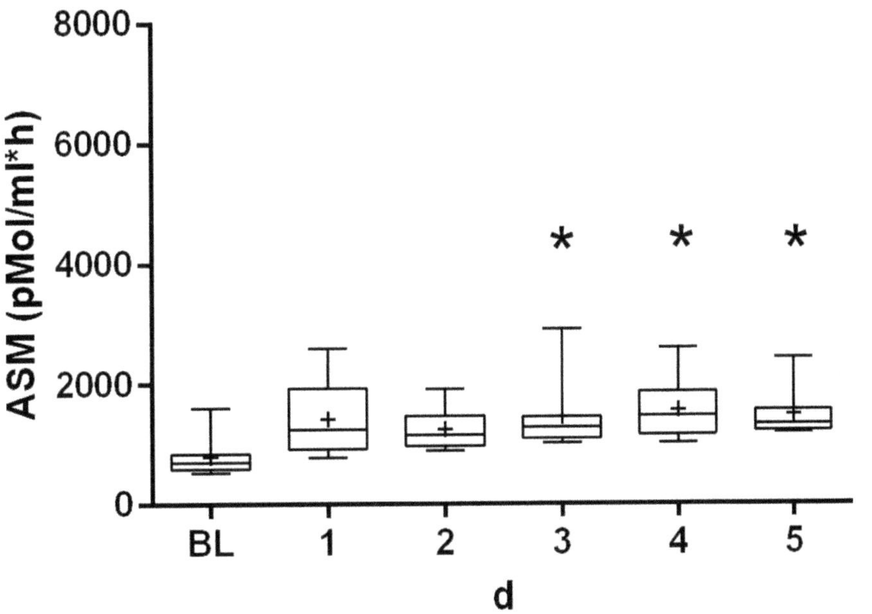

Figure 2. Kinetics of acid sphingomyelinase serum activity in the control group. The box plots display the minima/maxima (whiskers), 25%/75% percentile (box), median (−) and mean (+) values. Statistically significant differences ($P<0.05$) between baseline (BL) and post-operative values are marked with an asterisk (*). ASM: acid sphingomyelinase activity; BL: baseline (before surgery); d: days.

Table 2. Biomarker level and severity of illness measures of all study patients.

Variabe	ICU admission	ICU group		Control group
	(N = 40)	SI (N = 19)	No SI (N = 21)	(N = 8)
ASM (pMol/ml•h)	2593 (2021–4396)	2755 (1897–4396)	2529 (2041–4618)	709 (598–841)
PCT (ng/ml)	3.19 (1.03–8.15)	2.1 (0.75–4.88)	4.17 (1.57–10.38)	0.16 (0.12–0.23)
CRP (mg/l)	121 (35–274)	153 (12–235)	90 (35–304)	2.35 (0.97–25)
Lactate (mMol/l)	1.7 (0.9–2.5)	1.4 (0.8–2.6)	1.7 (1.1–2.5)	-
mSOFA score	7 (4–8)	7 (4–8)	6.5 (4–9)	-
SAPS II	46 (36–57)	46 (34–57)	48 (37–61)	-
TISS	19 (13–24)	14 (10–19)	22 (14–26)	-

In the ICU group, biomarker levels were measured in all patients at intensive care unit admission. For the control group, the pre-operative biomarker levels are displayed. Data are shown as median with interquartile ranges. Systemic inflammation was defined as new onset of systemic inflammatory response syndrome plus a two-fold increase in PCT concentration compared to the value of the preceding day or exceeding a minimum of >2 ng/ml. ASM: acid sphingomyelinase serum activity; CRP: C-reactive protein; mSOFA: modified Sequential Organ Failure Assessment score (excluding central nervous system); PCT: procalcitonin; SAPS II: Simplified Acute and Physiology Score II; SI: systemic inflammation; TISS: Therapeutic Intervention Scoring System.

prospectively on a daily basis and stored at −20°Celsius. ASM on the day of ICU admission was analysed in all included patients but due to financial restraints consecutive measurements of ASM (from PCT_{before} until patients' discharge or death) were performed only in those patients with a PCT peak.

Data collection

We collected baseline characteristics of the patients including demographic information, comorbidities and type of surgery. Severity of illness was determined by calculating the Simplified Acute and Physiology Score II (SAPS II) [16], Therapeutic Intervention Scoring System (TISS) [17] and a modified Sequential Organ Failure Assessment Score (mSOFA) [18] (excluding central nervous system). Serum samples for the analysis of PCT and ASM (10 ml of either central venous or arterial blood) were prospectively collected on a daily basis in addition to routine laboratory including white blood cell count (WBC), lactate, C-reactive protein (CRP) serum levels. The patients' management was left at the discretion of the attending ICU physician. Patients were followed up until discharge from the ICU or death.

Measurements of ASM serum activity

Plasma was obtained and centrifuged at 3000 g for 5 minutes (Sorvall -Super TRI, Kendro Laboratory Products GmbH, Langenselbold, Germany) and stored at −20°C until assayed. Analytical determination of ASM depended on detection of radio-

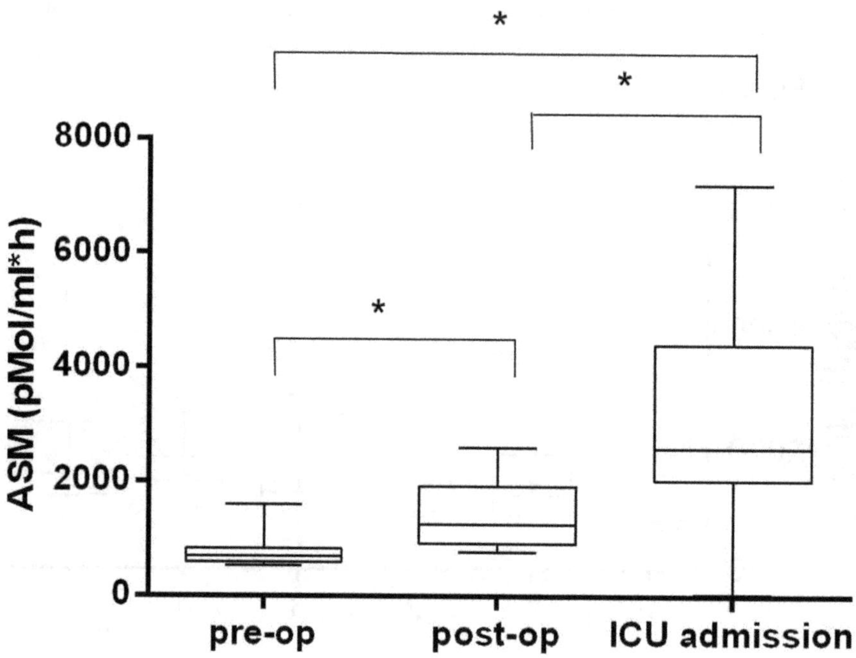

Figure 3. Acid sphingomyelinase serum activity in control and ICU patients. This figure indicates median pre- and post-operative acid sphingomyelinase serum activity of the control group and median acid sphingomyelinase serum activity of the ICU group on admission. Statistical significant differences between groups ($P<0.05$) are marked with an asterisk (*). The box plots display the minima/maxima (whiskers), 25%/75% percentile (box), and median (−) values. ASM: acid sphingomyelinase serum activity.

Table 3. Biomarker level and severity of illness measures in patients with systemic inflammation (N = 19) according to PCT time points.

Variable	Time point	All (N = 19)	Survivor (N = 9)	Non-survivor (N = 10)	*P* Value*
Procalcitonin	PCT_{before}	0.46 (0.29–2.08)	0.37 (0.19–1.38)	0.65 (0.42–2.78)	0.07
	PCT_{peak}	4.43 (2.54–11.74)	4.14 (2.42–21.43)	4.43 (2.81–10.65)	>0.99
	PCT_{low}	0.48 (0.43–1.09)	0.45 (0.41–0.72)	0.59 (0.44–1.12)	0.57
ASM	PCT_{before}	2782 (1991–3903)	2777 (1835–3244)	2874 (2278–4528)	0.40
	PCT_{peak}	3233 (1968–2907)	2501 (1953–3878)	3855 (1987–5122)	0.23
	PCT_{low}	2261 (2063–2907)	2205 (1596–2496)	2611 (2235–4402)	***0.03***
CRP	PCT_{before}	130 (87–220)	157 (74–210)	127 (80–233)	0.23
	PCT_{peak}	145 (95–256)	124 (77–237)	182 (111–295)	0.25
	PCT_{low}	98 (66–203)	70 (57–138)	141 (78–228)	***0.04***
Lactate	PCT_{before}	1.6 (1.1–3.8)	1.6 (0.9–3.05)	1.8 (1.3–4.5)	0.62
	PCT_{peak}	1.6 (1–3.2)	1.4 (1.1–3.2)	1.8 (1–3.9)	0.59
	PCT_{low}	1.1 (0.9–1.6)	1.1 (0.8–1.6)	1.1 (0.9–2.3)	0.54
mSOFA	PCT_{before}	7 (5–11)	7 (6–11)	7 (4–11)	0.67
	PCT_{peak}	8 (5–11)	8 (6–12)	6 (3–11)	0.39
	PCT_{low}	4 (2–6)	4 (3–7)	4 (1–6)	0.37
SAPS II	PCT_{before}	48 (37–50)	46 (37–49)	49 (29–55)	0.54
	PCT_{peak}	44 (37–51)	44 (40–46)	46 (30–58)	0.59
	PCT_{low}	41 (35–48)	39 (32–43)	43 (38–53)	0.17
TISS	PCT_{before}	21 (17–24)	22 (18–23)	20 (15–30)	0.88
	PCT_{peak}	18 (15–23)	18 (15–23)	20 (8–24)	0.73
	PCT_{low}	17 (6–23)	16 (9–19)	18 (0–26)	0.85

Time points were the day before the PCT peak (PCT_{before}), the day of the PCT peak (PCT_{peak}) and again lowered PCT (PCT_{low}).
**P* value for comparison of survivors vs. non-survivors. Systemic inflammation was defined as new onset of systemic inflammatory response syndrome plus a two-fold increase in PCT concentration compared to the value of the preceding day or exceeding a minimum of >2 ng/ml. ASM: acid sphingomyelinase serum activity, CRP: C-reactive protein concentration, mSOFA: modified Sequential Organ Failure Assessment Score (excluding central nervous system); PCT: procalcitonin; SAPS II: Simplified Acute and Physiology Score II; TISS: Therapeutic Intervention Scoring System.

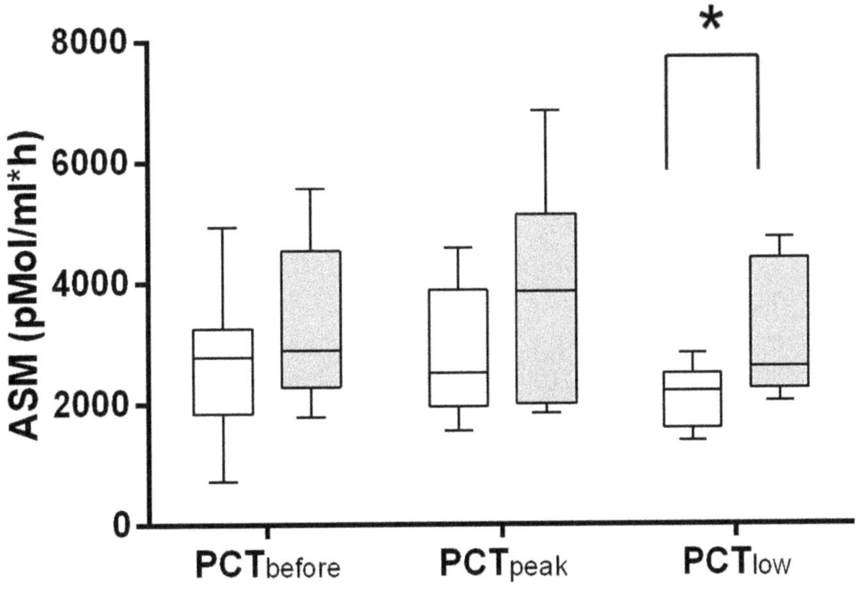

Figure 4. Acid sphingomyelinase serum activity in ICU patients with SIRS. Clear boxes represent survivors (n = 9) and grey boxes non-survivors (N = 10). Statistically significant difference ($P<0.05$) between survivors and non-survivors at PCT_{low} (*) for acid sphingomyelinase serum. The box plots show the minima/maxima (whiskers), 25%/75% percentile (box), and median (—) values. ASM: acid sphingomyelinase serum activity.

Table 4. Receiver operating characteristics curve analysis for patients with systemic inflammation at PCT_{low} (N = 19).

Variable	*P* Value	AUC	Optimal cut-off	Sensitivity (%)/Specifity (%)	LR
ASM (pMol/ml•h)	0.03	0.79	<2098	40/90	4
PCT	0.55	0.58	-	-	-
CRP	0.04	0.77	0.77	60/90	6
Lactate	0.52	0.58	-	-	-

At the two other time points, receiver operating characteristics curves were not significantly different from 0.5. Systemic inflammation was defined as new onset of systemic inflammatory response syndrome plus a two-fold increase in PCT concentration compared to the value of the preceding day or exceeding a minimum of > 2 ng/ml. ASM: acid sphingomyelinase serum activity; AUC: area under the curve; LR: likelihood ratio; CRP: C-reactive protein; PCT: procalcitonin.

labeled [14C]-Phosphorycholin that was generated by [14C]-sphingomyelin cleavage in aequimolar amounts to ceramide [19]. Protein quantity was determined by bicinchoninacid (BCA)-assays. 300 μg of purified protein were used in a total volume of 10 μl per assay. 100 μl ASM buffer and 40 μl of [14C]-substrate were added and incubated for at least 2 hours at 37°C. Reaction was stopped by adding 750 μl chloroforme/methanol (2:1) and 300 μl of destilled water. After 4 minutes of centrifugation by 14.000×g revolutions per minute, 300 μl of the upper aqueous phase were pipetted and filled into a scintillation test tube. 4 ml of scintillation fluid were added (Aquasafe 300 plus, Zinsser Analytic, Frankfurt), and β-count of radio-labeled [14C]-Phosphorycholin was measured (LS 6000LL, Beckman Coulter GmbH, Krefeld, Germany). ASM was calculated as pmol/ml•h.

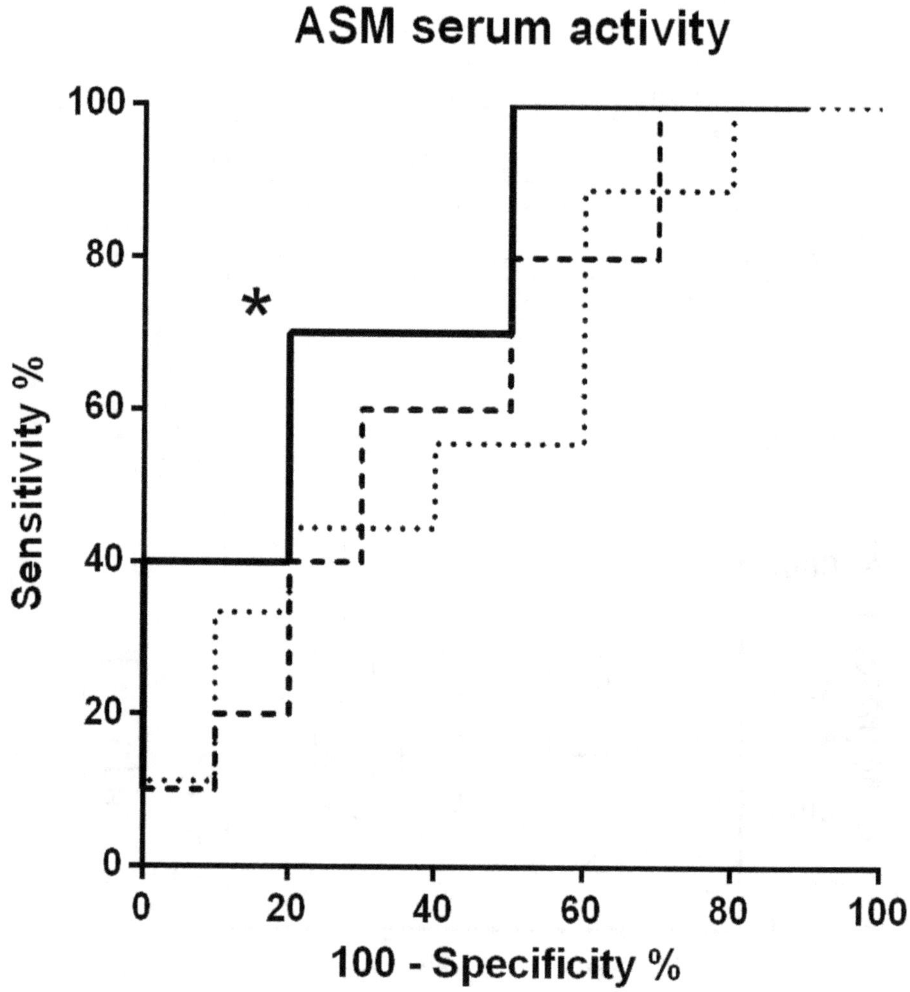

Figure 5. Receiver operating characteristics curve (ROC) analysis of acid sphingomyelinase serum activity. ROC analyses were performed at all three time points: PCT_{before} (fine dashed line), PCT_{peak} (dashed line), and PCT_{low} (solid line). ROC curves statistically significant different from 0.5 are marked with an asterisk (*). ASM: acid sphingomyelinase serum activity.

PCT measurements

PCT measurements were performed using a commercially available immunoluminometric assay (Elecsys BRAHMS PCT, BRAHMS-Diagnostica, Berlin, Germany) according to the manufacturer's instructions via the automated Kryptor platform (BRAHMS AG, Hennigsdorf, Germany). The direct measuring range of the assay is from 0.02–100 ng/ml, with automated dilution extending the upper range to 1.000 ng/ml. The functional assay sensitivity is 0.06 ng/ml, and the sample volume needed is 50 μl.

Statistical analysis

Means ± standard deviations (SD) or medians with interquartile ranges (IQR) are reported as appropriate. Differences in continuous variables between survivors and non-survivors were compared with the nonparametric Mann-Whitney test. Predictive values of serum ASM, PCT, CRP, WBC, body temperature and severity of illness measures regarding ICU mortality were evaluated. Discriminatory power (ability to distinguish between patients who die and those who survive) of laboratory tests and severity of illness scores were tested at all 3 time points to produce receiver operating characteristic (ROC) curves. The area under curve (AUC), with 95% confidence intervals (CI) and cut-offs for sensitivity and specificity were calculated in prediction of ICU mortality. A P value below 0.05 was considered statistically significant. Statistical analyses were performed with SPSS 17.0 (SPSS Inc., Chicago, IL, USA) and Prism 5 (GraphPad Software Inc., San Diego, CA, USA).

Results

Patient characteristics

A study flow chart is given in Figure 1. A total of 48 patients were included during the study period of whom 8 patients undergoing uncomplicated major abdominal surgery served as the control group. 40 patients fulfilled high-risk criteria and were included in the ICU group. Finally, 19 patients in the ICU group had new onset of SIRS *plus* a PCT peak (one patient with two episodes). Table 1 shows patients' baseline characteristics.

ASM, PCT and CRP levels in the control group

Figure 2 shows the pre- and post-operative kinetics of ASM in the control group. Median ASM measured before surgery was 709 pMol/ml•h (598–841 pMol/ml•h) and was significantly higher post-operatively (1320 pMol/ml•h; IQR: 1108–1565 pMol/ml•h). PCT and CRP both showed regular post-operative kinetics (data not shown).

ASM, PCT, CRP and lactate levels in the ICU group

ASM, PCT, CRP, lactate levels and severity of illness measures at ICU admission are shown in Table 2. Median ASM upon ICU admission in the ICU group was significantly higher than both baseline and post-operative values in the control group (Figure 3). In 21 patients of the ICU group, no newly developed SIRS plus a PCT peak were observed and median ASM upon ICU admission was not different when compared to the other 19 patients with PCT peak ($P = 0.8695$). Table 3 summarizes the course of biomarker level in the 19 patients with new onset of SIRS plus a PCT peak. Median PCT level at PCT_{before} was 0.46 ng/ml, increased markedly on PCT_{peak} to 4.43 ng/ml and subsequently returned to nearly baseline values at PCT_{low}. ASM showed no statistical significant differences between these three time points. Also, there was no difference in ASM in these patients between ICU admission and PCT_{before} ($P = 0.8995$). There were no significant changes in CRP, lactate levels and severity of illness measures (table 3).

Survivors vs. non-survivors

Among the 19 patients with SIRS and a PCT peak, 9 patients (47.4%) died during their ICU stay as opposed to 6 of the 21 patients without PCT peak who died (27.3%). With PCT_{low} as the baseline of ASM (equalling 100%), ASM increased only in non-survivors (by 34%), whereas in survivors a decline (by 10%) of ASM was detected even at PCT_{peak}. ASM declined in all patients at PCT_{low} (91% vs. 79%), but remained significantly higher in non-survivors when compared to survivors ($P = 0.03$; Table 3 and Figure 4).

ROC analysis for ICU mortality in the ICU group

ROC analyses were performed at all four time points for all measured laboratory parameters. Only at PCT_{low}, the areas under receiver operating curves (AUC) for ASM in prediction of ICU mortality were significantly different from 0.5 (AUC: 0.79, $P = 0.03$) with a sensitivity of 40% and specificity of 90% at an optimal cut-off value of 2098 pMol/ml•h, (likelihood ratio: 4). For CRP, the sensitivity was 60% and specificity 90% at an optimal cut-off value of 77.1 mg/L (Table 4).

Discussion

This prospective pilot cohort study evaluated the role of ASM as a potential early diagnostic and prognostic marker in a mixed ICU population at high risk of developing systemic inflammation. We found that ASM was generally increased in a mixed ICU population as compared to patients who underwent uncomplicated surgery. ASM was not found to be an early marker before the clinical onset of systemic inflammation as defined by fulfilling clinical SIRS criteria plus a PCT increase. However, ASM remained elevated in the presence of a low PCT level in non-surviving patients after systemic inflammation.

To our best knowledge, only two clinical studies have yet evaluated the role of ASM in patients with systemic inflammation. In a retrospective study of 12 severely septic patients, Claus et al. were able to show that sphingolytic activity was significantly increased compared to 13 healthy volunteers and that a further increase during the clinical course was proportional to the severity of illness (as indicated by a higher SOFA score on the day of maximal ASM) and paralleled by fatal outcome [12]. Drobnik et al. accordingly reported that ASM as reflected by the ceramide/sphingomyelin ratio was higher in septic patients compared to healthy controls and associated with a poor clinical outcome [20]. While both studies included patients with established sepsis, we evaluated for the first time the kinetics of ASM in ICU patients before systemic inflammation became clinically evident as defined by SIRS criteria plus a PCT increase. We evaluated the potential of ASM to serve as an early marker of inflammation as compared to established biomarkers such as PCT and CRP during the course of disease, and used a pragmatic approach including patients at high risk for developing systemic inflammation. In the 19 ICU patients who developed systemic inflammation during their ICU stay, there were no significant increases in ASM on the day before patients developed new SIRS plus a PCT peak elevation (PCT_{before}). ASM levels were also not significantly different between patients with or without systemic inflammation upon ICU admission. Thus, ASM may not be a marker to indicate inflammation at an earlier stage than PCT.

In the control group, we observed a significant increase in median ASM after surgery parallel to a post-operative PCT and

CRP increase. This increase reflects a "post-trauma" effect that is most likely explained by a lysosomal release of ASM resulting from tissue damage during surgery. However, the pre-operative and median post-operative ASM levels in the control group were still significantly lower as compared to the ICU patients.

We were also able to show the potential of ASM as prognostic marker for mortality. Although we could not detect an association to severity of illness measures, ASM remained elevated in non-surviving patients while PCT and lactate levels were lowered or within the normal range again. ROC analysis revealed a discriminative power for ASM in predicting ICU mortality at PCT_{low} (see figure 5). It is not clear whether ASM is useful in guiding risk stratification of the critically ill patient, as an AUC of 0.79 indicates that sensitivity and specifity are not in a range where a clinically reliable discrimination between survivors and non-survivors can be derived. Other pro- and anti-inflammatory cytokines like Interleukin [IL]-10, IL-8, IL-6, IL-1β, or Tumor necrosis factor-α were shown to hold similar AUC [21]. Thus, it is most likely that the one particular biomarker for predicting outcome of patients with systemic inflammation may not exist due to the complexity of the immune response. One may speculate that ASM increases as a result of inflammation, as various inflammatory stimuli lead to activation of ASM mediated lipid signalling, including oxidative stress [22,23], induction by or of cytokines [24,25], platelet activating-factor (PAF)-mediated pulmonary oedema formation during acute lung injury [26] and ceramide accumulation in ischemia/reperfusion injury in mitochondria [27]. Due to the various pathophysiological properties of ASM in mediation of inflammation and apoptosis, we may also speculate that non-declining or continuously increased ASM in critically ill patients with systemic inflammation plays a putative causative role with respect to adverse outcome.

Our study has some limitations which have to be mentioned. The main limitation is the low number of patients included and that it was conducted as a single center study. Therefore, our results should be interpreted with caution as there is a high likelihood of a type II error. However, this study should be regarded in the context of a single center, pilot study aiming to gain more insight into the clinical usefulness of ASM kinetics in the course of systemic inflammation. A further limitation is that we did not perform consecutive ASM measurements in the ICU patients without systemic inflammation. This was due to financial restraints of this pilot study. Measurements of ASM are not yet comparable with established laboratory for PCT or CRP that are easier and cheaper to conduct. It is also likely that the time interval at which ASM was measured did not accurately capture an early change in ASM kinetics (24 hours range between measurement at PCT_{before} and PCT_{peak}). Future studies on ASM kinetics may address this potential limitation choosing an even closer measurement interval. Lastly, the potential of using ASM as a prognostic marker after systemic inflammation in clinical practice warrants further improvement of the assay to become more widely available.

Conclusions

Our study showed that patients who underwent uncomplicated surgery exhibited a significant post-operative increase in ASM. In a mixed ICU population, ASM was significantly higher compared to these patients. While ASM did not indicate the onset of systemic inflammation earlier than PCT in our group of patients, it was able to predict ICU mortality in patients after systemic inflammation in the presence of low PCT level. ASM may hold potential as a tool for risk stratification of these patients, but the clinical value has to be further evaluated in larger studies.

Supporting Information

File S1 **Table S1,** Procalcitonin (ng/ml) values of the included patients, sorted by survivors and non-survivors. Time points were the day before the PCT peak (PCT_{before}), the day of the PCT peak (PCT_{peak}) and again lowered PCT (PCT_{low}). **Table S2,** Acid sphingomyelinase (pMol/ml*h) values for the included patients, sorted by survivors and non-survivors. Time points were the day before the PCT peak (PCT_{before}), the day of the PCT peak (PCT_{peak}) and again lowered PCT (PCT_{low}). **Table S3,** C-reactive protein (mg/L) values of the included patients, sorted by survivors and non-survivors. Time points were the day before the PCT peak (PCT_{before}), the day of the PCT peak (PCT_{peak}) and again lowered PCT (PCT_{low}). **Table S4,** Lactate (mMol/L) values of the included patients, sorted by survivors and non-survivors. Time points were the day before the PCT peak (PCT_{before}), the day of the PCT peak (PCT_{peak}) and again lowered PCT (PCT_{low}). **Table S5,** Modified SOFA-Score (points) values of the included patients, sorted by survivors and non-survivors. Time points were the day before the PCT peak (PCT_{before}), the day of the PCT peak (PCT_{peak}) and again lowered PCT (PCT_{low}). **Table S6,** SAPS-Score (points) values of the included patients, sorted by survivors and non-survivors. Time points were the day before the PCT peak (PCT_{before}), the day of the PCT peak (PCT_{peak}) and again lowered PCT (PCT_{low}). **Table S7,** TISS-Score (points) values of the included patients, sorted by survivors and non-survivors. Time points were the day before the PCT peak (PCT_{before}), the day of the PCT peak (PCT_{peak}) and again lowered PCT (PCT_{low}). **Table S8,** Acid sphingomyelinase activity, Procalcitonin (PCT), C-reactive protein (CRP), Lactate, modified SOFA-Score (mSofa), SAPS II Score and TISS Score of the included patients on the day of intensive care unit (ICU) admission. **Table S9,** Patients' characteristics and outcomes of the included patients. **Table S10,** Patients' characteristics and outcomes of included patients with systemic inflammatory response syndrome (SIRS) plus Procalcitonin (PCT) peak. **Table S11,** Patients' characteristics and outcomes of included patients without systemic inflammatory response syndrome (SIRS) plus Procalcitonin (PCT) peak.

Author Contributions

Conceived and designed the experiments: MK GE NW SS. Performed the experiments: SWM MR. Analyzed the data: MK GE MR SWM DS GZ IF SS NW. Contributed to the writing of the manuscript: MK GE MR SWM DS GZ IF SS NW.

References

1. Angus DC, Linde-Zwirble WT, Lidicker J, Clermon G, Carcillo J, et al. (2001) Epidemiology of severe sepsis in the United States: analysis of incidence, outcome, and associated costs of care. Crit Care Med 7: 1303–1310.
2. Rivers E, Nguyen B, Havstad S, Ressler J, Muzzin A, et al. (2001) Early goal-directed therapy in the treatment of severe sepsis and septic shock. NEJM 19: 1368–1377.
3. Wacker C, Prkno A, Brunkhorst FM, Schlattmann P (2013) Procalcitonin as a diagnostic marker for sepsis: a systematic review and meta-analysis. Lancet Infect Dis 13: 426–35.
4. Prkno A, Wacker C, Brunkhorst FM, Schlattmann P (2013) Procalcitonin-guided therapy in intensive care unit patients with severe sepsis and septic shock - a systematic review and meta-analysis. Crit Care 17: R291.

5. Reinhart K, Brunkhorst FM, Bone HG, Bardutzky J, Dempfle CE, et al. (2010) Prevention, diagnosis, treatment, and follow-up care of sepsis. First revision of the S2k Guidelines of the German Sepsis Society (DSG) and the German Interdisciplinary Association for Intensive and Emergency Care Medicine (DIVI). Anaesthesist 59: 347–370.
6. Meisner M, Adina H, Schmidt J (2006) Correlation of procalcitonin and C-reactive protein to inflammation, complications, and outcome during the intensive care unit course of multiple-trauma patients. Crit Care 10: R1.
7. Castelli GP, Pognani C, Meisner M, Stuani A, Bellomi D, et al. (2004) Procalcitonin and C-reactive protein during systemic inflammatory response syndrome, sepsis and organ dysfunction. Crit Care 4: R234–242.
8. Herrmann W, Ecker D, Quast S, Klieden M, Rose S, et al. (2000) Comparison of procalcitonin, sCD14 and interleukin-6 values in septic patients. Clin Chem Lab Med 38: 41–46.
9. Uzzan B, Cohen R, Nicolas P, Cucherat M, Perret GY (2006) Procalcitonin as a diagnostic test for sepsis in critically ill adults and after surgery or trauma: a systematic review and meta-analysis. Crit Care Med 34: 1996–2003.
10. Jenkins RW, Canals D, Hannun YA (2009) Roles and regulation of secretory and lysosomal acid sphingomyelinase. Cell Signal 21: 836–46.
11. Grassmé H, Riethmüller J, Gulbins E (2007) Biological aspects of ceramide-enriched membrane domains. Prog Lipid Res 46: 161–70.
12. Claus RA, Bunck AC, Bockmeyer CL, Brunkhorst FM, Lösche W, et al. (2005) Role of increased sphingomyelinase activity in apoptosis and organ failure of patients with severe sepsis. FASEB J. 19: 1719–1721.
13. Jbeily N, Suckert I, Gonnert FA, Acht B, Bockmeyer CL, et al. (2013) Hyperresponsiveness of mice deficient in plasma-secreted sphingomyelinase reveals its pivotal role in early phase of host response. J Lipid Res 54: 410–424.
14. Levy MM, Fink MP, Marshall JC, Abrahams E, Angus D, et al. (2003) 2001 SCCM/ESICM/ACCP/ATS/SIS International Sepsis Definitions Conference. Crit Care Med 4: 1250–1256.
15. Kornhuber J, Tripal P, Reichel M, Muhle C, Rhein C, et al. (2010) Functional Inhibitors of Acid Sphingomyelinase (FIASMAs): a novel pharmacological group of drugs with broad clinical applications. Cell Physiol Biochem 26: 9–20.
16. Le Gall JR, Lemeshow S, Saulnier F (1993) A new simplified acute physiology score (SAPS II) based on a European/North American multicenter study. JAMA 270: 2957–2963.
17. Cullen DJ, Civetta JM, Briggs BA, Ferrara LC (1974) Therapeutic Intervention Scoring System: a method for quantitative comparison of patient care. Crit Care Med 2: 57–60.
18. Vincent JL, Moreno R, Takala J, Willatts S, De Mendonça A, et al. (1996) The SOFA (Sepsis-related Organ Failure Assessment) score to describe organ dysfunction/failure. On behalf of the Working Group on Sepsis-Related Problems of the European Society of Intensive Care Medicine. Intensive Care Med 22: 707–710.
19. Edelmann B, Bertsch U, Tchikov V, Winoto-Morbach S, Jakob M, et al. (2011) Caspase-8 and caspase-7 sequentially mediate proteolytic activation of acid sphingomyelinase in TNF-R1-receptosomes. EMBO-J 30: 379–394.
20. Drobnik W, Liebisch G, Audebert FX, Frohlich D, Gluck T, et al. (2003) Plasma ceramide and lysophosphatidylcholine inversely correlate with mortality in sepsis patients. J Lipid Res 44: 754–761.
21. Bozza FA, Salluh JI, Japiassu AM, Soares M, Assis EF, et al. (2007) Cytokine profiles as markers of disease severity in sepsis: a multiplex analysis. Crit Care 11: R49.
22. Castillo SS, Levy M, Wang C, Thaikoottathil JV, Khan E, et al. (2007) Nitric oxide-enhanced caspase-3 and acidic sphingomyelinase interaction: a novel mechanism by which airway epithelial cells escape ceramide-induced apoptosis. Exp Cell Res 313: 816–823.
23. Corda S, Laplace C, Vicaut E, Duranteau J (2001) Rapid reactive oxygen species production by mitochondria in endothelial cells exposed to tumor necrosis factor-alpha is mediated by ceramide. Am J Resp Cell Mol Biol 24: 762–768.
24. Garcia-Ruiz C, Colell A, Mari M, Morales A, Calvo M, et al. (2003) Defective TNF-alpha-mediated hepatocellular apoptosis and liver damage in acidic sphingomyelinase knockout mice. J Clin Invest 111: 197–208.
25. Tokuda H, Kozawa O, Harada A, Uematsu T (1999) Extracellular sphingomyelinase induces interleukin-6 synthesis in osteoblasts. J Bio Chem 172: 262–268.
26. Göggel R, Winoto-Morbach S, Vielhaber G, Imai Y, Lindner K, et al. (2004) PAF-mediated pulmonary edema: a new role for acid sphingomyelinase and ceramide. Nat Med 10: 155–160.
27. Gudz TI, Tserng KY, Hoppel CL (1997) Direct inhibition of mitochondrial respiratory chain complex III by cell-permeable ceramide. J Biol Chem 272: 24154–24158.

Permissions

All chapters in this book were first published in PLOS ONE, by The Public Library of Science; hereby published with permission under the Creative Commons Attribution License or equivalent. Every chapter published in this book has been scrutinized by our experts. Their significance has been extensively debated. The topics covered herein carry significant findings which will fuel the growth of the discipline. They may even be implemented as practical applications or may be referred to as a beginning point for another development.

The contributors of this book come from diverse backgrounds, making this book a truly international effort. This book will bring forth new frontiers with its revolutionizing research information and detailed analysis of the nascent developments around the world.

We would like to thank all the contributing authors for lending their expertise to make the book truly unique. They have played a crucial role in the development of this book. Without their invaluable contributions this book wouldn't have been possible. They have made vital efforts to compile up to date information on the varied aspects of this subject to make this book a valuable addition to the collection of many professionals and students.

This book was conceptualized with the vision of imparting up-to-date information and advanced data in this field. To ensure the same, a matchless editorial board was set up. Every individual on the board went through rigorous rounds of assessment to prove their worth. After which they invested a large part of their time researching and compiling the most relevant data for our readers.

The editorial board has been involved in producing this book since its inception. They have spent rigorous hours researching and exploring the diverse topics which have resulted in the successful publishing of this book. They have passed on their knowledge of decades through this book. To expedite this challenging task, the publisher supported the team at every step. A small team of assistant editors was also appointed to further simplify the editing procedure and attain best results for the readers.

Apart from the editorial board, the designing team has also invested a significant amount of their time in understanding the subject and creating the most relevant covers. They scrutinized every image to scout for the most suitable representation of the subject and create an appropriate cover for the book.

The publishing team has been an ardent support to the editorial, designing and production team. Their endless efforts to recruit the best for this project, has resulted in the accomplishment of this book. They are a veteran in the field of academics and their pool of knowledge is as vast as their experience in printing. Their expertise and guidance has proved useful at every step. Their uncompromising quality standards have made this book an exceptional effort. Their encouragement from time to time has been an inspiration for everyone.

The publisher and the editorial board hope that this book will prove to be a valuable piece of knowledge for researchers, students, practitioners and scholars across the globe.

List of Contributors

Maru Aregawi, Michael Lynch and Ryan Williams
World Health Organization, Global Malaria Program, Geneva, Switzerland

Worku Bekele, Henok Kebede and Fatoumata Nafo-Traore
World Health Organization, Country Office, Addis Ababa, Ethiopia

Daddi Jima, Hiwot Solomon Taffese, Meseret Aseffa Yenehun, Abraham Lilay, Kesetebirhan Admasu and Tedros Adhanom Gebreyesus
Federal Ministry of Health, Addis Ababa, Ethiopia

Madeleine Thomson
International Research Institute for Climate and Society (IRI), Earth Institute, Columbia University, New York, New York, United States of America

Marc Coosemans
Institute of Tropical Medicine, Antwerp, Belgium

Erin Sadler
Department of General Surgery, University of Toronto, Toronto, Ontario, Canada

Brigette Hales
Quality and Patient Safety, Sunnybrook Health Sciences Centre, Toronto, Ontario, Canada

Blair Henry
Bioethics, Sunnybrook Health Sciences Centre, Toronto, Ontario, Canada

Wei Xiong
Trauma, Emergency and Critical Care Program, Sunnybrook Health Sciences Centre, Toronto, Ontario, Canada

Jeff Myers and Lesia Wynnychuk
Palliative Care, Sunnybrook Health Sciences Centre, Toronto, Ontario, Canada

Ru Taggar
Quality and Patient Safety, Chief Nursing and Health Professions Executive, Sunnybrook Health Sciences Centre, Toronto, Ontario, Canada

Daren Heyland
Department of Critical Care Medicine, Queen's University, Kingston, Ontario, Canada

Robert Fowler
Department of Critical Care Medicine, Sunnybrook Health Sciences Centre, Toronto, Ontario, Canada; Department of Medicine, University of Toronto, Toronto, Ontario Canada

Shaohui Zong, Li Du, Ye Fang and Taihang Gao
Department of Spine Osteopathia, the First Affiliated Hospital of Guangxi Medical University, Nanning, Guangxi, P.R. China

Gaofeng Zeng
College of Public Hygiene of Guangxi Medical University, Nanning, Guangxi, P.R. China

Jingmin Zhao
Department of Orthopaedics Trauma and Hand Surgery, the First Affiliated Hospital of Guangxi Medical University, Nanning, Guangxi, P.R. China

Takahisa Kawano
Department of Emergency Medicine, University of Fukui Hospital, Yoshida county, Fukui Prefecture, Japan

Kei Nishiyama
Department of Primary Care and Emergency Medicine, Kyoto University Graduate School of Medicine, Kyoto city, Kyoto Prefecture, Japan

Hiroyuki Hayashi
Department of General Medicine, University of Fukui Hospital, Yoshida county, Fukui Prefecture, Japan

Anders Berglund, Mats Ekelund and Lars Nyman
Pfizer Inc., Sollentuna, Sweden

Mark A. Fletcher
Pfizer Inc., Paris, France

Zheng Liu, Pengfei Lv and Cheng Chi
Department of Orthopaedics, Peking University Shougang Hospital, Beijing, China

Qi Fei, Bingqiang Wang, Yong Yang, Fan Zhao, Jisheng Lin and Zhao Ma
Department of Orthopaedics, Beijing Friendship Hospital, Capital Medical University, Beijing, China

Hiroyuki Kubota, Kenji Oishi and Takuya Akiyama
Yakult Honsha European Research Center for Microbiology ESV, Gent-Zwijnaarde, Belgium
Yakult Central Institute, Tokyo, Japan

Takafumi Sakai, Hiroshi Makino and Eiji Ishikawa
Yakult Central Institute, Tokyo, Japan

Agata Gawad
Yakult Honsha European Research Center for Microbiology ESV, Gent-Zwijnaarde, Belgium

Mônica Andrade de Carvalho, Hélio Tedesco Silva Junior and José Osmar Medina Pestana
Unidade de Transplante, Disciplina de Nefrologia, Universidade Federal de São Paulo, São Paulo, SP, Brazil

Flávio Geraldo Rezende Freitas and Antônio Toneti Bafi
Unidade de Transplante, Disciplina de Nefrologia, Universidade Federal de São Paulo, São Paulo, SP, Brazil
Disciplina de Anestesiologia, Dor e Terapia Intensiva. Universidade Federal de São Paulo, São Paulo, SP, Brazil

Flávia Ribeiro Machado
Disciplina de Anestesiologia, Dor e Terapia Intensiva. Universidade Federal de São Paulo, São Paulo, SP, Brazil

Claudia Fischer, Hester F. Lingsma and Ewout W. Steyerberg
Department of Public Health, Centre for Medical Decision Making, Erasmus MC, Rotterdam, the Netherlands

Perla J. Marang-van de Mheen
Department of Medical Decision Making, Leiden University Medical Centre, Leiden, the Netherlands

Dionne S. Kringos and Niek S. Klazinga
Department of Public Health, Amsterdam Medical Centre, Amsterdam, the Netherlands

Xiaoping Liu
Department of General Surgery, Nanfang Hospital, Southern Medical University, Guangzhou, Guangdong, P.R. China
Department of Gastrointestinal Surgery, The first affiliated hospital of Gannan medical university, Gannan medical university, Ganzhou, Jiangxi, P.R. China

Da Wang, Liansheng Zheng, Tingyu Mou, Hao Liu and Guoxin Li
Department of General Surgery, Nanfang Hospital, Southern Medical University, Guangzhou, Guangdong, P.R. China

Lisa Forsberg, Lars Navér and Katarina Wide
Department of Pediatrics, Karolinska University Hospital, Stockholm, Sweden
Department of Clinical Science, Intervention and Technology (CLINTEC), Karolinska Institutet, Stockholm, Sweden

Lars L. Gustafsson
Department of Laboratory Medicine, Division of Clinical Pharmacology, Karolinska Institutet, Stockholm, Sweden

Muhammad Ashraf Majrooh, Seema Hasnain, Javaid Akram and Arif Siddiqui
Allama Iqbal Medical College, Lahore, Pakistan

Zahid Ali Memon
Population Survives International - Greenstar, Karachi, Pakistan

Yu-Jen Yu, I-Wen Wu, Chin-Chan Lee, Chio-Yin Sun and Heng-Jung Hsu
Department of Nephrology, Chang Gung Memorial Hospital, Keelung, Taiwan
College of Medicine, Chang Gung University, Tao-Yuan, Taiwan

Chun-Yu Huang and Kuang-Hung Hsu
Laboratory for Epidemiology, Department of Health Care Management, Chang Gung University, Tao-Yuan, Taiwan

Mai-Szu Wu
Department of Nephrology, Chang Gung Memorial Hospital, Keelung, Taiwan
Division of Nephrology, Taipei Medical University Hospital, Taipei, Taiwan

School of Medicine, Taipei Medical University, Taipei, Taiwan

Jing Chen and Sarah M. McGhee
School of Public Health, The University of Hong Kong, Hong Kong, China

Carlos K. H. Wong
Department of Family Medicine and Primary Care, The University of Hong Kong, Hong Kong, China

Polly K. P. Pang and Wai-Cho Yu
Department of Medicine and Geriatrics, Princess Margaret Hospital, Hong Kong, China

Damian Hedinger, Julia Braun, Ueli Zellweger and Matthias Bopp
Epidemiology, Biostatistics and Prevention Institute, University of Zurich, Zurich, Switzerland

Vladimir Kaplan
District Hospital Freiamt Muri, Muri, Switzerland

Chih-Kuang Liang and Yu-Te Lin
Center for Geriatrics and Gerontology, Kaohsiung Veterans General Hospital, Kaohsiung, Taiwan
Division of Neurology, Department of Medicine, Kaohsiung Veterans General Hospital Kaohsiung, Taiwan
Aging and Health Research Center, National Yang Ming University, Taipei, Taiwan

Chin-Liang Chu
Center for Geriatrics and Gerontology, Kaohsiung Veterans General Hospital, Kaohsiung, Taiwan
Aging and Health Research Center, National Yang Ming University, Taipei, Taiwan
Department of Psychiatry, Kaohsiung Veterans General Hospital, Kaohsiung, Taiwan

Ming-Yueh Chou
Center for Geriatrics and Gerontology, Kaohsiung Veterans General Hospital, Kaohsiung, Taiwan
Aging and Health Research Center, National Yang Ming University, Taipei, Taiwan
Department of Family Medicine, Kaohsiung Veterans General Hospital, Kaohsiung, Taiwan

Ti Lu
Department of Psychiatry, Kaohsiung Veterans General Hospital, Kaohsiung, Taiwan

Chien-Jen Hsu
Department of Orthopaedics, Kaohsiung Veterans General Hospital, Kaohsiung, Taiwan

Liang-Kung Chen
Aging and Health Research Center, National Yang Ming University, Taipei, Taiwan
Center for Geriatrics and Gerontology, Taipei Veterans General Hospital, Taipei, Taiwan

Seitetsu L. Lee and Issei Komuro
Department of Cardiovascular Medicine, The University of Tokyo, Tokyo, Japan

Hideki Hashimoto
Department of Health and Social Behavior, The University of Tokyo, Tokyo, Japan

Takahide Kohro
Department of Clinical Informatics, Jichi Medical University, Tochigi, Japan

Hiromasa Horiguchi
Department of Clinical Data Management and Research, Clinical Research Center, National Hospital Organization Headquarters, Tokyo, Japan

Daisuke Koide
Department of Clinical Epidemiology and Systems, The University of Tokyo, Tokyo, Japan

Kiyohide Fushimi
Department of Health Policy and Informatics, Tokyo Medical and Dental University, Tokyo, Japan

Tsutomu Yamazaki
Clinical Research Support Center, The University of Tokyo, Tokyo, Japan

Hideo Yasunaga
Department of Clinical Epidemiology and Health Economics, The University of Tokyo, Tokyo, Japan

Malik Coulibaly, Elisabeth Thio and Issa Siribié
Projet MONOD ANRS 12206, Centre de Recherche Internationale pour la Santé , Site ANRS Burkina, Université de Ouagadougou, Ouagadougou, Burkina Faso

Nicolas Meda
Projet MONOD ANRS 12206, Centre de Recherche Internationale pour la Santé , Site ANRS Burkina, Université de Ouagadougou, Ouagadougou, Burkina Faso
Centre Muraz, Bobo Dioulasso, Burkina Faso

Caroline Yonaba and Ludovic Kam
Service de Pédiatrie, CHU Yalgado Ouédraogo, Ouagadougou, Burkina Faso

Sylvie Ouedraogo, Fla Koueta and Diarra Ye
Service de Pé diatrie Mé dicale, CHU Charles de Gaulle, Ouagadougou, Burkina Faso

Malika Congo
Laboratoire de Bactériologie - Virologie CHU Yalgado Ouédraogo, Ouagadougou, Burkina Faso

Mamoudou Barry
Service de laboratoire, CHU Charles de Gaulle, Ouagadougou, Burkina Faso

Stéphane Blanche
Groupe hospitalier Necker- Enfants malades, Paris, France

Phillipe Van De Perre
Inserm U1058, Université Montpellier 1, Montpellier, France

Valériane Leroy
Inserm, U897, Institut de Santé Publique, Epidémiologie et Développement (ISPED), Université de Bordeaux, Bordeaux, France

Tsira Chakhaia and Medea Gegia
University Research Co., LLC. Branch in Georgia, USAID Georgia TB Prevention Project, Tbilisi, Georgia

Matthew J. Magee
Division of Epidemiology and Biostatistics, School of Public Health, Georgia State University, Atlanta, Georgia, United States of America
Departments of Epidemiology and Global Health, Rollins School of Public Health, Emory University, Atlanta, Georgia, United States of America

Russell R. Kempker
Division of Infectious Diseases, Department of Medicine, School of Medicine, Emory University, Atlanta, Georgia, United States of America

Leila Goginashvili and Ucha Nanava
National Center for Tuberculosis and Lung Disease, Tbilisi, Georgia

Henry M. Blumberg
Division of Infectious Diseases, Department of Medicine, School of Medicine, Emory University, Atlanta, Georgia, United States of America
Departments of Epidemiology and Global Health, Rollins School of Public Health, Emory University, Atlanta, Georgia, United States of America

Evelyn D. Olthof and Geert J. A. Wanten
Intestinal Failure Unit, Department of Gastroenterology and Hepatology, Radboud University Medical Center, Nijmegen, The Netherlands

Michelle W. Versleijen
Department of Nuclear Medicine, Netherlands Cancer Institute - Antoni van Leeuwenhoek, Amsterdam, The Netherlands

Getty Huisman-de Waal
Intestinal Failure Unit, Department of Gastroenterology and Hepatology, Radboud University Medical Center, Nijmegen, The Netherlands
Scientific Institute for Quality of Healthcare, Radboud University Medical Center, Nijmegen, The Netherlands

Ton Feuth and Wietske Kievit
Department of Health Evidence, Radboud University Medical Center, Nijmegen, The Netherlands

Anne Kouvonen
Department of Social Research, University of Helsinki, Helsinki, Finland
University of Social Sciences and Humanities, Faculty in Wroclaw, Wroclaw, Poland
UKCRC Centre of Excellence for Public Health (Northern Ireland), Queen's University Belfast, Belfast, United Kingdom

Aki Koskinen, Lauri Kokkinen and Ari Väänänen
Finnish Institute of Occupational Health, Helsinki and Tampere, Finland'

Pekka Varje
Finnish Institute of Occupational Health, Helsinki and Tampere, Finland'
Department of Philosophy, History, Culture and Art Studies, University of Helsinki, Helsinki, Finland

Roberto De Vogli
Department of Public Health Sciences, School of Medicine, University of California Davis, Davis, United States of America
Department of Epidemiology and Public Health, University College London, London, United Kingdom

Joan Puig-Barberà
Fundación para el Fomento de la Investigación Sanitaria y Biomédica de la Comunitat Valenciana (FISABIO), Valencia, Spain
Centro de Salud Pú blica de Castelló n, Castellón, Spain

Juan García-de-Lomas
Instituto Valenciano de Microbiología, Valencia, Spain

Javier Díez-Domingo
Fundación para el Fomento de la Investigación Sanitaria y Biomédica de la Comunitat Valenciana (FISABIO), Valencia, Spain

Alberto Arnedo-Pena and Montserrat Ruiz-García
Centro de Salud Pú blica de Castellón, Castellón, Spain

Ramó n Limón-Ramírez and Silvia Pérez-Vilar
Hospital de la Plana, Vila-real, Spain

José Luis Micó-Esparza
Hospital Aranau de Vilanova, Valencia, Spain

Miguel Tortajada-Girbés
Hospital Doctor Peset, Valencia, Spain

Concha Carratalá-Munuera
Hospital San Juan, Alicante, Spain
Cátedra de Medicina de Familia, Departamento de Medicina Clínica, Universidad Miguel Hernández, San Juan, Alicante, Spain

Rosa Larrea-Gonzá lez and Juan Manuel Beltrán-Garrido
Hospital General de Castellón, Castellón, Spain

Maria del Carmen Otero-Reigada and Joan Mollar-Maseres
Hospital Universitario y Politécnico La Fe, Valencia, Spain

Patricia Correcher-Medina
Hospital Lluis Alcanyis, Xativa, Spain

Germán Schwarz-Chavarri
Centro de Salud San Blas, Alicante, Spain

Vicente Gil-Guillén
Hospital de Elda, Elda, Spain

Mihajlo Jakovljevic
Department of Pharmacology and Toxicology; The Faculty of Medical Sciences, University of Kragujevac, Kragujevac, Serbia

Mirjana Jovanovic
Department of Psychiatry; The Faculty of Medical Sciences, University of Kragujevac, Kragujevac, Serbia

Nemanja Rancic
Centre for Clinical Pharmacology; Medical Faculty Military Medical Academy, University of Defense, Belgrade, Serbia

Benjamin Vyssoki
Department of Psychiatry and Psychotherapy; Medical University of Vienna, Vienna, Austria

Natasa Djordjevic
Department of Pharmacology and Toxicology; The Faculty of Medical Sciences, University of Kragujevac, Kragujevac, Serbia

Anna Alassaad
Department of Medical Sciences, Uppsala University, Uppsala, Sweden
Uppsala University Hospital, Uppsala, Sweden

Maria Bertilsson
Uppsala Clinical Research Center, Uppsala, Sweden

Ulrika Gillespie
Uppsala University Hospital, Uppsala, Sweden

Johan Sundström
Department of Medical Sciences, Uppsala University, Uppsala, Sweden
Uppsala Clinical Research Center, Uppsala, Sweden

Margareta Hammarlund-Udenaes
Department of Pharmaceutical Sciences, Uppsala University, Uppsala, Sweden

Håkan Melhus
Department of Medical Sciences, Uppsala University, Uppsala, Sweden

Matthias Kott, Gunnar Elke, , Dirk Schädler, Günther Zick, Inéz Frerichs and Norbert Weiler
Department of Anesthesiology and Intensive Care Medicine, University Medical Center Schleswig-Holstein, Campus Kiel, Kiel, Germany

Maike Reinicke
Department of Anesthesiology and Intensive Care Medicine, University Medical Center Schleswig-Holstein, Campus Kiel, Kiel, Germany
Institute of Immunology, University Medical Center Schleswig-Holstein, Campus Kiel, Kiel, Germany

Supandi Winoto-Morbach and Stefan Schütze
Institute of Immunology, University Medical Center Schleswig-Holstein, Campus Kiel, Kiel, Germany

Index

P

R

S

T

U

V

W

www.ingramcontent.com/pod-product-compliance
Lightning Source LLC
LaVergne TN
LVHW080700210926
848485LV00003B/401